Advances in
Small Animal Total Joint Replacement

Advances in
Small Animal
Total Joint
Replacement

Edited by

Jeffrey N. Peck, DVM, Diplomate American College of Veterinary Surgeons

Denis J. Marcellin-Little, DEDV, Diplomate American College of Veterinary Surgeons, European College of Veterinary Surgeons, American College of Veterinary Sports Medicine and Rehabilitation

WILEY-BLACKWELL

A John Wiley & Sons, Inc., Publication

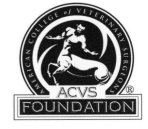

Editorial offices: 2121 State Avenue, Ames, Iowa 50014-8300, USA
The Atrium, Southern Gate, Chichester, West Sussex, PO19 8SQ, UK
9600 Garsington Road, Oxford, OX4 2DQ, UK

For details of our global editorial offices, for customer services and for information about how to apply for permission to reuse the copyright material in this book please see our website at www.wiley.com/wiley-blackwell.

Library of Congress Cataloging-in-Publication Data

Advances in small animal total joint replacement / edited by Jeffrey N. Peck, Denis J. Marcellin-Little.
       p. ; cm.
    Includes bibliographical references and index.
    ISBN 978-0-470-95961-9 (hardback : alk. paper) – ISBN 978-1-118-46271-3 (ePDF/eBook) – ISBN 978-1-118-46272-0 (ePub) – ISBN 978-1-118-46273-7 (eMobi)
    I. Peck, Jeffrey N.   II. Marcellin-Little, Denis J. (Denis Jacques), 1964–
    [DNLM: 1. Arthroplasty, Replacement–veterinary.   2. Surgery, Veterinary–methods.   3. Pets–surgery. SF 911]
    636.089′705–dc23
                                       2012019773

A catalogue record for this book is available from the British Library.

Cover design by Matt Kuhns

Set in 9.5 on 11.5 pt Palatino by Toppan Best-set Premedia Limited

Printed and bound in Singapore by Markono Print Media Pte Ltd

Disclaimer

1   2013

Dedication

This book is dedicated to Kathy and Kayla, and to the memory of Cody Ruderman, who reminded me that our most serious complications should be our greatest impetus for advancement.

Jeffrey N. Peck

This book is dedicated to Terry, Arianne, and Julien, and to all loving owners of dogs and cats.

Denis J. Marcellin-Little

Contents

Contributors

Matthew Allen, Vet MB, PhD
Associate Professor
College of Veterinary Medicine
The Ohio State University
Columbus, OH

Michael Conzemius, DVM, PhD, Diplomate
ACVS
Professor
College of Veterinary Medicine
University of Minnesota
St. Paul, MN

Loïc M. Déjardin, DVM, MS, Diplomate ACVS
Associate Professor
College of Veterinary Medicine
Michigan State University
East Lansing, MI

David J. DeYoung, DVM, Diplomate ACVS,
ACVA
Adjunct Professor
College of Veterinary Medicine
North Carolina State University
Raleigh, NC

Reunan P. Guillou, Doc. Vet.
Assistant Professor
College of Veterinary Medicine
Michigan State University
East Lansing, MI

Ola L.A. Harrysson, PhD
Associate Professor
Fitts Department of Industrial and Systems
Engineering
North Carolina State University
Raleigh, NC

Kei Hayashi, DVM, PhD, Diplomate ACVS
Associate Professor
College of Veterinary Medicine
University of California–Davis
Davis, CA

Michael P. Kowaleski, DVM, Diplomate ACVS,
ECVS
Associate Professor
Cummings School of Veterinary Medicine
Tufts University
North Grafton, MA

William D. Liska, DVM, Diplomate ACVS
Surgeon
Gulf Coast Veterinary Specialists
Houston, TX

Kenneth Mann, PhD
Professor of Orthopedic Surgery
Director of the Musculoskeletal Science Research
Center
Department of Orthopedic Surgery
Upstate Medical University
State University of New York
Syracuse, NY

Denis J. Marcellin-Little, DEDV, Diplomate
ACVS, ECVS, ACVSMR
Professor
College of Veterinary Medicine
North Carolina State University
Raleigh, NC

Jeffrey N. Peck, DVM, Diplomate ACVS
Surgeon
Affiliated Veterinary Specialists
Maitland, FL

Melvyn Pond, BVMS, MRCVS, Diplomate ACVS
Surgeon
New Haven Hospital for Veterinary Medicine
Milford, CT

Mariana Quina, DVM
Surgical Resident
Affiliated Veterinary Specialists
Maitland, FL

Simon C. Roe, BVSc, PhD, Diplomate ACVS
Professor
College of Veterinary Medicine
North Carolina State University
Raleigh, NC

Kurt S. Schulz, DVM, MS, Diplomate ACVS
Surgeon
Peak Veterinary Referral Center
Williston, VT

Greg Van Der Meulen, BSME
Director of Research and Development
BioMedtrix, LLC
Boonton, NJ
Ketchum, ID

Foreword

The editors have asked me to write about my experience and thoughts on canine total hip replacements. I have often said that humans were the research animal for dogs when it came to total hip replacements. Although total hip replacements were being implanted in humans in the 1940s by surgeons such as Dr. Austin Moore, it was not until the late 1950s and early 1960s that Sir John Charnley's work on implant design, materials, and fixation with polymethylmethacrylate (PMMA) bone cement made the procedure popular and widely used in humans. In 1957, Dr. Harry Gorman at The Ohio State University (OSU) worked on an experimental hip prosthesis in canines. These implants were cementless and the project was testing a design that was to be used humans. The femoral head was held in the acetabulum by a constraining metal ring, which was fixed to the pelvis with screws. This design was flawed and failed in most patients. However, Dr. Richard Rudy did tell me about one dog he implanted with this hip replacement that lasted for 13 years. It was not until 1974 when Dr. William Hoefle reported on a cemented total hip replacement in one dog that some people again began to think about doing this surgery in veterinary patients.

In early August 1976, 1 month after I started working at OSU, Dr. R. Bruce Hohn implanted the Veterinary College's first Richards II Canine Cemented Total Hip Replacement. His second hip replacement occurred a few weeks later and I jumped at the chance to scrub with him on that hip. From that point on, we each did hip replacements at OSU. We wanted to document our technique, clinical results, postoperative care, and complications in a manner that would be most beneficial to the profession. Thus, we did not rush to publish our results but took time to reflect on what we learned. Our complication rate was high (20%) and by today's standards would be unacceptable, but we found that as we accumulated cases and critically evaluated each complication, avoidable causes were identified. There was a marked reduction in complications in the last 2 years of this study. By continuing this evaluation even today, complication rates are minimized and now occur in approximately 7% of the cases.

Starting in 1977, an annual continuing education course was taught at OSU that included in the faculty both veterinarians and MDs from around the country who were implanting total hips. This gave valuable insight that was incorporated into the techniques used at OSU and around the world. These courses gave us an opportunity to exchange ideas and to teach the most current technique to veterinarians. It was not long before many veterinary surgeons were offering total hip replacements to their clients and patients.

When it became known that we were doing total hip replacements at OSU, there were those who said it was unnecessary to do this in dogs because excision arthroplasty (femoral head and neck ostectomy) worked well. We found that the easiest way for us to show the benefits of total hip replacement is to compare hip extended radiographs of a dog with a replaced hip and one with an excision arthroplasty taken 6 months after surgery. The total-hip dog will have well-developed muscle mass, while the excision-arthroplasty dog's muscles are atrophied. The direct connection of the femoral head to the pelvis is important for the dog's muscles and limb function to reach their full potential.

Our first major publication on the subject was a technique paper in a 1981 volume of *Veterinary Surgery*. The paper, documenting the results of the first 5 years of 221 consecutive clinical cases (216 of which had follow-ups for varying periods), did not come out until 1983. Since then, many more publications by myself and others have further expanded our understanding of canine total hip replacements. Total hip replacements have become a well-accepted technique for resolving discomfort and poor function resulting from canine hip diseases.

It became obvious to me as I worked with the Richards system that changes in implant design and instrumentation would be of benefit, so I discussed this with the company representatives. They declined to make changes. Thus, when in 1989 I was contacted about a new modular hip replacement system, I agreed to work on it. This collaboration resulted in the development of the BioMedtrix Canine Cemented Hip Replacement System. This company has been very receptive to changing the implants and instruments when clinical findings indicated that something was not working as well as it could, even if that was in just a few patients, or when a need was found that was not addressed by the system at a given time.

In an effort to improve what was offered to the patient, I was part of the group that worked on the cementless hip system for BioMedtrix. I saw the cemented and cementless systems as complementary to each other and felt they would expand the options a surgeon had available. I have not found one system to be overall superior to the other, but there are some cases where one system will work better for a given patient. In some cases, they can even be combined into a hybrid hip replacement. The surgeon who wants to provide the best possible service to the client and patient will be well versed in all aspects of both the cemented and cementless total hip replacement systems.

In human medicine, total hip replacement is considered the most consistently reproducible surgery with the most predictable results. This should also be true in veterinary medicine. It takes strict attention to detail, technique, and patient selection and care. The success rate of 95% dogs returning to normal to near-normal function is found no matter which implant is used. It is up to the surgeon to choose the best implants for a given patient.

Marvin L. Olmstead, DVM, MS
Emeritus Professor, The Ohio State University
Emeritus Diplomate, American College
of Veterinary Surgeons
Surgeon, Oregon Veterinary Referral Associates

Foreword

This textbook constitutes a summary of the current stage of arthroplasty in veterinary surgery. The foreword written by Marvin Olmstead provides us with a historical perspective of the landmark work of the pioneers of arthroplasty in veterinary medicine over the last quarter of the twentieth century. Not only was the technique developed by these individuals, but they also pushed arthroplasty beyond the barriers of the time and made total hip replacement the treatment of choice for veterinarians, as well as pet owners. It is important for the next generation of orthopedic surgeons to be aware of the steps that got us to this point and shoulder the responsibility of advancing the science and art of arthroplasty in the future.

As veterinary orthopedic surgeons, we have the responsibility to critically assess implant and patient performance and continue to develop implants and techniques to improve the outcomes for our patients. The ultimate goal of total joint replacement is to relieve pain, improve the patient's quality of life by returning function, and improve the client's relationship with their pet. In addition, the prosthesis should last the lifetime of the patient. Success toward meeting these goals has been measured using a variety of standards, most often retrospective studies involving assessment of patient function, as well as client satisfaction.

While clinical assessment is the most important outcome assessment, and was paramount to achieving improvements during the early stages of cemented total hip replacement in dogs, additional advancement could only be achieved using more finite criteria for implant performance. It was clear that patient function did not always correlate with radiographic assessment. In the mid-1980s, a retrieval analysis program was started at North Carolina State University (NCSU), offering us the opportunity to assess cemented implants, and the surrounding cement and bone harvested following the death of canine patients. The program provided the opportunity to assess mechanical stability of the implant–cement and cement–bone interfaces, establish the nature of the cells in fibrous membranes, and search for the presence of particulate debris. Serial sectioning of femurs with intact implants and cement revealed cement cracks or an incomplete cement mantle that provided channels for wear debris to gain access to the cement–bone interface leading to osteolysis. Over a period of years, serial radiographic assessment and retrieval analysis pointed out many of the failure mechanisms associated with bone cement and cementing techniques. These were addressed with varying degrees of success in dogs over the past decade. Every attempt has been made to link failures back to patient selection and surgical technique, and in some cases implant materials or design. Critical assessment of failures is the most direct path to improving implant longevity. However, to call them failures while the dog is running and jumping may not be appropriate; perhaps it is best to use the term "early indicators of impending problems." Changes leading to loss of implant stability are generally slow and insidious. They may take years, or in some cases, they may transpire at a frighteningly fast rate. In addition to clinical performance, serial radiographic assessment is the best clinical evidence of the implant performance over time and helps the surgeon reconstruct the causes of the failure. The important fact is to recognize the mechanisms of failure and take steps to minimize them or prevent them from occurring in future cases.

In 1986, an opportunity presented itself from David Hungerford, an orthopedic surgeon at Johns Hopkins University. He proposed to develop a cementless total hip system for clinical and research use in dogs in conjunction with surgeons at NCSU. The vision was to create a state-of–the-art cementless total hip system complete with accurate instrumentation. The system was to be used in research animals as well as clinical patients and to be implanted by the same team of veterinary surgeons. Having surgeons familiar with the hip system, implantation technique, performance, and assessment would enhance the quality of the research arm of the program. The same standards would be used for clinical and research animals and serial radiographic assessment would be used throughout the clinical and research studies, as well as retrieval analysis. This was the critical step that resulted in the development of the Canine PCA Total Hip System by Howmedica Inc. Multiple research studies were completed over a 15-year period, including a long-term prospective clinical trial. Research projects included the study of a variety of implant types and surface coatings and provided the team with extensive knowledge and experience that was applied to clinical patients. In retrospect, one significant decision was the training and use of an independent and unbiased observer to read all radiographic assessments made on the research studies, as well as clinical patients. A member of our team, Rick Schiller, was responsible for the reading, documentation, and interpretation of the radiographic

studies for all research and clinical animals. Many of the research studies were subsequently reviewed by a third-party consultant, Tom Gruen. The extensive clinical and research experience gained using the Canine PCA Total Hip System laid the foundation for the development of the BioMedtrix BFX Cementless Total Hip System nearly 20 years later. Concurrently, others had evolved an interest in cementless fixation leading to the development of the Zurich Cementless Total Hip Replacement System in the 1990s by Pierre Montavon and Slobodan Tepic in Zurich, Switzerland. Multi-center clinical studies were led by Randy Boudrieau in the United States and Aldo Vezzoni in Europe.

Another critical initiative in the advancement of canine hip arthroplasty was the initiation of a series of conferences, "Contemporary Issues in Canine Total Joint Replacement," held in 1999, 2000, 2001, 2005, and 2008. This conference was established with the goal to advance the science and art of canine total joint replacement. The objectives were to promote open discussion and debate on issues in total joint replacement using a variety of implant systems, actively engage surgeons and engineers in dialogue, emphasize optimal surgical technique for primary and revision arthroplasty procedures, and provide a forum for all participating surgeons to share their personal experiences. Significant changes were achieved as a result of the participation and contribution of surgeons attending these interactive conferences.

The first conference focused on the indications for hip replacement, patient selection, patient care, and surgical technique of cemented implants. The second conference in 2000 concentrated on surgical technique including canal and acetabular preparation, implant positioning and complications, revisions, and radiographic assessment. The 2001 conference expanded to include the clinical experience using a variety of cemented and cementless implants from the United States as well as Europe, including the CFX, PCA, Zurich Cementless, and the Biomécanique implant systems. This meeting proved to be a pivotal moment for cementless applications. The presentations on the clinical experience with the Zurich Cementless and the Canine PCA stimulated intense discussions and revealed how much interest there was in the positive results of cementless implants, and the desire to move in that direction was established. The next conference was not held until 2005, 2 years following the release of the BFX system. The entire meeting was dedicated entirely on the BFX cementless system, refinement of the operative technique, and resolving early complications. The last conference held in 2008 focused on refining the CFX and BFX operative procedures and instrumentation into a single system, the Universal Hip System. Input was provided by surgeons based on their experiences with the system over the past 3 years. These discussions led to the later refinement of the operative technique into a common Universal technique for CFX and BFX systems. Key observations and input from surgeons including Teresa Schiller, Denis Marcellin-Little, Loïc Déjardin, Melvin Pond, Michael Kowaleski, and Bill Liska were instrumental in refining the surgical technique, resulting in a reduction of early surgical complications. This conference also for the first time expanded to include micro hip implants and total knee and total elbow replacement. The 3-year

gap between 2005 and 2008 was a very productive time for the advancement of total joint replacement in dogs.

It is my hope that this textbook will not only provide a valuable reference source for surgeons, but remind them just how far we have come in a relatively short time and excite them about the possibilities for the future. Through continued critical assessment including basic research and prospective clinical studies, we will continue to make strides to achieve our goal. The format of interactive conferences to share ideas and experience is also critical in achieving consensus and direction.

David J. DeYoung, DVM,
Diplomate ACVS, ACVA
Professor Emeritus, Orthopedic Surgery,
College of Veterinary Medicine,
North Carolina State University
Dean Emeritus, School of Veterinary Medicine,
Ross University

Foreword

The American College of Veterinary Surgeons (ACVS) Foundation is excited to present *Advances in Small Animal Total Joint Replacement* in the book series entitled *Advances in Veterinary Surgery*. The ACVS Foundation is an independently charted philanthropic organization devoted to advancing the charitable, educational, and scientific goals of the American College of Veterinary Surgeons. Founded in 1965, the ACVS sets the standards for the specialty of veterinary surgery. The ACVS, which is approved by the American Veterinary Medical Association, administers the board certification process for Diplomates in veterinary surgery and advances veterinary surgery and education. One of the principal goals of the ACVS Foundation is to foster the advancement of the art and science of veterinary surgery. The Foundation achieves these goals by supporting investigations in the diagnosis and treatment of surgical diseases; increasing educational opportunities for surgeons, surgical residents, and veterinary practitioners; improving surgical training of residents and veterinary students; and bettering animal patients' care, treatment, and welfare. This collaboration with Wiley-Blackwell will benefit all who are interested in veterinary surgery by presenting the latest evidence-based information on a particular surgical topic.

Advances in Small Animal Total Joint Replacement is edited by Drs. Jeffrey N. Peck and Denis J. Marcellin-Little, both Diplomates of the American College of Veterinary Surgeons and prominent small animal orthopedic surgeons in the field of total joint replacement. They have assembled the leaders in the field of joint replacement, presenting a historical perspective of joint replacement in veterinary surgery, the relevant issues regarding implant materials, the common sites of total joint replacement, including the hip, knee, and elbow, emerging arthroplasties sites, and the use of custom prostheses. The ACVS Foundation is proud to partner with Wiley-Blackwell in this important series and is honored to present this book in the series.

Mark D. Markel
Chair, Board of Trustees
ACVS Foundation

Preface and Acknowledgments

Joint replacement for companion animals has been available for approximately four decades. Fortunately, over time, several pioneers have pushed the boundaries of our knowledge, technology, and capabilities. Several of these early pioneers, such as Hap Paul, Dave Nunamaker, and Tom Turner, were veterinarians who embraced the "One Medicine" philosophy and were involved in the early development of both human and veterinary joint prostheses.

Until the 1990s, joint replacement in veterinary surgery had mostly been limited to the hip and was available at only a small number of institutions. As we grew to expand the breadth of joint replacements available to our patients, we have been enduring the same growing pains and made errors similar to our human surgeon counterparts. Most often, we start out by creating highly constrained prostheses with restricted kinematic function. As our understanding of the kinematics and biomechanics of the normal joint grows, so does the likelihood of repeatable, successful long-term outcomes.

In addition to expanding the armamentarium of available joint replacements, there has also been a substantial increase in the number of surgeons performing joint replacement procedures worldwide. In order to maximize the success of any new procedure, it is critical that the surgeon's knowledge and skill exceed what is necessary to simply perform the procedure. A deeper level of understanding is necessary to minimize the incidence of complications and to manage them when they occur. Furthermore, a larger population of knowledgeable surgeons will accelerate the rate at which we can improve on existing designs and procedures.

This book's aim is to facilitate the advancement of joint replacement in veterinary surgery by pooling the existing body of information and providing a solid foundation of knowledge to joint replacement surgeons. That knowledge is necessary to provide optimal patient care, to conduct clinical research, and to educate future surgeons.

Acknowledgments

We thank all implant manufacturers for their support. We thank Terry Marcellin-Little for her assistance with the Index, and Dr. William D. Liska for the radiograph used on the cover.

Jeffrey N. Peck
Denis J. Marcellin-Little

Advances in
Small Animal
Total Joint
Replacement

1

The History of Joint Replacement in Veterinary Surgery

Mariana Quina and Jeffrey N. Peck

Total joint replacement has gained an important place in veterinary orthopedic surgery. There are currently commercially available prosthetic components and instrumentation for canine and feline total hip replacement, canine total elbow replacement, and canine total knee replacement. Although many different implant systems have been developed for experimental use, descriptions of the implants in this chapter are limited to the commercially available systems.

Total hip replacement

Total hip replacement became commercially available in the dog in 1974 (Hoefle 1974). The implant system used was a cemented, fixed-head, stainless steel femoral component and polyethylene acetabular cup that was available in three sizes (Richards Manufacturing, Memphis, TN; Figure 1.1). The Richards II canine total hip prosthesis was the only commercially available canine system until 1990. Design modifications to the implants were made in the late 1970s in order to decrease the tendency for luxation, provide more consistent placement of the acetabular component, and

reduce the possibility of damage to the femoral component during preparation of the femur. These changes included a 20-degree cutaway on the dorsal aspect of the acetabular component, establishment of a guide system for placement of the acetabular component, several minor changes to the femoral component design, and introduction of a femoral component trial prosthesis to be used during preparation of the femur.

In 1979, Leighton reported on the use of the Richards II system in nine experimental dogs. Each of the three available sizes of prostheses was implanted in three dogs each. Of the nine dogs, there was one failure due to infection resulting in acetabular component loosening. The remaining eight dogs reportedly had good or excellent function 1 year after surgery. Use of the Richards II system was reported in a clinical setting with good success (Lewis and Jones 1980; Olmstead et al. 1983). Lewis and Jones performed 20 total hip replacements in 15 dogs and reported the results with a minimum of 1-year follow-up. The most common complication was loosening of the acetabular component, the femoral component, or both. Causes of aseptic loosening were not clearly identified or understood at the time of the Lewis

Advances in Small Animal Total Joint Replacement, First Edition. Edited by Jeffrey N. Peck and Denis J. Marcellin-Little.
© 2013 John Wiley & Sons, Inc. Published 2013 by John Wiley & Sons, Inc.

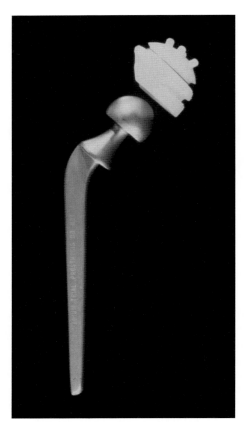

Figure 1.1 The Richards II canine total hip prosthesis. (Image courtesy of David DeYoung)

publication. Contributing factors to implant loosening that were identified included infection, inadequate preparation of the bone prior to cement placement, undersizing of implants, and improper positioning of the implants. Other complications included failure of the femoral component via bending or breakage at the stem–neck angle and luxation. Only six of the hips did not have post-operative complications. Four of the 20 hips were eventually explanted. Of the remaining 16, 75% were considered to have excellent outcome.

Olmstead et al. (1983) reviewed 221 total hip replacements over a 5-year period. Follow-up information was available for 216 of the cases. The minimum follow-up period for inclusion in the study was 4 weeks, and of the 149 hips that were not lost to follow-up at study completion, none had an evaluation period shorter than 25 weeks. At the final evaluation, 91% were reported to have satisfactory function, with owners reporting increased activity levels, improved muscle mass, and elimination of pain. Of the dogs with bilateral hip dysplasia, unilateral hip replacement resulted in enough improvement in clinical signs that surgery on the contralateral side was not deemed necessary for 80% of dogs. Complications included luxation, infection, aseptic loosening of the acetabular component, femoral fracture, and sciatic neurapraxia. The overall complication rate was 20%, with 58% of cases with complications eventually achieving a satisfactory outcome. Evaluation of follow-up radiographs, as well as what constituted a satisfactory outcome, was not discussed.

In June 1990, the BioMedtrix CFX® system (BioMedtrix, Boonton, NJ), a modular cemented total hip prosthesis and instrumentation set, was introduced (Olmstead 1995). The most significant change in this modular system compared with the fixed-head system was the introduction of a two-piece femoral component. The femoral component consists of a stem and a head secured together via a locking taper mechanism. This change allowed for three different neck lengths for each stem. The original CFX femoral stem was made of titanium alloy (TiAlVn) and was available in five sizes. The head was made of cobalt-chrome and available in three sizes. New instrumentation was also introduced, including power reaming of the femur and acetabulum to increase accuracy and the ease of the procedure. Olmstead (1995) reported preliminary clinical results for 52 total hip replacements using this system. Follow-up ranged from 2 months to 15 months (mean: 6 months) and consisted of owner questionnaires regarding the dogs' function following total hip replacement. Only two complications were reported, one luxation and one iatrogenic intrapelvic hematoma causing urethral compression, both of which were resolved successfully with additional surgical intervention. In 2004, Liska reported on 730 consecutive hip replacements using the BioMedtrix CFX system, with a mean follow-up of 3.9 years.[1] Complications included both craniodorsal and ventral luxation, infection, aseptic loosening, femur fracture, sciatic neuropraxia, pulmonary embolism, incision granuloma, extraosseous cement granuloma, medullary infarction, and osteosarcoma. The procedure was considered successful in 96% of cases. The Liska study included the most comprehensive description of outcome and complications to date. While several of these complications had been described in case reports (Roe et al. 1996; Marcellin-Little et al. 1999a,b; Sebestyen et al. 2000; Bergh et al. 2006), this large study was the most comprehensive to date and it allowed a direct comparison of the rate of all complications. The BioMedtrix CFX system is discussed in detail in Chapter 7.

The original total hip replacement femoral implants were made of stainless steel. Newer generations of femoral implants were made of titanium alloy. Titanium is resistant to corrosion and is highly biocompatible, making it an attractive material for surgical implants. However, under certain conditions, particularly when used as a cemented stem, titanium alloys are more susceptible to severe abrasive corrosive wear than stainless steel or cobalt-chrome alloys (Agins et al. 1988). This is primarily associated with the elastic modulus mismatch between cement and titanium and the proclivity of titanium alloys to generate wear debris under such condition (see Chapters 3 and 6). Lee et al. (1992) found an unusually large amount of metal debris in the tissues around titanium alloy prostheses showing early failure as well as larger polyethylene particles in tissues from failed titanium alloy than from cobalt-chrome or stainless steel prostheses. These particles lead to wear debris, which stimulates macrophage recruitment and cytokine release and result in bone resorption and, therefore, aseptic loosening (Goldring et al. 1983).

Uncemented total hip replacement techniques have been developed to avoid the use of cement, which, despite improvements in cementing techniques, continues to be implicated in irreversible infections and aseptic loosening (DeYoung et al. 1992; Marcellin-Little et al. 1999b). Skurla et al. (2005) investigated aseptic loosening in 38 total hip replacements from 29 client-owned dogs. The duration of implantation ranged from 8 months to over 11 years and all were postmortem retrieval specimens. Nine of the femoral components were grossly loose and 15 were mechanically loose, for a total of 63.2% loose implants. Stem loosening occurred more commonly at the cement–implant interface than at the cement–bone interface. No significant difference was found in loosening rates for implants retrieved in the short term (defined as less than 3 years) and in the long term. Edwards

et al. (1997) also reviewed aseptic loosening in 11 total hip replacements in 10 dogs. Loosening of the femoral component occurred at the cement–implant interface at a mean of 30 months postoperatively. Radiographic changes associated with aseptic loosening included asymmetrical periosteal reaction along the femoral diaphysis, radiolucent zone at the stem–cement interface, altered implant position, and femur fracture. They found that aseptic loosening was significantly more common when the distal tip of the femoral component was in contact with the cortical endosteum than when there was no contact.

The clinical use of the PCA Canine Total Hip system (Howmedica, Mahwah, NJ) was reported, but was not commercially produced for the veterinary market (DeYoung et al. 1992; Marcellin-Little et al. 1999a). However, the PCA system is considered the predecessor for the BioMedtrix BFX® system. DeYoung et al. (1992) described the PCA implant design as well as the surgical technique for implantation. The femoral component of this system was available in four sizes, each made of cast cobalt-chromium alloy with porous coating at the proximal one-third of the stem. The modular femoral head allowed for two different femoral neck lengths and to be used interchangeably with the stems and acetabular components. The acetabular component was a cast cobalt-chromium alloy with a backing of three layers of beads and an ultrahigh-molecular-weight polyethylene insert. Two polyethylene insert depths were also available. Both the acetabular and femoral components were a press-fit with long-term stability imparted by porous bone ingrowth. A preliminary study was done on 60 experimental hips followed by 40 clinically affected hips in 32 client-owned dogs. The overall success rate for the 100 total hips was 98%. There were six complications including three luxations, two fissure fractures of the femur, and one displacement of the acetabular component due to improper positioning. Only two of the hips were eventually explanted. Marcellin-Little et al. (1999b) reported on 50 consecutive total hip replacements in 41 dogs. Mean long-term follow-up was 63 months. Radiographically, all cups and stems had bone ingrowth fixation and no evidence of osteolysis, late stem subsidence, or cup tilting. At the long-term follow-up, 74% of hips had normal function. Of those with abnormal function, three had luxations and the remainder had unrelated problems causing abnormal hind limb gait.

The Zurich Cementless Total Hip Replacement system (Kyon, Zurich, Switzerland) has been available since the late 1990s (Guerrero and Montavon 2009). In this system, the femoral components are made of titanium and titanium alloy and the acetabular component is lined with ultrahigh-molecular-weight polyethylene. The femoral stem in this system is anchored to the medial cortex of the femur with locking screws. This design is intended to decrease complications resulting from subsidence, as well as micromotion at the bone–implant interface. Stress shielding of the bone is also meant to be minimized.[2] This prosthesis is discussed in detail in Chapter 7. The BioMedtrix BFX system is an uncemented total hip replacement system designed to be interchangeable with the BioMedtrix CFX system. It was commercially introduced in 2003. The femoral and acetabular components of the BFX system are press-fit and designed to allow porous ingrowth for long-term stability. This prosthesis is discussed in detail in Chapter 7.

The dog has been used as a model for human total hip replacement for decades. Total hip replacement in the dog as a model for the development of a prosthesis for human use was first reported in 1957 (Gorman 1957). Gorman implanted a cementless, stainless steel prosthesis in over 50 dogs. The acetabular component was stabilized using three toggle bolts and the femoral component was simply inserted into the femoral canal without fixation, although the first-generation stem was transfixed to the medullary canal (Figure 1.2). The femoral head was retained within the acetabular component by a retaining rim to prevent luxation. The author reported generally positive results.

Chen et al. (1983) performed total hip replacement in 13 dogs. The cementless femoral component was square in cross section and with a titanium core and a 2-mm outer layer of unalloyed 50% fiber titanium composite. Seven dogs were implanted with a cementless acetabular component of ultrahigh-molecular-weight polyethylene and a cylindrical outer surface, coated with unalloyed titanium fiber. The remaining six dogs were implanted with cemented acetabular components. Bone ingrowth occurred in all porous-coated

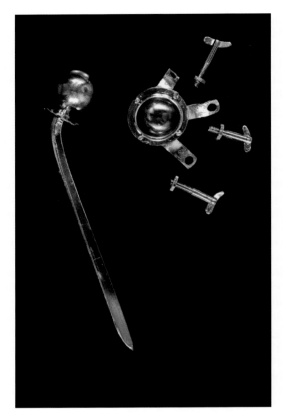

Figure 1.2   The Gorman total hip prosthesis was used in canine patients as a model for human total hip replacement. (Image courtesy of David DeYoung)

implants; however, no mechanical testing was performed in this study to evaluate the strength characteristics of the implants. All of the animals walked without functional deficits and all femoral stems and acetabular cups were stable at 6 months postoperatively.

Gitelis et al. (1982) studied the effects of weight bearing on the bone–cement interface in cemented total hip replacements in two groups of six dogs. A cobalt-chrome femoral component and ultrahigh–molecular-weight polyethylene acetabular component were implanted using acrylic cement. In one group, immediate weight bearing with unrestricted activity was allowed, while in the second group amputation distal to the knee was performed in order to prevent weight bearing. Three of the dogs in the weight-bearing group had postoperative luxation. These dogs were eliminated from the study and replaced with three new dogs. Endosteal bone remodeling with a fibrous membrane located between the endosteal surface of the bone and cement was found in both weight-bearing and nonweight-bearing dogs. The study found that early postoperative weight bearing was not a factor in bone remodeling at the bone–cement interface and surrounding bone.

Dowd et al. (1995) investigated the role of implant motion, titanium alloy, cobalt-chrome alloy, and polyethylene particles in the process of osteolysis and aseptic loosening. Forty dogs had total hip replacements and were assigned to the control group or one of five experimental groups. The control group had a standard prosthesis implanted. The prosthesis was modified for the experimental groups to create a motion model, a gap model, and three particulate debris models (a titanium model, a cobalt-chrome model, and a high-density polyethylene model). Two dogs had intraoperative femur fracture during implantation and were excluded from the study. One dog had a postoperative luxation, underwent open reduction, and remained in the study. All dogs had a clinically normal gait by 2 weeks after surgery. After 12 weeks, the femurs were harvested. All control implants were stable with no obvious motion between the implant and bone. All of the experimental implants had some degree of motion and the femoral prosthesis was easily separated from the femur. Histological and biochemical assessment of the periprosthetic tissues from the control group had relatively acellular periprosthetic tissue with low levels of biochemical activity. In contrast, assessment of the motion group as well as all three particulate debris groups showed increased numbers of macrophages as well as increased levels of biochemical mediators of bone resorption consistent with osteolysis.

Among the most interesting uses of the canine model for human total hip replacement was the use of Robodoc, an industrial robot adapted for used in surgery (Paul et al. 1992). The purpose of this study was to determine whether robotic preparation of the femoral canal would result in improved implant–bone contact and fewer intraoperative cracks or fissures compared to hand broaching for a cementless total hip prosthesis. The clinical portion of this study included 25 canine patients with robotic femoral canal preparation and 15 patients with manual femoral canal preparation. Robotic preparation resulted in a higher implant–bone contact than manual preparation and resulted in no fissures or cracks.

Total elbow replacement

The first clinical case of total elbow replacement in small animals was reported in 1964 (Whittick et al. 1964). A custom-manufactured, hinged, constrained stainless steel prosthesis was implanted in a cat with comminuted fractures of the distal humerus and proximal radius and ulna. Due to inherent constraints of the implant design the cat had limited range of motion of the elbow postoperatively, but the results were considered acceptable. Three months postoperatively, the cat was estimated to use its leg at 80% of normal function and was able to resume its normal activities, including running and climbing trees.

Unlike total hip replacement and total knee replacement, there is no comparable human model for elbow osteoarthritis in dogs. In addition, the elbow presents the additional challenge of being a three-bone joint, with the inherent risks this poses to implant loosening. Nevertheless, the high incidence of end-stage elbow osteoarthritis in dogs with relatively few treatment options has encouraged several groups to work toward total or partial elbow (unicompartmental) replacement.

Since the late 1990s, a constrained hinged system, a four-component nonconstrained system, and a semiconstrained system have been designed, tested, and abandoned prior to publishing any results due to high complication rates (see Chapters 11 and 12; Conzemius 2009). The TATE Total Elbow (BioMedtrix) consists of a preassembled, prealigned combined humeral and radioulnar implant. Preliminary trials using the TATE Total Elbow were reported by Acker and Van Der Meulen in 2008. The system was implanted in six client-owned dogs with elbow pain secondary to end-stage osteoarthritis.[3] Complications included an epicondylar fracture with pin migration, ulnar nerve transection, and implant malpositioning with a humeral crack. At the time of the report, none of the dogs had required explantation. The TATE prosthesis is discussed in detail in Chapter 12.

The BioMedtrix (Iowa State) Canine Elbow has been used clinically for more than 10 years. Conzemius and colleagues initially reported on its use in six normal dogs in 1998 and again in 2001. The 1998 prototype system was a cemented snap-fit semiconstrained system that yielded suboptimal results, with loosening of the radioulnar component in five of six dogs (Conzemius and Aper 1998). The system was modified to an unconstrained, cemented, two-component system consisting of a stainless steel humeral component and an ultrahigh-molecular-weight polyethylene radioulnar component (Conzemius et al. 2001). Three of six dogs in the later report had excellent results, with normal use of the operated limb 1 year after surgery (Conzemius 2009). Modifications to the BioMedtrix elbow were made based on these results, and the system was implanted in 20 client-owned dogs with severe radiographic elbow osteoarthritis and daily lameness from elbow pain unresponsive to medical management (Conzemius et al. 2003). The revised system was still an unconstrained, cemented, two-component system made from the same materials as previously. This system and its current (third-generation) design are described in detail in Chapter 12.

Total knee replacement

Dogs have been used as preclinical models for human total knee replacement for over 30 years (Bobyn et al. 1982; Turner et al. 1989; Sumner et al. 1994; Allen et al. 2009). Bobyn et al. (1982) investigated biological fixation in a canine total knee prosthesis in six beagle dogs. A custom-designed, unconstrained prosthesis with a wide bearing surface and a single radius of curvature was selected in order to facilitate fabrication and surgical implantation. The cobalt alloy femoral component had a porous-surfaced central stem with two small pins on either side to provide immediate rotational and translational stability. The tibial component was made of ultrahigh-molecular-weight, high-density polyethylene with a pentagonal projection at the base and a central stem with V-shaped circumferential grooves allowing for tissue ingrowth. The keel at the base was designed to fit into a similarly shaped recess in the tibial plateau in order to provide rotational and translational stability. Four of the six dogs regained normal function in the leg, including the ability to run and jump without lameness or gait abnormality. Of the two with residual deficits, one had a pronounced lameness and the other ambulated with the leg externally rotated. Four dogs were explanted, one each at 3, 6, 9, and 12 months. All four had loosening of the tibial component. Significant bony proliferation was present and a thin layer of fibrous tissue was present between the implant and the bone, suggesting micromotion during loading with eventual loosening. None of the four had loosening of the femoral component; however, there was substantial bone remodeling present. The authors concluded that the stability of the femoral implants was a positive achievement and that further changes to both components were needed. Turner et al. (1989) evaluated bone ingrowth into a porous-coated tibial component of a canine total knee replacement model. An unconstrained total condylar-type prosthesis was designed to model the available human prostheses and implanted in six dogs. The cobalt-chromium alloy femoral component was textured with cobalt-chromium alloy beads and cemented in place. The tibial component was composed of an ultrahigh-molecular-weight polyethylene articular surface bonded to a 1-mm-thick perforated titanium reinforcement plate and 2-mm-thick pad of 50% dense fiber porous metal composite with three cylindrical pegs. These pegs, along with a caudal screw, provided the initial stabilization for the tibial implant. After 6 months, extensive bone ingrowth was identified in all six tibial components. Fibrous tissue ingrowth was present in the areas of the pad that did not have bone ingrowth, suggesting that there was either a gap present at implantation or postoperative relative motion between the implant and bone. Unlike the Bobyn study, bony proliferation was not present in the dogs in this study. The authors concluded that precise attention to surgical technique to create intimate contact between the implant and bone, as well as implant design modifications to decrease the incidence of implant-bone relative motion, would be needed to improve the results for clinical total knee replacement. The development of jigs and cutting guides has improved the precision, and thus the fit, of knee prostheses.

Canine total knee replacement in a clinical setting is still relatively new. In 2007, Liska et al. described the use of a custom total knee replacement in a dog with a nonunion of the medial femoral condyle. The cobalt chrome femoral component and ultrahigh-molecular-weight polyethylene tibial component of the BioMedtrix system (Canine Total Knee, BioMedtrix) were used along with a titanium and porous tantalum augment to the femoral component to address the femoral bone defects present. The outcome in this case was successful. Seventeen months postoperatively, the dog had returned to his normal activities, including moose hunting, with lameness occurring only after strenuous exercise (see Chapter 14). The BioMedtrix Canine Total Knee system that is currently commercially available is a modular hybrid press-fit and cemented system. This prosthesis is discussed in detail in Chapter 10.

Conclusion

Regardless of the joint being replaced, continued progress in the arena of joint replacement for companion animals will require a consistent means of outcomes assessment. Further, the need for improvement will only be recognized by a critical evaluation of outcomes, and what is meant by a "successful" or "unsuccessful" outcome. A low revision rate does not equal a high success rate, unless it is clear to the reader that the prostheses are functioning at the level expected. We anticipate that, in the future, validated joint scores will be a key component of the decision making for patients with severe joint disease and the outcome assessment of total joint prostheses.

Endnotes

1. Liska WD. Cemented total hip replacement: Experience in USA with the BioMedtrix prosthesis. In: *Proceedings of the Pre-congress of the European Society of Veterinary Orthopaedics and Traumatology*. Munich, Germany, 2004.
2. Tepic S, Montavon PM. Concepts of cementless Zürich prosthesis. In: *Proceedings of the Pre-congress of the European Society of Veterinary Orthopaedics and Traumatology*. Munich, Germany, 2004.

3. Acker R, Van Der Meulen G. TATE Elbow preliminary trials. In: *Proceedings of the 35th Annual Conference of the Veterinary Orthopedic Society*. Big Sky, MT, 2008.

References

Agins HJ, Alcock NW, Bansal M, et al. Metallic wear in failed titanium-alloy total hip replacements. J Bone Joint Surg Am 1988;70:347–356.

Allen MJ, Leone KA, Lamonte K, et al. Cemented total knee replacement in 24 dogs: Surgical technique, clinical results, and complications. Vet Surg 2009;38: 555–567.

Bergh MS, Gilley RS, Shofer FS, et al. Complications and radiographic findings following cemented total hip replacement: A retrospective evaluation of 97 dogs. Vet Comp Orthop Traumatol 2006;19:172–179.

Bobyn JD, Cameron HU, Abdulla D, et al. Biologic fixation and bone modeling with an unconstrained canine total knee prosthesis. Clin Orthop Relat Res 1982;166:301–312.

Chen PQ, Turner TM, Ronnigen H, et al. A canine cementless total hip prosthesis model. Clin Orthop Relat Res 1983;176:24–33.

Conzemius MG. Nonconstrained elbow replacement in dogs. Vet Surg 2009;38:279–284.

Conzemius MG, Aper RL. Development and evaluation of semiconstrained arthroplasty for the treatment of elbow osteoarthritis in the dog. Vet Comp Orthop Traumatol 1998;11:54a.

Conzemius MG, Aper RL, Hill CM. Evaluation of a canine total-elbow arthroplasty system: A preliminary study in normal dogs. Vet Surg 2001;30:11–20.

Conzemius MG, Aper RL, Corti LB. Short-term outcome after total elbow arthroplasty in dogs with severe, naturally occurring osteoarthritis. Vet Surg 2003;32: 545–552.

DeYoung DJ, DeYoung BA, Aberman HA, et al. Implantation of an uncemented total hip prosthesis: Technique and initial results of 100 arthroplasties. Vet Surg 1992;21:168–177.

Dowd JE, Schwendeman LJ, Macaulay W, et al. Aseptic loosening in uncemented total hip arthroplasty in a canine model. Clin Orthop Relat Res 1995;319: 106–121.

Edwards MR, Egger EL, Schwarz PD. Aseptic loosening of the femoral implant after cemented total hip arthroplasty in dogs: 11 cases in 10 dogs (1991–1995). J Am Vet Med Assoc 1997;211:580–586.

Gitelis S, Chen PQ, Andersson GBJ, et al. The influence of early weight-bearing on experimental total hip arthroplasties in dogs. Clin Orthop Relat Res 1982;169:291–302.

Goldring SR, Schiller AL, Roelke M, et al. The synovial-like membrane at the bone-cement interface in loose total hip replacements and its proposed role in bone lysis. J Bone Joint Surg Am 1983;65:575–584.

Gorman HA. A new prosthetic hip joint; experiences in its use in the dog, and its probable application to man. Mil Med 1957;121(2):91–93.

Guerrero TG, Montavon PM. Zurich cementless total hip replacement: Retrospective evaluation of 2nd generation implants in 60 dogs. Vet Surg 2009;38:70–80.

Hoefle WD. A surgical procedure prosthetic total hip replacement in the dog. J Am Anim Hosp Assoc 1974;10:269–276.

Lee JM, Salvati EA, Betts F, et al. Size of metallic and polyethylene debris particles in failed cemented total hip replacements. J Bone Joint Surg 1992;74-B: 380–384.

Leighton RL. The Richard's II canine hip prosthesis. J Am Anim Hosp Assoc 1979;15:73–76.

Lewis RH, Jones JP. A clinical study of canine total hip arthroplasty. Vet Surg 1980;9:20–23.

Liska WD, Marcellin-Little DJ, Eskelinen EV, et al. Custom total knee replacement in a dog with femoral condylar bone loss. Vet Surg 2007;36:293–301.

Marcellin-Little DJ, DeYoung BA, Doyens DH, et al. Canine uncemented porous-coated anatomic total hip arthroplasty: Results of a long-term prospective evaluation of 50 consecutive cases. Vet Surg 1999a;28: 10–20.

Marcellin-Little DJ, DeYoung DJ, Thrall DE, Merrill CL. Osteosarcoma at the site of bone infarction associated with total hip arthroplasty in a dog. Vet Surg 1999b;28:54–60.

Olmstead ML. The canine cemented modular total hip prosthesis. J Am Anim Hosp Assoc 1995;31:109–124.

Olmstead ML, Hohn RB, Turner TM. A five-year study of 221 total hip replacements in the dog. J Am Vet Med Assoc 1983;183:191–194.

Paul HA, Bargar WL, Mittlestadt B, et al. Development of a surgical robot for cementless total hip arthroplasty. Clin Orthop Relat Res 1992;286:57–66.

Roe SC, DeYoung D, Weinstock D, Kyles A. Osteosarcoma eight years after total hip arthroplasty. Vet Surg 1996;25:70–74.

Sebestyen P, Marcellin-Little DJ, DeYoung BA. Femoral medullary infarction secondary to canine total hip arthroplasty. Vet Surg 2000;29:227–236.

Skurla CP, Pluhar GE, Frankel DJ, et al. Assessment of the dog as a model for human total hip replacement. J Bone Joint Surg Br 2005;87:120–127.

Sumner DR, Berzins A, Turner T, et al. Initial in vitro stability of the tibial component in a canine model of cementless total knee replacement. J Biomechanics 1994;27(7):929–939.

Turner TM, Urban RM, Sumner DR, et al. Bone ingrowth into the tibial component of a canine total condylar knee replacement prosthesis. J Orthop Res 1989;7: 893–901.

Whittick WG, Bonar CJ, Reeve-Newson JA. Two unusual orthopaedic prostheses. Can Vet J 1964;5:56–60.

2 Implant Materials: Structural

Simon C. Roe

Selecting the best metal for a joint prosthesis is a very complex decision. There is considerable history in both human and veterinary prosthesis production that supports the "classic" choices, but new metals and manufacturing techniques, combined with new design concepts, can lead to innovative approaches. The final choice will be dictated by balancing design, metallurgy, manufacturing, biological, and economic factors. This balance requires input from specialists in the many aspects of the process. In this chapter, the principles associated with metallurgy and manufacturing will be summarized. The common metals used in joint prostheses—stainless steel, cobalt-chromium alloys, titanium and its alloys—will be covered. The information in these sections is a summary from a number of texts on biomaterials, metals, and joint replacement fundamentals (Crowninshield and Anderson 1985; Lemons 1991; Helsen and Breme 1998; Leng 2006; Wright and Maher 2007). A brief review of tantalum, a newer metal being used in human joint prostheses that may become more available in the veterinary field, is included. The chapter concludes with a description of the materials and processing techniques used for the implant systems currently available in the veterinary market.

General metallurgy

There are a number of metals commonly used for hip implants. Most of the metals that have become common in the medical field were developed for the aerospace, marine, or chemical industries. As they were developed and refined, and the various aspects of their physical and chemical properties were understood, they were evaluated for medical use. Their desirability was dependent on the intended use. For joint prostheses, the important factors are as follows:

1. Mechanical properties: strength, modulus, ductility, hardness, fatigue resistance
2. Biological properties: corrosion resistance, biocompatibility, toxicity of elements and particulates released
3. Manufacturing processes: cast, forged, machined, surface treatments, coatings

Advances in Small Animal Total Joint Replacement, First Edition. Edited by Jeffrey N. Peck and Denis J. Marcellin-Little.
© 2013 John Wiley & Sons, Inc. Published 2013 by John Wiley & Sons, Inc.

4. Business considerations: cost and availability of materials and manufacturing cost

Metals and their alloys have a very closely packed structure, with strong multidirectional bonds, which impart their strength. At a nanostructural level, 70%–75% of the volume is filled with atoms. The multidirectional bonds also convey to metals their ability to plastically deform. The bonds are able to "flow" within the structure with little loss of strength. Alloys are made by combining elements within the primary metal molecules. These additional elements are added to improve the physicochemical properties so that the final "solution" can meet the desired design criteria. The specific roles of the alloying elements will be presented for each of the metals discussed.

Many of the mechanical and biological properties are influenced by the manufacturing process. Metals start in molten form and, through various processes, end up as solid implants. The first step—transitioning from liquid to solid—is an important factor for the final properties. As the metal cools, crystals form and coalesce to form grains. The strength and fatigue properties of the metal can be enhanced by ensuring the grain size stays small. This is influenced by the rate of cooling—generally, the more rapid the cooling, the smaller the grain size—and by the relative sizes and affinities of the atoms of the composing elements. There are a number of ways in which the atoms can arrange themselves, which results in different phases within the microstructure. These can be beneficial (e.g., chromium in steel) or detrimental (e.g., carbon in steel), so the concentrations must be well controlled. Impurities often end up at the grain boundaries, and can influence crack propagation and corrosion.

Fabricating shapes

There are several methods for creating metal components. The appropriate approach for a particular component will be influenced by the complexity of the shape, the desired mechanical properties, the preferred metal or alloy, the number of parts needed, and the costs of processing. The steps include forming the desired shape, postprocessing

manipulations of the microstructure, and surface treatments.

Moderately complex shapes can be formed by investment casting. A wax mold of the part is covered with ceramic slurries to build a heat-resistant cast. The wax is melted and the cavity filled with molten metal. The rate of cooling is controlled to optimize grain size but prevent gas retention voids from forming.

Forging involves heating the metal precursor and then pressing it into its shape using a mold and a large amount of force. For a femoral stem, this may involve a series of molds that progressively build on the complexity of the part until it has reached its desired shape. Because heat and pressure are combined, the grain size is often reduced, and the final part will be stronger than one formed by investment casting.

Many of the metals that are suitable for joint implants are very difficult to machine because they are very hard, and become harder as they are "worked." As such, usually only small or simple shapes are produced by machining. Computer-controlled systems have greatly increased the capability for producing more complex shapes. These systems are also used to finish parts that were primarily formed by casting or forging.

A number of techniques have been developed to improve the mechanical properties of metals both prior to forming the part and afterward. Hot working involves heating the metal to near-melting and extruding it into a basic form. Forging is a type of hot working. These processes aim to reduce grain size and internal stresses but they do not change strength and hardness. After processing, annealing is used in a similar fashion. The part is heated and the rate of cooling controlled to optimize microstructure. Hot isostatic pressing (HIP'ing) is frequently used to consolidate voids in cast products, particularly Ti alloys. The metal part is heated to just below its melting point, and high pressures (>1000 atm) applied. This will increase the fatigue life and corrosion resistance of the part.

Cold working of metal involves rolling or drawing bulk material to reduce its dimensions without heating. The grain size is reduced and the microstructure is made more uniform. This process will increase the yield strength and reduce ductility. It is used most frequently with stainless steel, a metal that is not frequently used in joint prostheses.

Adding porous coatings

The primary forms of porous coating are beads and fiber wire/mesh. Adding porous coatings can affect the overall implant mechanical properties. These are usually hand applied to the implant surface and adhered by sintering or diffusion bonding. Sintering involves heating the coating and part to 90%–95% of its melting temperature so that the coating material bonds strongly with the base material. However, this can result in growth of the grains of the microstructure, resulting in a reduction of the yield and tensile strength of the part. Also, if there are impurities, they may melt and leave voids. This will also reduce the fatigue resistance. Diffusion bonding is another method used to bond the porous coating to the base part. It uses less heat and adds significant pressure to promote a strong bond. This results in less effect on the base metal. Porous coatings also cause a stress concentration, or notch effect at the points where they attach to the part, which reduces the fatigue life of the implant. More details about porous coatings and bone ingrowth and ongrowth are provided in Chapter 3.

Metals used for implant fabrication

Stainless steel

Stainless steel is not used in prosthesis parts as it is not strong enough, nor does it have ideal fatigue properties. It is, however, used in many orthopedic applications and in the management of complications associated with joint replacement. In most medical applications, 316L grade 2 stainless steel is used, which is defined by the American Society for Testing and Materials (ASTM) F138 standard. The alloying elements are chromium (17%–20%), nickel (10%–17%), molybdenum (2%–4%), with carbon levels specifically kept below 0.03% for the "L" designation, and minor amounts of manganese, phosphorus, sulfur, and silicon. Chromium is important as it forms a surface oxide that imparts corrosion resistance. This is enhanced

by etching the finished implants in a strong nitric acid bath. The chromium also helps stabilize the ferritic phase elements. However, medical-grade stainless steel is in the austenitic phase, which the nickel helps stabilize. This imparts better mechanical properties and corrosion resistance. It is important that carbon levels are kept low as higher levels result in an altered grain structure and variable chromium distribution, making the material more prone to corrosion-related fracture. All standard implants, other than wire, are machined from stock that has been cold worked to increase the yield and tensile strengths. The amount of cold working is selected so that the material retains some ductility.

Cobalt-chromium alloy

Cobalt-chromium alloys are commonly used for joint prostheses because they have very high strength and fatigue resistance. The most usual alloying elements are chromium (27%–30%), molybdenum (5%–7%), and nickel (2.5%). If the parts are formed by investment casting, the material is defined by the ASTM F75 standard. HIP'ing can be used to reduce grain size and improve mechanical properties.

Components can also be made by forging. The nitrogen levels in the alloy are increased to strengthen the material. This alloy and its processing are defined by the ASTM F799 standard. This method of fabrication results a reduced grain size and thus, the yield and tensile strengths are double that of ASTM F75, and ductility is 50% greater. Similar to stainless steel, chromium imparts corrosion resistance by passively forming an oxide layer on the surface. Because the material is so hard, it is difficult to machine. However, this feature results in very good wear resistance, so it is commonly used as a prosthetic head component. To reduce wear of the adjacent polyethylene, the surface of the heads must be highly polished.

Titanium

Commercially pure (CP) titanium (ASTM F67) is used in some orthopedic applications as it is very biocompatible, but it has low yield and tensile strength, so is not used in load-bearing components.

The most popular titanium alloy is a titanium-aluminum-vanadium mixture. Aluminum is at 5.5%–6.5% and vanadium at 3.5%–4.5%. The common designation is Ti6Al4V (ASTM F136). The alloy molecules stabilize the titanium and impart high fatigue resistance. The modulus of titanium is half that for steel and cobalt—116 GPa c.f. 190 GPa and 210 GPa. The tensile strength is lower than the cobalt alloys and similar to steel. Because of the lower hardness, it is not as resistant to wear, so it is not used commonly for the femoral head. This material is very notch sensitive, so sites that have extreme changes in geometry may be points of stress concentration. This may be an issue with adding of porous coatings, so processes that are less "geometric," such as plasma spraying, are preferred.

Components can be produced by forging, casting, or machining. Strain hardening occurs with cold working. Microhardening occurs during machining, so this approach requires considerable care. HIP'ing improves fatigue strength.

Concern over the possibility of vanadium toxicity has led to the development of newer alloys. The primary one for medical applications has niobium as the crystal stabilizing element and zirconium instead of vanadium. This alloy (Ti13Nb13Zr—ASTM F1713) has a lower modulus than, but similar strength to, Ti6Al4V.

Tantalum

This section was summarized from Patil et al. (2009). Tantalum is a metal that can be fabricated with porosity and mechanical characteristics similar to bone. It is made by depositing tantalum onto a vitreous carbon scaffold that was created from a polyurethane foam. The resulting pore size range from 500 to 600 μm and the volume porosity is 75%–80%. It has a modulus of 3 GPa, which is similar to that generally given for subchondral (2 GPa) and cancellous (1.5 GPa) bone. Its yield strength is higher than cancellous bone, enabling it to contribute to the strength of a construct. The porosity results in excellent bone ingrowth, and this can be improved by adding calcium-phosphate coatings.

Tantalum has been used in reconstructive surgery following tumor excision, failed or challenging joint replacement, and complex spinal fusions in humans (Fernandez-Fairen et al. 2008; Patil et al. 2009; Khan et al. 2012). Some human primary hip and knee systems have used tantalum as the metal for the cup and tibial component (Fernandez-Fairen et al. 2008; Patil et al. 2009). The polyethylene is injection molded so that it penetrates into the porous metal, making a very secure bond. This monobloc design means that liner cannot be replaced, and if bone ingrowth occurs, revision of a tantalum cup can be difficult. It is more commonly used for complicated revisions, or joint replacement in areas that underwent radiation therapy.

Materials used in veterinary joint replacement systems

There are a variety of metals used in the manufacture of joint prostheses for the veterinary market. A detailed description is provided in Table 2.1.

The standard BFX® (BioMedtrix Inc., Boonton, NJ) femoral stem is cast cobalt-chromium, with a sintered bead porous ingrowth surface. However, recently, a machined, plasma-sprayed, titanium alloy stem has been made available, and is in limited clinical use. The topography of the bead and plasma-sprayed surfaces are displayed in Figure 2.1. The titanium stem is less stiff, particularly in its distal tip.

The BioMedtrix prosthetic head is machined from wrought cobalt-chromium, and then polished to a very smooth finish to reduce polyethylene wear (Figure 2.2). The standard CFX® (BioMedtrix Inc.) stem is also cast cobalt-chromium. A matte surface is created to enhance bonding with polymethylmethacrylate. Similar materials and methods are used in the manufacture of the knee and elbow prostheses from BioMedtrix.

The Helica® (Veterinary Instrumentation Ltd., Sheffield, U.K.) prosthetic femoral and acetabular components are machined from titanium alloy, and have a macro thread for initial stability. The

Table 2.1 Implant materials, manufacturing methods, and specifications for veterinary joint replacement prostheses

Product	Component	Material	Manufacturing method	Bone ingrowth surface	Cement fixation surface	Articular surface
BFX Hip[a]	Femoral stem: CoCr	ASTM F75 Cobalt-chrome	Cast cobalt-chrome Machine taper, hand finish stem	Sintered CoCr beads (250 μm)	NA	NA
	Femoral stem: Ti Acetabular cup	ASTM F136 Ti6Al4V EL1	Machined titanium	Plasma-sprayed titanium particles	NA	NA
	Shell	ASTM F1472 Ti6Al4V	Machined titanium	Sintered Ti beads (250 μm)	NA	NA
	Insert	ASTM F648 UHMWPE	Machined polyethylene	NA	NA	16 μin Ra max
	Femoral head	ASTM F799 Wrought CoCr	Machined cobalt-chrome from wrought bar stock	NA	NA	2.0 μin RA max
CFX Hip[a]	Femoral stem: CoCr	ASTM F75 Cobalt-chrome	Cast cobalt-chrome Machine taper, hand finish stem	NA	Bead blast Matte finish	NA
		ASTM F799 Wrought cobalt-chrome	Machined cobalt-chrome for smaller stems (nano, micro, #4,#4/5,#5)	NA	Bead blast Matte finish	NA
	Acetabular cup	ASTM F648 UHMWPE	Machined polyethylene	NA	Radial and circumferential grooves	16 μin Ra max
Canine Total Knee[a]	Femoral	ASTM F75 Cobalt-chrome	Cast cobalt-chrome Hand finish articular surface	Sintered CoCr beads (250 μm)	If required, beads would provide cement fix surface	4 μin Ra max
	Tibial all-poly	ASTM F648 UHMWPE	Machined polyethylene	NA	Undersurface grooves and central stem	16 μin Ra max
	Tibial metal-backed tray Tray	ASTM F75 Cobalt-chrome	Cast cobalt-chrome Machined insert pocket	Sintered CoCr beads (250 μm)	NA	NA
	Insert	ASTM F648 UHMWPE	Machined polyethylene	NA	NA	16 μin Ra max

15

Table 2.1 *Continued*

Product	Component	Material	Manufacturing method	Bone ingrowth surface	Cement fixation surface	Articular surface
TATE Total Elbow[a]	Humeral	ASTM F799 Wrought cobalt-chrome	Machined cobalt-chrome	Sintered CoCr beads (250 µm)	NA	4 µin Ra max
	Radial-ulnar Base	ASTM F799 Wrought cobalt-chrome	Machined cobalt-chrome	Sintered CoCr beads (250 µm)	NA	NA
	Insert	ASTM F648 UHMWPE	Machined polyethylene	NA	NA	16 µin Ra max
Helica Hip[b]	Femoral stem	ASTM F136 Ti6Al4V	Machined titanium	Sand blasted; roughness = 0.04 mm; average porosity 35%; Macro thread	NA	NA
	Acetabular cup Shell	ASTM F136 Ti6Al4V	Machined titanium	Sand blasted; roughness = 0.04 mm; macro thread	NA	NA
	Insert	ASTM F648 UHMWPE	Tampered	NA	NA	NP
	Femoral head	ASTM F1586 316L stainless steel	Machined	NA	NA	TiN coating[e] Plasma steam
Zurich Cementless Hip[c]	Femoral stem	ASTM F136 Ti6Al4V	Machined titanium	Micropeened Plasma sprayed	NA	NA
	Screws	ASTM F136 Ti 6Al 4V	Machined titanium	TiN coating[e]	NA	NA
	Acetabular cup Shell	ASTM F67 CP titanium, grade 4	Machined titanium	Plasma sprayed	NA	NA
	Liner	ASTM F648 UHMWPE	Machined polyethylene	NA	NA	NP
	Femoral head and neck	ASTM F136 Ti6Al4V	Machined titanium	NA	NA	Amorphous diamond-like coating[f,g]

Table 2.1 *Continued*

Product	Component	Material	Manufacturing method	Bone ingrowth surface	Cement fixation surface	Articular surface
VI Hip[d]	Femoral stem	ASTM F75 Cobalt-chrome	Cast cobalt-chrome Machine taper, hand finish stem	NA	Alumina grit blast to smooth finish	NA
	Acetabular cup	ASTM F648 UHMWPE	Machined polyethylene	NA	Radial and circumferential grooves	NP
	Femoral head	ISO 5832 part 1 316L stainless steel	Machined from stainless steel bar stock	NA	NA	Manual polish

[a]Information provided by Chris Sidebotham, BioMedtrix Inc, Boonton, NJ.
[b]Information provided by Manssur Arbaian, Innoplant, Hannover, Germany.
[c]Information from Kyon website (http://www.kyon.ch) and Dr. Jeff Peck, FL.
[d]Information provided by John Lapish, Veterinary Instrumentation, Sheffield, U.K.
[e]TiN: titanium nitride; hard ceramic coating to improve smoothness and wear performance.
[f]Amorphous diamond-like coating: hard coating to improve smoothness and wear performance.
[g]Product prior to 2010 had a TiN coating.
NA: not applicable; NP: not provided.

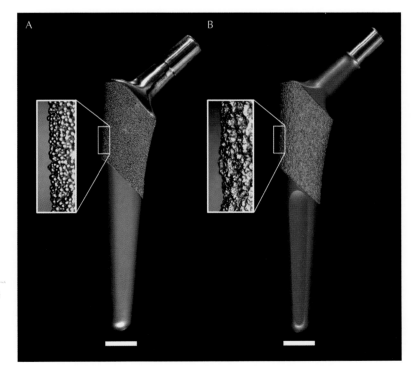

Figure 2.1 Photograph of the BFX® femoral stems. The cobalt-chromium stem (A) has a sintered bead ingrowth surface. The titanium stem (B) has a plasma-sprayed ingrowth surface in the same region. The bars are 10 mm. The insets show the beaded and plasma-sprayed surfaces at 40× magnification. For reference, the beads have a diameter of 0.25 mm.

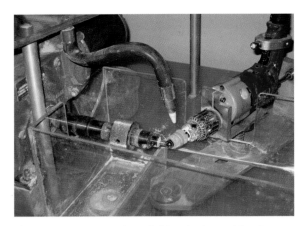

Figure 2.2 Apparatus for polishing the femoral head component. (Courtesy of Chris Sidebotham, BioMedtrix Inc.)

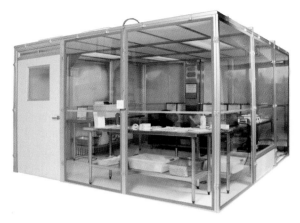

Figure 2.3 Example of a clean room for final processing and packaging of implants. (Courtesy of Chris Sidebotham, BioMedtrix Inc.)

surface is sand blasted to enhance ongrowth/ingrowth. The head is machined from 316L stainless steel, which is then coated with titanium nitride (TiN) to produce a very hard, wear-resistant bearing surface.

The Zurich Cementless Hip® (Kyon, Zurich, Switzerland) uses titanium alloy for the stem. It is machined, then micropeened (to improve fatigue resistance) and plasma sprayed to optimize the ongrowth surface. The screws are also titanium alloy, and are coated with TiN to reduce the possibility of cold welding. The shell of the cup is machined from CP titanium, grade 4, and is plasma sprayed. The head and neck component is machine from titanium alloy, and then coated with amorphous diamond-like carbon to create a smooth, hard, bearing surface. Earlier versions of the head and neck component were coated with TiN.

The femoral stem from Veterinary Instrumentation is cast cobalt-chromium, with sand blasting to a smooth finish. The head is machined from 316L stainless steel and is polished to ensure low wear.

After the final manufacturing steps, implants are moved to a clean room for final processing (Figure 2.3). They are degreased, cleaned by ultrasound, and packaged. Gamma irradiation is the standard sterilization process.

References

Crowninshield RD, Anderson PJ. Mechanical properties and manufacturing techniques for orthopaedic implants. In: Advanced Concepts in Total Hip Replacement, Harris WH (ed.). Thorofare, NJ: Slack, 1985, pp. 179–189.

Fernandez-Fairen M, Sala P, Dufoo M Jr., et al. Anterior cervical fusion with tantalum implant: A prospective randomized controlled study. Spine (Phila Pa 1976) 2008;33:465–472.

Helsen JA, Breme HJ. Metals As Biomaterials. West Sussex, England: John Wiley & Sons, 1998.

Khan FA, Rose PS, Yanagisawa M, et al. Surgical technique: Porous tantalum reconstruction for destructive nonprimary periacetabular tumors. Clin Orthop Relat Res 2012;470:594–601.

Lemons JE. Metals and alloys. In: Total Joint Replacement, Petty W (ed.). Philadelphia: WB Saunders, 1991, pp. 21–27.

Leng Y. Biomedical metallic materials. In: Introduction to Biomaterials, Shi D (ed.). Beijing, China: Tsinghua University Press, 2006, pp. 110–139.

Patil N, Lee K, Goodman SB. Porous tantalum in hip and knee reconstructive surgery. J Biomed Mater Res B Appl Biomater 2009;89:242–251.

Wright T, Maher SA. Biomaterials. In: Orthopaedic basic science: Biology and Biomechanics of the Musculoskeletal System, 3rd ed. Einhorn TA, O'Keefe RJ, Buckwalter JA (eds.). Rosemont, IL: American Academy of Orthopaedic Surgeons, 2007, pp. 65–85.

3 Implant Materials: Surface Coating

David J. DeYoung and Denis J. Marcellin-Little

Implants were developed for cementless fixation for both the acetabular and femoral components in an effort to address the fixation failures with cemented total hip prostheses. In spite of this fact, both cemented and cementless prostheses appear necessary and are widespread in veterinary applications mainly due to the size and breed variability of canine patients. In addition to the vast differences in femoral bone morphology and bone quality, the presence of advanced hip dysplasia in most canine patients undergoing total hip replacement presents the veterinary orthopedic surgeon with significant challenges. While many dogs are aptly suited for press-fit cementless components, most small- and giant-breed dogs are not due to their femoral size and shape. They require a cemented femoral stem.

In light of a better understanding of the mechanisms of failure of total hip components over the past 20 years, new implants, both cemented and cementless (press-fit and screw fixation), have been developed for veterinary applications. Concurrent with the improvements in prostheses, more focus has been placed on improved cementing techniques, including better bone preparation. Also, enhancements to the surface of the cemented stem have been made in an attempt to improve the implant–cement interface. These enhancements include roughening the surface of the stem, polishing the surface smooth, and precoating the stem with polymethylmethacrylate (PMMA).

The use of porous-coated devices has gained considerable acceptance as a method of achieving long-term implant fixation. Over the past 35 years, much attention has been focused on the area of surface coatings and bone ingrowth. A wealth of knowledge has been gained, much of which was determined using the dog as an *in vivo* model. Many surface coatings have been developed to enhance biological fixation of these implants to bone, providing long-term fixation. Long-term fixation to bone is dependent on achieving initial stability of the implant during surgery either by press-fit or by screw fixation. In both instances, bone ingrowth and bone ongrowth are necessary for achieving long-term stability. Much of the initial stability depends on implant design and bone preparation; however, several newer surface treatments have been shown to enhance surface friction and contribute significantly to the initial stability. The most common implant surface treatments for cementless components include sintered

Advances in Small Animal Total Joint Replacement, First Edition. Edited by Jeffrey N. Peck and Denis J. Marcellin-Little.
© 2013 John Wiley & Sons, Inc. Published 2013 by John Wiley & Sons, Inc.

beads or powder, fiber metal mesh, and plasma spray coatings. More recent developments include porous metal surfaces with increased porosity and optimal pore sizes when compared with previous coatings. Other surface treatments such as bisphosphonates and hydroxyapatite are bioactive coatings that affect the local environment and enhance the process of osseointegration.

Surface treatment of cemented femoral stems

Roughened surface, PMMA precoated, and smooth polished surface

Surface treatment of cemented femoral components is a very controversial topic in implant design. Surface alterations include roughening the surface by bead or grit blasting, polishing the surface smooth, or precoating of the stem with PMMA. Various studies report long-term success, as well as high failure rates, with rough and with PMMA-precoated stems (Mohler et al. 1995; Howie et al. 1998; Sporer et al. 1999; Schmalzried et al. 2000; Vail et al. 2003; Duffy et al. 2006; Lachiewicz et al. 2008). Although a great deal of controversy exists, it is an important issue because it influences the stem fixation to bone cement, generation of particulate cement debris, lysis of bone, and manufacturing cost (Mohler et al. 1995; Vail et al. 2003). The conflicting data reported may be related more to the cementing technique, in particular defects in the cement mantle, and to patient selection than to the actual surface treatment (Shepard et al. 2000; Vail et al. 2003). In the end, it serves to emphasize the importance of the implant–bone cement interface, including bone preparation, proper cementing technique, the use of a stem centralizer, and appropriate handling of the stem prior to insertion.

The surface treatments of roughening or precoating the stem with PMMA have resulted from the desire to achieve permanent fixation of the stem to the cement mantle. The concept of a roughened surface is to enhance the mechanical strength of the implant–bone cement interface (Bundy and Penn 1987; Davies and Harris 1994). Finite element analysis has predicted that bonding of the implant to the cement will significantly reduce mantle stresses well below the level of cement fatigue

strength (Chang et al. 1998). A permanent bond would result in a motionless interface that minimizes debonding, cement cracking, and cement debris generation resulting from motion (Mohler et al. 1995; Huiskes et al. 1998). The concept of precoating the stem with PMMA emanates from the fact that the interface strength between the implant and the bone cement is diminished in a surgical environment as compared with a controlled manufacturing environment. Under manufacturing conditions, the PMMA coating can be applied to the implant following meticulous preparation of its surface and at temperatures conducive to the curing process (Raab et al. 1982). At the time of surgical implantation, the unreacted monomer in the bone cement may soften the surface layer of the PMMA-precoated stem, effectively creating a level of chemical bonding between the two cement applications (Raab et al. 1982).

Alternatively, the rationale behind the smooth polished stem emanates from the belief that no cemented stem will remain permanently bonded (Vail et al. 2003). Once debonded, the smooth tapered stem will subside into the cement mantle and minimize the generation of cement debris resulting from motion of the stem against the cement (Vail et al. 2003). Clinical reports support this claim (Firestone et al. 2007; Ling et al. 2009). Several investigators have concluded that in the presence of a good cement mantle and good cementing technique, there is little difference between a roughened surface stem and polished stems (Shepard et al. 2000; Vail et al. 2003; Duffy et al. 2006). However, others have demonstrated potentially undesirable consequences of increased surface roughness on implant longevity in cemented stems, including rapid bone destruction following stem debonding (Sporer et al. 1999). The investigators concluded that if debonding of the stem does occur, a stem with a smooth surface is preferable (Sporer et al. 1999).

Surface treatment of cementless femoral stems and acetabular cup

Sintered beads, fiber metal mesh, plasma spray, porous tantalum

Cementless acetabular and femoral components depend on the ingrowth of bone into a textured

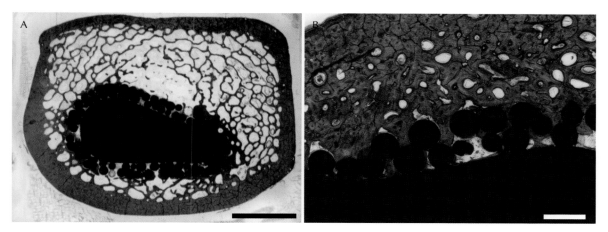

Figure 3.1   (A) Transverse histological section through the shaft of a canine femur with a porous-coated press-fit stem. The section is stained with toluidine blue. The femur was collected 12 months after surgery. Struts of cancellous bones link the endosteal surface to the stem. The cortical bone does not appear to be osteopenic or atrophic. The horizontal bar measures 5 mm. (B) Transverse histological section through the shaft of a canine femur collected 24 months after surgery. The section is stained with toluidine blue. Osseointegration onto and into the beaded region of the stem is visible. The horizontal bar measures 1 mm.

surface for long-term stability (Figure 3.1; Cameron et al. 1976; Bobyn et al. 1980; Cook et al. 1985). This biological means of fixation requires that the initial stability of the implants be achieved through press-fit or screw fixation. As in fracture fixation, bone contact and initial stability must be achieved in order for bone growth and remodeling to occur into the porous surface of the implant. Optimal fixation by bone ingrowth is dependent on good bone contact with the porous-coated surface (Cook et al. 1988). The stability achieved by press-fit at the time of implantation is dependent on multiple design characteristics of the implant, including the geometric shape of the implant and the texture or resistance offered by the porous surface against the bone bed. The fit and fill of the femoral stem in the femoral canal is important to minimize micromotion and subsidence (Rashmir-Raven et al. 1992). Gaps of 1.5–2.0 mm between the porous surface and the host bone can be bridged by bone, but may require up to 12 weeks (Bobyn et al. 1981). The same applies for the acetabular component. The design of the implant and instrumentation, as well as the bone preparation, should result in a press-fit free of micromotion and gaps, and be able to withstand immediate load bearing on the day of surgery. Preparation of the bone bed requires exact instrumentation and a thorough understanding of the application of the instrumentation by the surgeon (DeYoung et al. 1992).

Fortunately for veterinary orthopedic surgery, much of the basic research on porous surfaces, bone ingrowth, the ability of bone to grow across gaps, and the enhancement of ingrowth has been conducted in dogs using transcortical plugs as well as with total hip systems. Studies have included both mechanical and histological evaluations (Bobyn et al. 1980, 1987, 1999b; Turner et al. 1986; Jasty et al. 1993; Schiller et al. 1993).

Commercially available porous implants are made of either cobalt-chromium alloy or titanium. Porous metallic coatings consist of cobalt-chromium alloy or titanium spherical beads or powder, fiber metal mesh, or porous tantalum applied to a solid metal substrate. The bead coatings are applied to the substrate with a binder that holds the beads in place and catalyzes the surface fusion of the beads to each other and to the substrate during the sintering process, creating a highly interconnected system of pores (Figure 3.2). By altering the sintering process and the bead size, the average pore size and average volume porosity of the coating can be controlled. If the sintering process results in too much particle interconnectivity by increasing the "neck" size between particles, then the interconnection pore size is reduced and may restrict bone ingrowth. If the interconnectivity is too large, the structural strength of the coating will be decreased. An average volume porosity of 30%–40% for spherical bead coatings

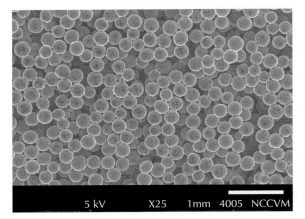

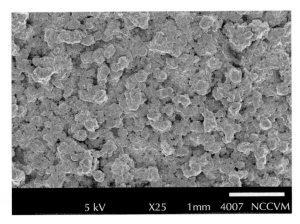

Figure 3.2 Scanning electron micrograph of sintered cobalt-chromium beads covering the surface of a canine BFX stem. Three layers of beads cover the stem. The horizontal bar measures 1 mm.

Figure 3.3 Scanning electron microscopy image of the plasma-sprayed surface of a canine BFX stem. The surface texture is visible. The horizontal bar measures 1 mm.

represents a compromise between maintaining strength of the coating and adequate pore size for bone ingrowth (Haddad et al. 1987).

A study of pore size using cobalt-chromium alloy cylindrical plugs implanted in the femoral cortex of dogs found that a pore size of 50–400 μm provided the best results during mechanical testing at 8 weeks (Bobyn et al. 1980). In a canine study using a cobalt-chromium alloy beaded, porous-coated hip prosthesis with an average pore size of 200–250 μm and 35%–40% volume porosity, the same investigator reported that, histologically, the porous region was ingrown with bone around the majority of the implant circumference (Bobyn et al. 1987). Using loaded porous-coated acetabular components with pore sizes of 140, 200, and 450 μm, excellent and uniform bone ingrowth was seen histologically in dogs at 3 months (Jasty and Harris 1988). Basically, no differences in ingrowth were seen between the groups with the various pore sizes. The mean bone ingrowth for the 140-, 200-, and 450-μm groups was 7.5%, 13.0%, and 13.3%, respectively. These studies confirmed that bone ingrowth into a wide range of pore sizes will occur in the dog. Biological fixation of porous-surfaced implants is a process influenced by a variety of factors in addition to pore size, including biocompatibility, implant geometry, material properties, and stability and proximity of the porous surface to the bone, as well as postoperative loading conditions (Turner et al. 1986).

Other popular porous coatings in use include fiber metal mesh coatings, plasma sprayed, and porous tantalum. Fiber metal mesh coatings are fabricated to form metallurgical bonds between the mesh wires and the substrate through a process of solid-state diffusion bonding. An alternative to sintered beads or diffusion-bonded fiber metal is to plasma spray coatings onto titanium (Figure 3.3). An electric arc is used to ionize a gas, creating a plasma. Metal powder, usually titanium, is sprayed through the plasma stream and melted. Once the molten metal is deposited on the implant it resolidifies, creating the porous surface. By manipulating the process, the porosity of the coating can be controlled. Following the plasma spray process, titanium alloy implants retain 90% of their fatigue strength, compared with less than 50% for sintered beads or diffusion-bonded titanium (Bourne et al. 1994).

Although excellent results have been shown with all of these porous coatings, a relatively new coating material, porous tantalum, may offer some advantages. Tantalum is a low-modulus metal with excellent biocompatibility. The porous surface is manufactured by chemical vapor deposition of pure tantalum into and on a vitreous carbon scaffolding with an open-cell dodecahedron repeating pattern (Bobyn et al. 1999b; Levine et al. 2006). The resulting material has a resemblance to trabecular bone (Figure 3.4), and the trabecular pattern provides the structural strength for the low-modulus metal. The advantages offered by the resulting structure include a high volume porosity (70%–80%), low modulus of elasticity (3 MPa), and high frictional characteristics (Levine et al. 2006). The mean pore size of current tantalum-coated prostheses range from 400 to 600 μm. A transcortical study in dogs investigated the extent of filling of the tantalum pores by bone using two different pore sizes, 430 μm and 650 μm (Bobyn et al. 1999a). In the small-pore cylinders, 42% of the pore space was filled with bone at 4 weeks, 63% at 16 weeks, and 80% at 52 weeks. The large-pore cylinders averaged 13% at 2 weeks, 53% at 4 weeks, and 70% at 16 and 52 weeks. Mechanical push-out testing

of the small-pore implants yielded 18.5 MPa minimum shear fixation strength at 4 weeks. This figure is higher than that obtained by the same investigator using the same model with beaded cobalt-chromium implants with similar pore sizes. The maximum mean shear strength for the cobalt-chromium implants at 4 weeks was 9.3 MPa. The difference of 9.2 MPa was significant (Student's t-test; $p = 0.004$; Bobyn et al. 1980, 1999a). These studies document that high fixation strength occurs much earlier with porous tantalum. Subsequently, 22 tantalum porous acetabular components were implanted in 11 dogs for a period of 6 months. The polyethylene was compression molded directly into the fully porous tantalum shell (Figure 3.5). All components were determined to be stable by histology, high-resolution contact radiographs, and electron microscopy. Ingrowth depth ranged from 0.2 to 2 mm in all 22 acetabular components. Ingrowth was a mean of 16.8% for all sections and 25.1% at the cup periphery. This compares favorably with results of cobalt-chromium beaded, porous-surfaced cups (13.4%) and fiber metal mesh titanium porous-coated cups (21.5%) supported with bone screw fixation reported in by a different investigator (Jasty and Harris 1988; Jasty et al. 1993). In a separate study in dogs, similar ingrowth (12%) was reported for a cobalt-chromium beaded, porous-coated cup with a single fixation peg at 6 months (Schiller et al. 1993). In a study investigating bone ingrowth through a perforated titanium-backed acetabular shell in dogs, bone ingrowth through the perforations was reported to be 50%, 20%, and 44% at 2, 6, and 12 months, respectively (Lauer et al. 2009).

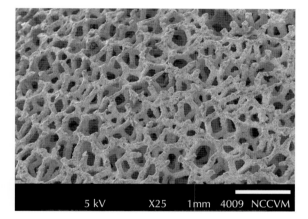

Figure 3.4 Scanning electron micrograph of a canine acetabular cup made of porous tantalum. The dodecahedron structure resembles trabecular bone. The porosity of the implant is approximately 75%. The horizontal bar measures 1 mm.

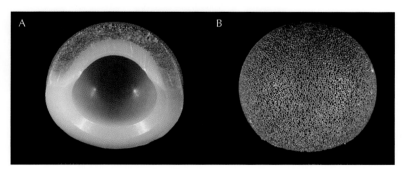

Figure 3.5 Front (A) and back (B) sides of a canine acetabular cup made of porous tantalum. The bearing surface of the cup is made of ultrahigh-molecular-weight polyethylene molded into the porous tantalum shell. The cup is courtesy of BioMedtrix (Boonton, NJ).

Regardless of the type of porous coating, other factors worthy of consideration include the extent of the stem that is porous coated longitudinally and whether or not the coating completely encircles the stem circumferentially. Regarding the longitudinal extent of the coating, less porous coating results in less cortical bone resorption (Engh and Bobyn 1988; Turner et al. 1986). The type of coating is less important than the extent of the coating on the stem (Turner et al. 1986). The current trend seems to be to only coat the proximal region of the femoral stem. Bone ingrowth into the porous surface creates a rigid interface between the bone and the implant resulting in stress shielding of the bone. A proximal porous coating concentrates the transfer of stress during loading to the proximal portion of the femur and helps preserve cortical bone surrounding the uncoupled or smooth portion of the stem. The smooth portion of the stem is surrounded by a periprosthetic cavity, outlined by a thin shell of trabecular bone, separated from the implant by fibrous tissue oriented parallel to the stem (Figure 3.6; Bobyn et al. 1995; DeYoung and Schiller 1992; Turner et al. 1986).

The periprosthetic cavity surrounding the smooth portion of the stem has been shown to serve as a pathway for the migration of particulate debris generated by the bearing surface and accumulated in the hip joint. Changes in intracapsular pressure can drive the debris into potential spaces remote from the joint space, provided that they communicate with the joint. Polyethylene has been shown to preferentially migrate along these smooth implant surfaces, both in long-term canine and human hip retrievals. Polyethylene particles have been identified within histiocytes and foreign-body giant cells located in the periprosthetic cavity, adjacent to the smooth regions of the stem (Bobyn et al. 1995). The migration of polyethylene wear debris from the joint to the implant–bone interface is a major cause of osteolysis and loosening of femoral stems (Kraemer et al. 1995). The migration of wear debris from the joint into the periprosthetic cavity has been shown to be blocked by the ingrowth of bone into a porous-coated surface (Bobyn et al. 1995; Kraemer et al. 1995; Emerson et al. 1999; von Knoch et al. 2000). These studies concluded that an ingrown circumferential porous coating effectively seals off the implant–bone interface from the joint space.

Biologically active coatings

Hydroxyapatite, bisphosphonate, microtexture, antibiotic, silver particles

Bone ingrowth into porous surfaces has been very successful in obtaining long-term biological fixation of implants to the surrounding bone.

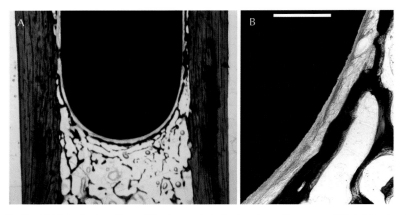

Figure 3.6 (A) Longitudinal histological section of the femoral shaft of a dog with a press-fit total hip implant. The section was made through the smooth portion of the distal stem tip and stained with toluidine blue. The distal portion of the stem is visible in the femoral canal and surrounded by a thin shell of bone. The space between the implant surface and the shell of bone forms the periprosthetic cavity and is filled with fibrous tissue. (B) On the detail, longitudinally oriented fibrous tissue is visible, filling the periprosthetic space. The horizontal bar measures 500 μm.

Circumstances including the age and condition of the patient, loading conditions, bone defects following revision, revision following infection, gaps at the implant–bone interface, micromotion, or bone morphology may benefit from an accelerated rate or quantity of bone ingrowth. To address some of these issues, much interest has evolved in the application of additional surface treatments to stimulate new bone formation and optimize initial implant fixation. Some of these applications stimulate new bone formation (hydroxyapatite, bisphosphonates, and microtexturing), while others are directed at prevention or elimination of bacteria in the local environment in order to facilitate fixation by bone (antibiotics and silver particles) in specific instances. Hydroxyapatite, bisphosphonates, antibiotics, and silver particles are biologically active chemicals or pharmaceuticals that can be bound to porous implant surfaces, while microtexturing is an additional surface treatment that has the ability to enhance bone ingrowth by stimulating osteoblasts.

Hydroxyapatite is an inorganic mineral structure that is by itself osteoconductive. It aids bone formation by releasing calcium and phosphate ions directly into the local environment surrounding the implant (van Blitterswijk et al. 1985; Ducheyne et al. 1990; Beck 2003). In addition, hydroxyapatite may become osteoinductive by binding and concentrating serum morphogenetic proteins, facilitating osteoblastic activity (Kilpadi et al. 2001; LeGeros 2002; Porter et al. 2002). Osteoblasts may attach directly to the surface and release osteoinductive factors (Beck 2003; Hermida et al. 2010). Hydroxyapatite coatings on porous-coated implants have been shown to enhance bone ingrowth and create a stronger interface with bone, both when press-fit and in a gap model (Soballe 1993; Tisdel et al. 1994; Dalton et al. 1995). Also, in an experimental study in dogs, hydroxyapatite prevented the peri-implant migration of polyethylene wear debris (Rahbek et al. 2001; Coathup et al. 2005). Hydroxyapatite coating was shown to be beneficial in a canine revision model (Soballe et al. 2003).

A coating of hydroxyapatite is commonly plasma sprayed directly onto either nonporous or porous-coated surfaces of either titanium, titanium alloy, or cobalt-chromium alloy to facilitate bone ongrowth or ingrowth. When applied to a nonporous surface, the substrate surface is roughened by grit blasting to increase the attachment strength (Sun et al. 2001). Softer titanium alloys provide better bonding strength than does the harder cobalt-chromium alloy (Sun et al. 2001). Also, hydroxyapatite coatings can be applied directly to porous surfaces to enhance bone ingrowth into pores. The recommended thickness of plasma-sprayed coating, based on mechanical testing of transcortical titanium alloy implants in dogs, is 50–75 μm (Wang et al. 1993).

Bisphosphonates are another class of biologically active substances, or in this instance drugs, that can be applied to a porous-coated surface to enhance bone formation and fixation (Bobyn et al. 2005, 2009; Tanzer et al. 2005). Zolendronic acid has received the most attention in recent investigations because it is a third-generation drug and is the most potent bisphosponate. Zolendronic acid reduces bone catabolism at the cellular level and by causing osteoclast apoptosis. Also, evidence exists that it may directly affect osteoblastic function (Fromigue and Body 2002).

Zolendronic acid, through its chemical affinity for calcium phosphate, chemically and physically bonds to hydroxyapatite-coated porous surfaces (Tanzer et al. 2005; Bobyn et al. 2009). The drug is then delivered directly into the local environment as an initial surge followed by a slower sustained delivery over many weeks (Tanzer et al. 2005). The targeted delivery of the drug through elution from the surface of the implant is preferred over systemic delivery that can lead to adverse remodeling throughout the entire skeletal system. A potential application of both hydroxyapatite and zolendronic acid in canine patients is during revision surgery where bone defects are present and the press-fit stability may be rather tenuous. These biologically active coatings could make the difference between success and failure to achieve early fixation under these circumstances or in any situation where initial press-fit stability may be compromised.

Manipulation of the roughness or surface topography of a porous coating is an interesting concept that offers great potential for enhancing bone ingrowth. The use of acid etching is a low-cost means of creating a microtextured surface on a geometrically complex porous coating. The advantage of the acid-etched surface is that it eliminates the possibility of debonding or dissolution. Surface roughness is described by the parameter R_a, the arithmetical mean roughness, and is often expressed in micrometers (μm).

The superimposition of a microtextured surface onto an existing porous-coated surface has been shown to increase bone formation by 60% using a canine intramedullary model (Hacking et al. 2003). Sintered bead porous-coated titanium rods etched in an acid solution to create a surface microtexture (R_a, $1.12 \pm 0.72\,\mu$m) were compared with control rods with a smooth surface texture (R_a, $0.09 \pm 0.02\,\mu$m; Figure 3.7). Twelve weeks

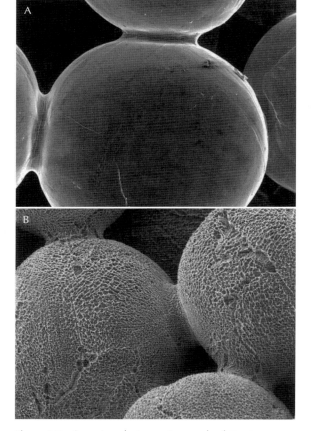

Figure 3.7 Scanning electron micrograph of titanium beads used for bone ingrowth. (A) The control implants are in an as-sintered condition. (B) The treated implants have been etched in a boiling acidic solution, creating an irregular surface. (Reproduced from Hacking et al. [2003], with permission and copyright of the British Editorial Society of Bone and Joint Surgery)

following intramedullary implantation in dogs, the extent of bone ingrowth into the control rods was $15.8\% \pm 12.3\%$, while bone ingrowth into the microtextured surface rods was $25.3\% \pm 16.5\%$. The 60% enhancement of bone ingrowth in the acid-etched implants was significant (paired analysis; $p = 0.001$). Studies looking at the effect of the surface microtexture of titanium on osteoblastic activity have determined that smooth implants with an R_a value less than $0.4\,\mu$m are generally surrounded by fibrous tissue, whereas implants with a R_a value of $1.0–6.7\,\mu$m have a positive effect on osteoblastic activity, resulting in bone formation (Hacking et al. 2003). Cell cultures of osteoblasts grown on microtextured surfaces have been shown to increase adherence and release of osteoinductive factors (Bowers et al. 1992; Kieswetter et al. 1996; Bigerelle et al. 2002).

Implant-related infections that result from intraoperative contamination or from hematogenous spread have devastating consequences. The ability to protect the implant surface against bacteria and the prevention of formation of biofilm would be highly desirable, especially if effective against antibiotic-resistant strains of bacteria. One potential method of preventing or mitigating periprosthetic infection is to render the implant surface bactericidal. The bonding of antibiotics and the application of a nanolayer of pure silver particles directly onto the surface of the implant are promising options.

Several early investigations have reported on the process and the efficacy of bonding vancomycin to titanium alloy to prevent bacterial colonization and biofilm formation *in vivo* (Jose et al. 2005; Antoci et al. 2007). Vancomycin was chosen because the chemical alteration that occurs during the bonding process does not affect its bactericidal properties. Also, since vancomycin acts at the bacterial cell wall, it is effective while remaining bonded to the implant surface. The chemical linkages between the titanium and the vancomycin extend the antibiotic away from the titanium surface and allow it to enter the bacterial cell wall. Unlike a coating that results in free release of antibiotic, the titanium-bonded vancomycin was not lost from the surface following incubation with bacteria. During the time period of the studies, the bonded vancomycin remained active following repeated bacterial challenges with *Staphylococcus*

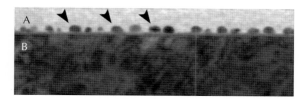

Figure 3.8   Electron micrograph of the surface of a silver-coated implant (HyProtect™, Bio-Gate, Nuremberg, Germany). A SiOxCy biocompatible plasma polymer (A) covers silver particles (arrowheads) affixed to the stainless steel substrate (B).

aureus for more than 6 weeks. The coating resisted abrasion following multiple press-fit insertions into the femurs of rats. Other studies have evaluated the effect of surface modification of titanium on the loading and release of vancomycin and gentamicin out into the periprosthetic area (Radin et al. 1997; Neut et al. 2011; Swanson et al. 2011).

A surface coating process currently utilized in a variety of medical and nonmedical applications is the physical vapor deposition of pure silver particles on the surface of materials, including medical devices. In an *in vitro* study investigating a silver coating for use in fracture fixation devices, silver particles 5–50 nm in diameter were applied to a 316 L stainless steel substrate and completely covered by a biocompatible plasma polymer, SiOxCy (Figure 3.8; Khalilpour et al. 2010). The total thickness of the coating was 30–50 nm. Moisture activates the silver particles to generate and release silver ions that migrate through and to the surface of the plasma polymer. The silver ions kill the bacteria on the surface of the implant. The coating exhibited excellent antimicrobial activity when tested *in vitro* against *Staphylococcus aureus*, *Staphylococcus epidermidis*, and methicillin-resistant *Staphylococcus aureus*. In an *in vivo* aspect of the study, the antimicrobial activity was sustained throughout the 28-day study duration. How long the coating remains effective beyond the 28 days could not be determined in this study. Adhesion strength or abrasion resistance of the coating was assessed by screwing coated threaded external fixator pins into cadaveric bone and examining the explanted pins with scanning electron microscopy. No morphological changes were seen in the coating of the explanted implants.

Other studies have investigated the use of a 2-μm-thick titanium/silver hard coating created by the simultaneous physical vapor deposition of both silver and titanium onto a titanium substrate (Ewald et al. 2006). The hard surface was created to improve the mechanical properties, especially shear due to abrasion, in a load-bearing implant–bone interface. The surface demonstrated highly effective antimicrobial properties and biocompatibility *in vitro*. However, in this preliminary study, load bearing tests were not conducted to evaluate the hypothesis that the hard coating would withstand shear better when compared with polymer coatings available at the time.

Silver-based antimicrobials offer the advantage that they are highly effective, nontoxic to cells including osteoblasts, and there are few bacterial organisms that are resistant when compared with antibiotic-modified surfaces (Ewald et al. 2006). The mechanism of action is based on the availability of free silver ions that bind with cellular structural proteins and enzymes, thereby interfering with cell membrane integrity and with energy production (Khalilpour et al. 2010). The mechanisms of action of the silver ions make it difficult for bacteria to acquire single point mutations.

References

Antoci V Jr., King SB, Jose B, et al. Vancomycin covalently bonded to titanium alloy prevents bacterial colonization. J Orthop Res 2007;25:858–866.

Beck GR Jr. Inorganic phosphate as a signaling molecule in osteoblast differentiation. J Cell Biochem 2003;90:234–243.

Bigerelle M, Anselme K, Noel B, et al. Improvement in the morphology of Ti-based surfaces: A new process to increase *in vitro* human osteoblast response. Biomaterials 2002;23:1563–1577.

van Blitterswijk CA, Grote JJ, Kuypers W, et al. Bioreactions at the tissue/hydroxyapatite interface. Biomaterials 1985;6:243–251.

Bobyn JD, Pilliar RM, Cameron HU, et al. The optimum pore size for the fixation of porous-surfaced metal implants by the ingrowth of bone. Clin Orthop Relat Res 1980;149:263–270.

Bobyn JD, Pilliar RM, Cameron HU, et al. Osteogenic phenomena across endosteal bone-implant spaces with porous surfaced intramedullary implants. Acta Orthop Scand 1981;52:145–153.

Bobyn JD, Pilliar RM, Binnington AG, et al. The effect of proximally and fully porous-coated canine hip stem design on bone modeling. J Orthop Res 1987;5: 393–408.

Bobyn JD, Jacobs JJ, Tanzer M, et al. The susceptibility of smooth implant surfaces to periimplant fibrosis and migration of polyethylene wear debris. Clin Orthop Relat Res 1995;311:21–39.

Bobyn JD, Stackpool GJ, Hacking SA, et al. Characteristics of bone ingrowth and interface mechanics of a new porous tantalum biomaterial. J Bone Joint Surg Br 1999a;81:907–914.

Bobyn JD, Toh KK, Hacking SA, et al. Tissue response to porous tantalum acetabular cups: A canine model. J Arthroplasty 1999b;14:347–354.

Bobyn JD, Hacking SA, Krygier JJ, et al. Zoledronic acid causes enhancement of bone growth into porous implants. J Bone Joint Surg Br 2005;87:416–420.

Bobyn JD, McKenzie K, Karabasz D, et al. Locally delivered bisphosphonate for enhancement of bone formation and implant fixation. J Bone Joint Surg Am 2009;91(Suppl. 6):23–31.

Bourne RB, Rorabeck CH, Burkart BC, et al. Ingrowth surfaces. Plasma spray coating to titanium alloy hip replacements. Clin Orthop Relat Res 1994;298:37–46.

Bowers KT, Keller JC, Randolph BA, et al. Optimization of surface micromorphology for enhanced osteoblast responses in vitro. Int J Oral Maxillofac Implants 1992;7:302–310.

Bundy KJ, Penn RW. The effect of surface preparation on metal/bone cement interfacial strength. J Biomed Mater Res 1987;21:773–805.

Cameron HU, Pilliar RM, Macnab I. The rate of bone ingrowth into porous metal. J Biomed Mater Res 1976;10:295–302.

Chang PB, Mann KA, Bartel DL. Cemented femoral stem performance. Effects of proximal bonding, geometry, and neck length. Clin Orthop Relat Res 1998;355:57–69.

Coathup MJ, Blackburn J, Goodship AE, et al. Role of hydroxyapatite coating in resisting wear particle migration and osteolysis around acetabular components. Biomaterials 2005;26:4161–4169.

Cook SD, Walsh KA, Haddad RJ, Jr. Interface mechanics and bone growth into porous Co-Cr-Mo alloy implants. Clin Orthop Relat Res 1985;193:271–280.

Cook SD, Thomas KA, Haddad RJ Jr. Histologic analysis of retrieved human porous-coated total joint components. Clin Orthop Relat Res 1988;234:90–101.

Dalton JE, Cook SD, Thomas KA, et al. The effect of operative fit and hydroxyapatite coating on the mechanical and biological response to porous implants. J Bone Joint Surg Am 1995;77:97–110.

Davies JP, Harris WH. Tensile bonding strength of the cement-prosthesis interface. Orthopedics 1994;17:171–173.

DeYoung DJ, Schiller RA. Radiographic criteria for evaluation of uncemented total hip replacement in dogs. Vet Surg 1992;21:88–98.

DeYoung DJ, DeYoung BA, Aberman HA, et al. Implantation of an uncemented total hip prosthesis. Technique and initial results of 100 arthroplasties. Vet Surg 1992;21:168–177.

Ducheyne P, Beight J, Cuckler J, et al. Effect of calcium phosphate coating characteristics on early postoperative bone tissue ingrowth. Biomaterials 1990;11:531–540.

Duffy GP, Lozynsky AJ, Harris WH. Polished vs rough femoral components in grade A and grade C-2 cement mantles. J Arthroplasty 2006;21:1054–1063.

Emerson RH Jr., Sanders SB, Head WC, et al. Effect of circumferential plasma-spray porous coating on the rate of femoral osteolysis after total hip arthroplasty. J Bone Joint Surg Am 1999;81:1291–1298.

Engh CA, Bobyn JD. The influence of stem size and extent of porous coating on femoral bone resorption after primary cementless hip arthroplasty. Clin Orthop Relat Res 1988;231:7–28.

Ewald A, Gluckermann SK, Thull R, et al. Antimicrobial titanium/silver PVD coatings on titanium. Biomed Eng Online 2006;5:22.

Firestone DE, Callaghan JJ, Liu SS, et al. Total hip arthroplasty with a cemented, polished, collared femoral stem and a cementless acetabular component. A follow-up study at a minimum of ten years. J Bone Joint Surg Am 2007;89:126–132.

Fromigue O, Body JJ. Bisphosphonates influence the proliferation and the maturation of normal human osteoblasts. J Endocrinol Invest 2002;25:539–546.

Hacking SA, Harvey EJ, Tanzer M, et al. Acid-etched microtexture for enhancement of bone growth into porous-coated implants. J Bone Joint Surg Br 2003;85:1182–1189.

Haddad RJ Jr., Cook SD, Thomas KA. Biological fixation of porous-coated implants. J Bone Joint Surg Am 1987;69:1459–1466.

Hermida JC, Bergula A, Dimaano F, et al. An in vivo evaluation of bone response to three implant surfaces using a rabbit intramedullary rod model. J Orthop Surg Res 2010;5:57.

Howie DW, Middleton RG, Costi K. Loosening of matt and polished cemented femoral stems. J Bone Joint Surg Br 1998;80:573–576.

Huiskes R, Verdonschot N, Nivbrant B. Migration, stem shape, and surface finish in cemented total hip arthroplasty. Clin Orthop Relat Res 1998;355:103–112.

Jasty M, Harris WH. Observations on factors controlling bony ingrowth into weight-bearing, porous, canine total hip replacements. In: Non-Cemented Total Hip Arthroplasty, Fitzgerald R (ed.). New York: Raven Press, 1988, p. 175.

Jasty M, Bragdon CR, Haire T, et al. Comparison of bone ingrowth into cobalt chrome sphere and titanium fiber mesh porous coated cementless canine acetabular components. J Biomed Mater Res 1993;27:639–644.

Jose B, Antoci V Jr., Zeiger AR, et al. Vancomycin covalently bonded to titanium beads kills Staphylococcus aureus. Chem Biol 2005;12:1041–1048.

Khalilpour P, Lampe K, Wagener M, et al. Ag/SiO(x) C(y) plasma polymer coating for antimicrobial protection of fracture fixation devices. J Biomed Mater Res B Appl Biomater 2010;94:196–202.

Kieswetter K, Schwartz Z, Hummert TW, et al. Surface roughness modulates the local production of growth factors and cytokines by osteoblast-like MG-63 cells. J Biomed Mater Res 1996;32:55–63.

Kilpadi KL, Chang PL, Bellis SL. Hydroxylapatite binds more serum proteins, purified integrins, and osteoblast precursor cells than titanium or steel. J Biomed Mater Res 2001;57:258–267.

von Knoch M, Engh CA Sr., Sychterz CJ, et al. Migration of polyethylene wear debris in one type of uncemented femoral component with circumferential porous coating: An autopsy study of 5 femurs. J Arthroplasty 2000;15:72–78.

Kraemer WJ, Maistrelli GL, Fornasier V, et al. Migration of polyethylene wear debris in hip arthroplasties: A canine model. J Appl Biomater 1995;6:225–230.

Lachiewicz PF, Kelley SS, Soileau ES. Survival of polished compared with precoated roughened cemented femoral components. A prospective, randomized study. J Bone Joint Surg Am 2008;90:1457–1463.

Lauer SK, Nieves MA, Peck J, et al. Descriptive histomorphometric ingrowth analysis of the Zurich cementless canine total hip acetabular component. Vet Surg 2009;38:59–69.

LeGeros RZ. Properties of osteoconductive biomaterials: Calcium phosphates. Clin Orthop Relat Res 2002;395:81–98.

Levine BR, Sporer S, Poggie RA, et al. Experimental and clinical performance of porous tantalum in orthopedic surgery. Biomaterials 2006;27:4671–4681.

Ling RS, Charity J, Lee AJ, et al. The long-term results of the original Exeter polished cemented femoral component: A follow-up report. J Arthroplasty 2009;24:511–517.

Mohler CG, Callaghan JJ, Collis DK, et al. Early loosening of the femoral component at the cement-prosthesis interface after total hip replacement. J Bone Joint Surg Am 1995;77:1315–1322.

Neut D, Dijkstra RJ, Thompson JI, et al. Antibacterial efficacy of a new gentamicin-coating for cementless prostheses compared to gentamicin-loaded bone cement. J Orthop Res 2011;29:1654–1661.

Porter AE, Hobbs LW, Rosen VB, et al. The ultrastructure of the plasma-sprayed hydroxyapatite-bone interface predisposing to bone bonding. Biomaterials 2002;23:725–733.

Raab S, Ahmed AM, Provan JW. Thin film PMMA precoating for improved implant bone-cement fixation. J Biomed Mater Res 1982;16:679–704.

Radin S, Campbell JT, Ducheyne P, et al. Calcium phosphate ceramic coatings as carriers of vancomycin. Biomaterials 1997;18:777–782.

Rahbek O, Overgaard S, Lind M, et al. Sealing effect of hydroxyapatite coating on peri-implant migration of particles. An experimental study in dogs. J Bone Joint Surg Br 2001;83:441–447.

Rashmir-Raven AM, DeYoung DJ, Abrams CF Jr., et al. Subsidence of an uncemented canine femoral stem. Vet Surg 1992;21:327–331.

Schiller TD, DeYoung DJ, Schiller RA, et al. Quantitative ingrowth analysis of a porous-coated acetabular component in a canine model. Vet Surg 1993;22:276–280.

Schmalzried TP, Zahiri CA, Woolson ST. The significance of stem-cement loosening of grit-blasted femoral components. Orthopedics 2000;23:1157–1164.

Shepard MF, Kabo JM, Lieberman JR. The Frank Stinchfield Award. Influence of cement technique on the interface strength of femoral components. Clin Orthop Relat Res 2000;381:26–35.

Soballe K. Hydroxyapatite ceramic coating for bone implant fixation. Mechanical and histological studies in dogs. Acta Orthop Scand Suppl 1993;255:1–58.

Soballe K, Mouzin OR, Kidder LA, et al. The effects of hydroxyapatite coating and bone allograft on fixation of loaded experimental primary and revision implants. Acta Orthop Scand 2003;74:239–247.

Sporer SM, Callaghan JJ, Olejniczak JP, et al. The effects of surface roughness and polymethylmethacrylate precoating on the radiographic and clinical results of the Iowa hip prosthesis. A study of patients less than fifty years old. J Bone Joint Surg Am 1999;81:481–492.

Sun L, Berndt CC, Gross KA, et al. Material fundamentals and clinical performance of plasma-sprayed hydroxyapatite coatings: A review. J Biomed Mater Res 2001;58:570–592.

Swanson TE, Cheng X, Friedrich C. Development of chitosan-vancomycin antimicrobial coatings on titanium implants. J Biomed Mater Res A 2011;97:167–176.

Tanzer M, Karabasz D, Krygier JJ, et al. The Otto Aufranc Award: Bone augmentation around and within porous implants by local bisphosphonate elution. Clin Orthop Relat Res 2005;441:30–39.

Tisdel CL, Goldberg VM, Parr JA, et al. The influence of a hydroxyapatite and tricalcium-phosphate coating on bone growth into titanium fiber-metal implants. J Bone Joint Surg Am 1994;76:159–171.

Turner TM, Sumner DR, Urban RM, et al. A comparative study of porous coatings in a weight-bearing total hip-arthroplasty model. J Bone Joint Surg Am 1986;68:1396–1409.

Vail TP, Goetz D, Tanzer M, et al. A prospective randomized trial of cemented femoral components with polished versus grit-blasted surface finish and identical stem geometry. J Arthroplasty 2003;18:95–102.

Wang BC, Lee TM, Chang E, et al. The shear strength and the failure mode of plasma-sprayed hydroxyapatite coating to bone: The effect of coating thickness. J Biomed Mater Res 1993;27:1315–1327.

4

Weight-Bearing Surfaces

Jeffrey N. Peck

The study of bearing surfaces, including the friction, wear, and lubrication of those surfaces, is called tribology. A variety of bearing surfaces and surface coatings has been used in joint replacement. The most common surfaces include plastic (polyethylene), metal, and ceramic. Improvements in the quality and function of these surfaces are geared toward the development of the ideal: low friction, low wear debris generation, damage resistance, and absence of toxicity. Unfortunately, progress on one front is often associated with a setback on another front or the development of an entirely new problem. This chapter describes the advantages and disadvantages of the most common weight-bearing surfaces used in total joint replacement, as well as the variety of articulating combinations of currently used bearing surfaces.

Osteolysis secondary to wear debris is the major limiting factor in the longevity of total joint prostheses in people. Consequently, measurement of wear and wear debris are used to compare among and between different prostheses and different types of bearing surfaces. Wear is most often a linear measurement, either in millimeter per year (mm/year) for clinical studies, or millimeter per

cycle (mm/cycle) for simulator studies (Livermore et al. 1990). Despite the relatively shorter life span of veterinary patients compared with human patients, annual wear rates are often accelerated in veterinary patients because of higher overall activity levels (i.e., increased number of cycles per unit of time). Measurement of the volume of wear debris, or volumetric wear, is generally determined by gravimetric means. Volumetric wear is based on the weight of the collected debris divided by the density of the material.

In 2000, Dowd correlated the development of wear debris-mediated osteolysis with linear wear rates. The Dowd study found that osteolysis did not occur with linear wear rates less than 0.1 mm/year. With linear wear rates of 0.1–0.2 mm/year, there was a 43% incidence of osteolysis, and with linear wear rates of 0.2–0.3 mm/year, the incidence of osteolysis increased to 80% (Dowd et al. 2000).

Polyethylene

The first widely used form of ethylene polymer that was utilized in joint replacement was

Advances in Small Animal Total Joint Replacement, First Edition. Edited by Jeffrey N. Peck and Denis J. Marcellin-Little.
© 2013 John Wiley & Sons, Inc. Published 2013 by John Wiley & Sons, Inc.

ultrahigh-molecular-weight polyethylene (UHMWPE). UHMWPE works well as a low-friction surface, but is prone to generation of wear debris and subsequent aseptic loosening. The generation of wear debris is accelerated by impingement or third-body wear. UHMWPE remains the most commonly used form of plastic bearing surface in veterinary and human joint replacements.

Hylamer is a form of UHMWPE exposed to gamma irradiation in air, and Poly II is UHMWPE with the addition of carbon fibers. *In vitro* studies suggested improved wear characteristics over UHMWPE; however, both of these products had inferior performance *in vivo*. Hylamer was found to have wear rates of 1.5 mm/year, *in vivo*, in one study (Livingston et al. 1997) and excessive eccentric wear in other studies (Chmell et al. 1996), and these findings were consistent with those of many other studies. The carbon fiber-reinforced UHMWPE, Poly II, was introduced in the 1970s, but was abandoned by the early 1980s. Less surface damage was found in materials that articulated with Poly II inserts, but the Poly II was more prone to abrasion and embedding of wear debris (Medel et al. 2008).

Highly cross-linked polyethylene

Highly cross-linked polyethylene (XLPE) is a highly dense form of UHMWPE. Cross-linking is thought to make the polyethylene more wear resistant. There are various ways to achieve cross-linking; however, heat and radiation are common to all methods. Irradiation is provided by either gamma rays or electron beams. With either method of irradiation, oxygen, which can be found in the polyethylene material itself, or within voids inside the polyethylene structure, is transformed into oxygen free radicals. The free radicals, particularly those within the amorphous portion of the polyethylene, lead to oxidative wear of the polyethylene. Radicals that are found within the crystalline portion of the polyethylene are more stable; however, the crystalline portion of polyethylene accounts for roughly 35% of the UHMWPE structure. Oxidation caused by oxygen radicals reduces cross-linking and can lead to cracking and delamination (Collier et al. 2003).

Several techniques have been utilized to both maintain material strength and minimize the presence of free radicals in irradiated polyethylene. In one study, the polyethylene was placed at high temperature and pressure that resulted in transition to a hexagonal phase polyethylene structure. This process is called high-pressure annealing (HPA). The hexagonal-phase structure permitted mobility of the crystalline phase of the polyethylene and allowed recombination of elemental oxygen to nearly eliminate the free radicals (Oral et al. 2008). In addition to nearly eliminating free radicals, the tensile strength of the XLPE was maintained in low to moderate cross-linked specimens, but highly cross-linked specimens suffered mechanical degradation. The HPA process eliminates the need of postirradiation melting, which adversely affects the material properties of the polyethylene.

Another method of eliminating free radicals from irradiated polyethylene is postirradiation melting. Melting virtually eliminates free radicals, but decreases the crystalline content of the polyethylene and adversely affects its mechanical properties (Lewis 2001). Tensile yield strength for cross-linked polyethylene that was annealed above melting temperature was lower than the tensile yield strength for cross-linked polyethylene annealed below its melting temperature (Collier et al. 2003).

One additional technique for reduction of free radicals in irradiated polyethylene is annealing the polyethylene with vitamin E, a free radical scavenger (Oral et al. 2006). Oral et al. reported good wear and material properties in vitamin E-stabilized, highly cross-linked UHMWPE.

Both gamma and electron beam radiation result in decreased tensile strength compared with non-irradiated UHMWPE. Loss in tensile strength is directly related to radiation dose. Overall, radiation doses above 5 Mrad results in decreased material toughness (Collier et al. 2003).

Metal

The most common metals used as bearing surfaces in total joint replacement include cobalt-chromium (CoCr), stainless steel, and titanium/titanium alloy. The use of stainless steel as a bearing surface is uncommon today.

The rate of polyethylene wear, as well as the generation of polyethylene and metallic wear debris, differs from metal to metal. The effect of metallic debris on the periprosthetic tissues, as well as systemic effects, also varies with the type of metal.

There is substantial variability in the reported rate of polyethylene wear (i.e., thinning of poly-ethylene induced by bearing contact with metal) with the different metals (Bankston et al. 1993; Pappas et al. 1995). There is also much variation in the volume of wear debris created by the different metals. CoCr generates the smallest amount of wear debris, followed by titanium and stainless steel. However, uncoated titanium or titanium alloys are rarely used as bearing surfaces. Weight-bearing surfaces of titanium implants are typically coated with titanium nitride (TiN) or, more recently, other hardening coatings to improve wear performance. These surface coatings are discussed below.

While the generation of wear debris from CoCr implants is low, the wear particles are cytotoxic to macrophages. The toxicity of the CoCr wear particles is greater than the toxicity of similarly sized particles from titanium alloys; however, the inflammatory reaction generated by titanium particles is more severe than the CoCr particles (Haynes et al. 1993). The degree of inflammation and stimulation of bone-resorbing mediators (e.g., PGE2, IL-1) may be more significant than toxicity in the development of aseptic loosening.

The method of fixation affects the size and number of wear particles, as well as the roughening of the metallic articulating surface. In general, the size and number of particles is greatest when a titanium bearing surface is used with a cemented prosthesis.

Surface coatings

The relatively soft pure titanium or titanium alloys (titanium-6aluminum-4vanadium) are not suitable bearing surfaces without the use of protective coating. Surface scratches, fretting, and the development of third-party wear are common with unprotected titanium or titanium alloy.

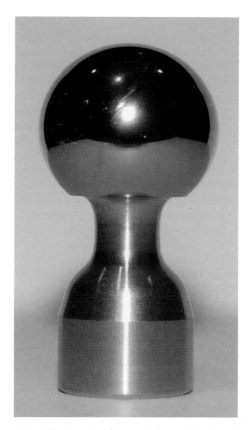

Figure 4.1 Titanium nitride-coated femoral head-neck component from an earlier generation of the Zurich Cementless Hip (Kyon, Zurich, Switzerland).

Additionally, free aluminum ions are potentially neurotoxic. The most common coating used over titanium or TiAlV alloys is a thin (8 μm) ceramic coating of TiN (Figure 4.1). In one study, the poly-ethylene wear rate when UHMWPE was coupled with a TiN coated head was 2% of the reported wear rate of a CoCr head with UHMWPE (Pappas et al. 1995). However, several case series report that TiN may be inadequate to prevent fretting and that TiN coating breakthrough is common (Raimondi and Pietrabissa 2000).

Another coating material is diamond-like carbon (DLC) or amorphous carbon film (Figure 4.2). There are many forms of DLC (amorphous carbon, nonhydrogenated amorphous carbon, tet-rahedral amorphous carbon, etc.), each with some-what different tribological properties (Roy and Lee 2007). DLC coatings have the advantages of

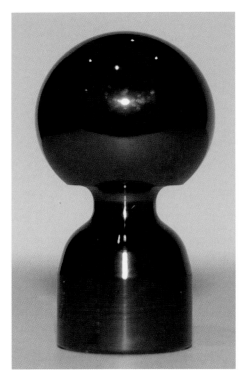

Figure 4.2   Current-generation femoral head-neck component coated with amorphous diamond-like carbon (Kyon, Zurich, Switzerland).

low friction, hardness, wear and corrosion resistance, are chemically inert, and extremely smooth. As with TiN coatings, results on the effectiveness of DLC in improvement of wear characteristics have been inconsistent. Femoral heads of stainless steel, CoCr, and TiAlV have been evaluated in wear simulators with and without DLC. DLC significantly improved the wear characteristics of a stainless steel head, but did not significantly improve the wear characteristics of CoCr (Dowling et al. 1997; Sheeja et al. 2005). The wear characteristics of TiAlV heads were improved, but not significantly better than other surface treatments, such as thermal oxidation (TO; Dong et al. 1999). Surface treatment with TO was developed by Dong et al. and was found to decrease polyethylene surface wear by a factor of 2.5. The TO surface treatment has not made its way into widespread clinical use.

Ceramic

Ceramic is harder than metal and produces non-reactive wear debris. However, ceramic is prone to cracking and ceramic-on-ceramic (COC) implants can have the undesirable side effect of audible squeaking. The use of ceramics in orthopedic surgery has evolved through three generations. In first-generation ceramics, large crystals adversely affected implant density and made ceramics more prone to cracks. Second-generation ceramics added oxides that decreased granule size and improved the mechanical properties of the ceramics (Bae and Baik 1993). Current, or third-generation, ceramics are processed utilizing hot isostatic pressing (HIP), which further reduces grain size and improves ceramic density (Rahaman et al. 2007). Based on retrieval data, current processing methods have dramatically reduced the incidence of ceramic fracture to 0.004% (Gerd 2000).

Ceramic acetabular components are generally metal backed. Because of the high elastic modulus of ceramic relative to bone, ceramic-only or cemented ceramic acetabular components have a high incidence of loosening due to modulus mismatch (300 times greater than cancellous bone). Due to the high elastic modulus, ceramics are not capable of deformation without breakage (Hannouche et al. 2005).

Alumina is the most common ceramic used in joint replacement surgery. It is a monophasic ceramic that is very stable, highly oxidized, and has excellent thermal conductivity. Alumina is also chemically and biologically inert. Further, alumina is hydrophilic, thus allowing fluid film lubrication of the prosthetic joint and reducing production of wear debris. Fluid film lubrication is a form of hydrodynamic lubrication where both articulating surfaces are nearly completely coated by a layer of liquid and the liquid is load bearing. Fluid film lubrication dramatically decreases wear. Volumetric wear rates for alumina are thousands of times less than those for UHMWPE. The wear debris that is produced is bioinert and generates minimal inflammatory response (Christel 1992).

Zirconium is a metal; however, oxidation of the surface of zirconium transforms the metal into a zirconia ceramic surface. Oxidized zirconium has wear characteristics that appear to be consistently superior to CoCrMo. Unlike alumina, which is monophasic, zirconia is triphasic and has the potential to transform *in vivo*. Yttrium is used to stabilize zirconia in the tetragonal phase. Transformation to another phase *in vivo* can result in crack formation. Zirconia also has low thermal conductivity, allowing for heat generation during activity (Hannouche et al. 2005).

Articulations

In an attempt to reduce or eliminate the problem of polyethylene wear debris, a variety of weight-bearing surface combinations have been developed and are in clinical use. These combinations include metal-on-polyethylene (MOP), metal-on-metal (MOM), metal-on-ceramic (MOC), COC, and ceramic-on-polyethylene (COP). Wood, glass, and acrylic have also historically been used as articulating surfaces, but are not in current use due to poor clinical performance (Pramanik et al. 2005).

MOP

MOP has been the gold standard for joint replacement and continues to be the most common form of weight-bearing articulation. The greatest persistent issue with long-term survivability of MOP implants is aseptic loosening or osteolysis. Since the primary cause of aseptic loosening is the presence of wear debris, elimination or minimizing the production of wear debris or eliminating the cytological reaction to wear debris has been the goal. Particle size of the wear debris appears to be the critical factor that determines the cytological response to wear products, with the critical size range of 0.2–0.8 μm necessary for macrophage activation (Ingham and Fisher 2000).

MOM

MOM prostheses appear to result in smaller volumes and smaller particle size wear debris compared with MOP prostheses. The small particle size of the metallic debris generates less tissue reaction and, consequently, less osteolysis surrounding the implant (Lee et al. 1992; Doorn et al.

1996). Simulator-produced volumetric wear was compared between MOM and COP prostheses and these results were compared with historically reported volumetric wear rates for MOP. When comparing volumetric wear rates using the same diameter (28 mm) head, the wear rates were $0.45\,mm^3/10^6$ cycles, $6.3\,mm^3/10^6$ cycles, and 60–$180\,mm^3$/year for MOM, COP (zirconia ceramic), and MOP, respectively (Goldsmith et al. 2000). The authors of the above study comment that the total number of particles produced by MOM articulations may be greater than the number produced by MOP articulations, but the particle size is much smaller. It is believed that smaller particles can be more readily transported away from the periprosthetic tissues and do not incite a significant inflammatory response. Studies consistently find wear rates of 20–100 times lower for MOM than for MOP prostheses (Silva et al. 2005). The Silva study reported an average linear wear rate of 0.004 mm/year, and their findings were similar to those reported in other studies.

Despite an apparent improvement in wear characteristics, MOM prostheses may be associated with other complications. There is concern about the development of allergic reactions (delayed-type hypersensitivity) secondary to metallosis, as well as concerns about the possibility of malignancies secondary to metallosis. A specific form of delayed-type hypersensitivity, known as aseptic lymphocyte-dominated vasculitis-associated lesion (ALVAL), may be responsible for failure of MOM prostheses (Langton et al. 2010). Concerns about malignancy have not been substantiated in modern MOM prostheses. One study compared serum levels of cobalt, chromium, and molybdenum in patients with MOM hip prostheses and in patients with MOP hip prostheses. Follow-up time, age, and health status were similar between groups. Patients with MOM prosthesis had significantly higher levels of cobalt and chromium compared with the MOP group (Savarino et al. 2002). A similar study by MacDonald et al. had the same findings. Additionally, the MacDonald study found that erythrocyte ion concentrations were increasing at the latest follow-up and that there was no difference in outcomes-based clinical function (Harris Hip Score, Western Ontario and McMasters Arthritis Index [WOMAC], and Short Form-12; MacDonald et al. 2003).

Serum and urine metal levels in patients with MOM prostheses are typically several times the normal level (i.e., the level in healthy patients without prostheses); however, they are below the levels considered to be dangerous in industrial metal workers. Local tissue levels of these metals, conversely, can exceed toxic levels and cause tissue necrosis (Cobb and Schmalzreid 2006). Despite these potential issues, MOM proponents consider them the procedure of choice for young, active patients. This is particularly the case if a large femoral head is used, as larger femoral heads generate greater wear debris.

MOC

MOC prostheses are relatively new phenomena in joint replacement. The development of MOC grew out of concerns over cracking in COC prostheses. In a recent hip simulator study, a HIP alumina femoral head and CoCrMo socket were tested over 5 million cycles. Gravimetric analysis did not detect any wear; however, a change in surface topography at the pole suggested the presence of wear. Additionally, frictional analysis suggested that fluid film lubrication occurred in parts of the walking cycle (Williams et al. 2009). Barnes et al. compared the wear characteristic of MOM bearings of similar hardness, MOM bearings of different hardness, and COM bearings. COM bearings produced the least metal wear debris and like-hardness MOM produced the greatest amount of metal wear debris. The Barnes study also found that, in general, differential-hardness bearings produce less damage and less surface wear than bearings of similar hardness (Barnes et al. 2008). This study further found that the harder the femoral head, the lower percentage of wear debris that was produced by the femoral head; thus, ceramic femoral heads contributed the least to wear debris production. The benefits of differential hardness appear to hold true only if the femoral head is harder than the acetabular liner.

COP

Urban et al. (2001) performed long-term follow-up (average: 18 years) on patients with total hip prostheses with alumina femoral heads and UHMWPE cemented cups. Linear wear rates in the Urban study were 0.034 mm/year, which compares favorably with MOP prostheses (reported range: 0.08–1 mm/year). Osteolysis was not present in any of the 64 implanted hips in the series. Higher COP linear wear rates were reported in studies using first- or second-generation ceramic implants (Sugano et al. 1995). As noted previously, first- and second-generation ceramics had high failure rates due to cracking. Increased ceramic wear debris was due to a design flaw that led to impingement in several early prostheses. The findings of the Urban study were consistent with other studies in which third-generation ceramic prostheses were implanted (Schuller and Marti 1990; Wroblewski et al. 1996).

COC

Compared with other bearing surface combinations, current-generation COC prostheses are reported to have the best overall wear rates. Linear wear rates of COC implants are reported between 0.001 and 0.003 mm/year (Ross and Brown 2010). In addition, the wear particles that are created are more biologically inert than MOM particles. If impingement is prevented by appropriate implant positioning, there is minimal risk of ceramic cracks. A single incidence of a bearing crack was reported in a large case series, with an overall incidence of 0.54%. The single case was actually a revision and had a trochanteric nonunion that increased the risk of impingement (Murphy et al. 2006). Similar findings were reported in a study with a minimum 18.5-year follow-up (Hamadouche et al. 2002). Similar to MOM proponents, proponents of COC implants advise COC joint replacements for young, active patients. Reports of "squeaking" are inconsistent and the incidence is unclear.

References

Bae SI, Baik S. Sintering and grain growth of ultrapure alumina. J Mater Sci 1993;28:4197–4204.

Barnes CL, DeBoer D, Corpe RS et al. Wear performance of large-diameter differential-hardness hip bearings. J Arthroplasty 2008;23(6):56–60.

Bankston AB, Faris PM, Keating EM et al. Polyethylene wear in total hip arthroplasty in patient-matched groups: A comparison of stainless steel, cobalt chrome and titanium-bearing surfaces. J Arthroplasty 1993;8(3):315–322.

Chmell MJ, Poss R, Thomas W et al. Early failure of Hylamer acetabular inserts due to eccentric wear. J Arthroplasty 1996;11(3):351–353.

Christel PS. Biocompatibility of surgical-grade dense polycrystalline alumina. Clin Orthop Relat Res 1992;282:10–18.

Cobb AG, Schmalzreid TP. The clinical significance of metal ion release from cobalt-chromium metal-on-metal total hip joint arthroplasty. Proc Inst Mech Eng [H] 2006;220(2):385–398.

Collier JP, Currier BH, Kennedy FE et al. Comparison of cross-linked polyethylene materials for orthopedic applications. Clin Orthop Relat Res 2003;414:289–304.

Dong H, Shi W, Bell T. Potential of improving tribological performance of UHMWPE by engineering the Ti6Al4V counterfaces. Wear 1999;225–229:146–153.

Doorn PF, Mirra JM, Campbell PA et al. Tissue reaction to metal on metal total hip prostheses. Clin Orthop Relat Res 1996;329:187–205.

Dowd JE, Sychterz CJ, Young AM, Engh CA. Characterization of long-term femoral-head-penetration rates. Association with and prediction of osteolysis. J Bone Joint Surg Am 2000;82:1102–1107.

Dowling DP, Kola PV, Donnelly K et al. Evaluation of diamond-like carbon-coated orthopaedic implants. Diam Relat Mater 1997;6:390–393.

Gerd W. Ceramic femoral head retrieval data. Clin Orthop Relat Res 2000;379:22–28.

Goldsmith AJ, Dowson D, Isaac GH et al. A comparative joint simulator study of the wear of metal-on-metal and alternative material combinations in hip replacements. Proc Inst Mech Eng [H] 2000;214(1):39–47.

Hamadouche M, Boutin P, Daussange J et al. Alumina-on-alumina total hip arthroplasty: A minimum 18.5-year follow-up study. J Bone Joint Surg Am 2002;84:69–77.

Hannouche D, Hamadouche M, Nizard R et al. Ceramics in total hip replacement. Clin Orthop Relat Res 2005;430:62–71.

Haynes DR, Rogers SD, Hay S et al. The differences in toxicity and release of bone-resorbing mediators induced by titanium and cobalt-chromium alloy wear particles. J Bone Joint Surg Am 1993;75(6):825–834.

Ingham E, Fisher J. Biological reactions to wear debris in total joint replacement. Proc Inst Mech Eng [H] 2000;214(1):21–37.

Langton DJ, Jameson SS, Joyce TJ et al. Early failure of metal-on-metal bearings in hip resurfacing and large-diameter total hip replacement. J Bone Joint Surg Br 2010;92:38–46.

Lee JM, Salvati EA, Betts F et al. Size of metallic and polyethylene debris particles in failed cemented total hip replacements. J Bone Joint Surg Br 1992;74:380–384.

Lewis G. Properties of cross-linked UHMWPE. Biomaterials 2001;22:371–401.

Livermore J, Ilstrup D, Morrey B. The effect of femoral head size on wear of the polyethylene acetabular component. J Bone Joint Surg Am 1990;72:518–528.

Livingston BJ, Chmell MJ, Spector M et al. Complications of total hip arthroplasty associated with the use of an acetabular component with a Hylamer liner. J Bone Joint Surg 1997;79:1529–1538.

MacDonald SJ, McCalden RW, Chess DG et al. Metal-on-metal versus polyethylene in hip arthroplasty: A randomized clinical trial. Clin Orthop Relat Res 2003;406(1):282–296.

Medel F, Kurtz SM, Klein G. Clinical, surface damage and oxidative performance of Poly II tibial inserts after long-term implantation. J Long Term Eff Med Implants 2008;18(2):151–156.

Murphy SB, Ecker TM, Tannast M. Two- to 9-year clinical results of alumina ceramic-on-ceramic THA. Clin Orthop Relat Res 2006;453:97–102.

Oral E, Christensen SD, Arnaz S et al. Wear resistance and mechanical properties of highly cross-linked UHMWPE doped with vitamin-E. J Arthroplasty 2006;21(4):580–591.

Oral E, Beckos CG, Moratoglu OK. Free radical elimination in irradiated UHMWPE through crystal mobility in phase transition to the hexagonal phase. Polymer 2008;49:4733–4739.

Pappas MJ, Makras G, Buechel FF. Titanium nitride ceramic film against polyethylene: A 48 million cycle wear test. Clin Orthop Relat Res 1995;317(1):64–70.

Pramanik S, Argawal AK, Rai KN. Chronology of total hip replacement and materials development. Trends Biomater Artif Organs 2005;19(1):15–26.

Rahaman MN, Yao A, Bal BS, et al. Ceramics for prosthetic hip and knee joint replacement. J Am Ceram Soc 2007;90(7):1965–1988.

Raimondi MT, Pietrabissa R. The in vivo wear performance of prosthetic femoral heads with titanium nitride coating. Biomaterials 2000;21(9):907–913.

Ross J, Brown TE. Return to athletic activity following total hip arthroplasty. Open Sport Med J 2010;4:42–50.

Roy RK, Lee KR. Biomedical applications of diamond-like coatings: A review. J Biomed Mater Res 2007;83:72–84.

Savarino L, Granchi D, Ciapetti G et al. Ion release in patients with metal-on-metal hip bearings in total joint replacement: A comparison with metal-on-polyethylene bearings. J Biomed Mater Res 2002;63:467–474.

Schuller HM, Marti RK. Ten-year socket wear in 66 hip arthroplasties. Ceramic versus metal heads. Acta Orthop Scand 1990;61:240–243.

Sheeja D, Tay BK, Nung LN. Tribological characterization of surface modified UHMWPE against DLC-coated Co-Cr-Mo. Surf Coat Technol 2005;190: 231–237.

Silva M, Heisel C, Schmalzried T. Metal-on-metal total hip replacement. Clin Orthop Relat Res 2005;430: 53–61.

Sugano N, Nishii T, Nakata K et al. Polyethylene sockets and alumina ceramic heads in cemented total hip arthroplasty. A ten-year study. J Bone Joint Surg Br 1995;77:548–556.

Urban JA, Garvin KL, Boese CK et al. Ceramic-on-polyethylene bearing surfaces in total hip arthroplasty seventeen to 21-year-results. J Bone Joint Surg Am 2001;83:1688–1694.

Williams SR, Wu JJ, Unsworth A et al. Tribological and surface analysis of 38Alumina-as-cast Co-Cr-Mo total hip arthroplasties. Proc Inst Mech Eng [H] 2009;223(8): 941–954.

Wroblewski BM, Siney PD, Dowson D et al. Prospective clinical and joint simulator studies of a new total hip arthroplasty using alumina ceramic heads and cross-linked polyethylene cups. J Bone Joint Surg Br 1996;78:280–285.

5 Methods of Immediate Fixation

Kei Hayashi and Kurt S. Schulz

Introduction

Recent review articles on human total joint arthroplasty identified implant loosening as the greatest current concern for this generally successful procedure (Corbett et al. 2010; Paxton et al. 2010; Huo et al. 2011). The initial mechanical stability of the implant is essential for long-term viability of the total joint replacement (Mai et al. 2010; Pérez and Seral-García 2012; Ruben et al. 2012). Numerous clinical and laboratory studies in the human literature have evaluated implant stability; however, information in veterinary literature is quite limited. Unfortunately, data from human literature are not always relevant to veterinary medicine due to differences in anatomy, biomechanics, and the required longevity of the prosthesis (Franklin et al. 2012). In addition, studies in human literature can be commercially driven and objective data on the initial stability of implants are often referenced as "manufacturer's test report" and not available for critical review. This chapter includes a general review of the mechanics of biomaterials involved in immediate implant fixation and the currently available veterinary information in total arthroplasty procedures. The ultimate test of appropriate fixation methods in veterinary total joint arthroplasty needs to be verified by long-term survival in randomized, controlled, prospective clinical studies.

Basic biomechanics and implant design

Important mechanical considerations in total joint arthroplasty include (1) the geometric and material design of the articulating surfaces and (2) the design of the interface between the implants and the surrounding bone (Hallab et al. 2004; Pruitt and Chakravartula 2011). Most total joint arthroplasty systems use ultrahigh-molecular-weight polyethylene (UHMWPE) as a bearing surface and a metal (either a titanium alloy or a cobalt-chromium alloy) for the remaining portion of the implant. The metal part of the implant is typically involved in fixation. The two most widely used methods for fixing the implant to the bone are (1) the use of polymethylmethacrylate (PMMA) cement (cemented application) or (2) the use of a press-fit and porous metal surface to allow osseo-integration (cementless application) (Charnley et

Advances in Small Animal Total Joint Replacement, First Edition. Edited by Jeffrey N. Peck and Denis J. Marcellin-Little.
© 2013 John Wiley & Sons, Inc. Published 2013 by John Wiley & Sons, Inc.

al. 2000; Eldridge and Learmonth 2000; Buechel and Pappas 2011).

Because of the difference in material properties of the bone and the implant, "an interface" is created where the two materials come into contact. In total joint arthroplasty, load is transferred from the implant to the surrounding bone at the bone–implant interface. In this situation, two closely related factors are major determinants of the immediate stability: (1) implant design (material properties such as stiffness, shape, and surface architecture) and (2) interface boundary mechanics (Beksac et al. 2006). The stiffness ratio of the implant to the bone will determine how much load is borne by each. Since the stiffness of implant is greater than that of bone, the implant carries most of the load, which can lead to stress shielding of the bone. The interface needs to withstand high stresses to create the load transition between the implant and the bone, which explains why the bone–implant interface is the most critical design feature for most implants (Hallab et al. 2004; Pruitt and Chakravartula 2011).

In addition to the implant design, another important determinant of interface stress is the character of the bond between the implant and the bone (Mann et al. 2008). Bonding characteristics can range from a completely bonded interface to a nonbonded interface with no friction. A bonded interface is the characteristic of a cemented implant system, while a nonbonded interface is a characteristic of smooth surface (no friction) cementless implant system. Most current cementless implant systems have surface designs to generate desired friction between the implant and the surrounding bone.

If the interface is bonded as with a cemented implant, shear stresses are generated at the interface to support the implant. In nonbonded situations, shear stresses cannot be generated due to the lack of friction at the interface, and compressive stresses must be generated to withstand the applied force. These compressive stresses can only be generated when the implant subsides into the bone. Even in a cemented implant system, if bonding between the implant and the cement, or the bone and the cement, is lost, the interface cannot withstand shear stresses. If shear stresses overcome the interfacial bond, then the implant will subside into the bone and generate compressive stresses responsible for bearing the applied load. Prevention of debonding depends both on the implant design and surgical experience with cement preparation (discussed later in this chapter).

Mechanical analyses suggest that the successful total arthroplasty implant design is a trade-off among many factors. Stiff implants may reduce interface motion, but may lead to stress shielding and more bone resorption. Increasing surface roughness of the implant may increase the friction coefficient of the implant–cement interface, but may also increase the localized stress concentrations within the cement. An alternative to a cement–implant interface is a press-fit and a porous-coated implant interface. The theory behind porous coating is that bone will grow into pores on the implant surface, which will eliminate the reliance on poor mechanical properties of the cement. However, porous-coated implants rely on a biological process (osseointegration) that is not as predictable as an immediate cemented interface. The interface bond develops over time and a porous-coated implant interface is much more dependent on precise surgical fit to obtain an ideal implant–bone interface (discussed later in this chapter). Currently available total arthroplasty implants are the result of design evolution through computational modeling, material engineering, and clinical experience.

Cemented systems

The benefits of modern cementing techniques in improving immediate implant stability have been reported in a clinical study (Ota et al. 2005), and these modern techniques are currently recommended for cemented canine total joint arthroplasty (Schulz 2000). Implant design has been evolving to improve implant–cement interface mechanics (Beksac et al. 2006). There are a few commercially available cemented total hip arthroplasty systems, as well as total elbow arthroplasty and total knee arthroplasty systems in North America (Figure 5.1).

Implant surface preparation techniques are designed to strengthen the cement–implant interface (Beksac et al. 2006). Methods of strengthening the interface of femoral stemmed components

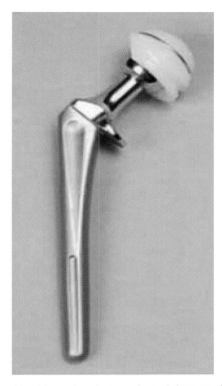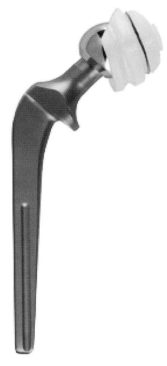

Figure 5.1 Cemented total hip arthroplasty implants (*left*: BioMedtrix CFX, Boonton, NJ; *right*: New Generation Devices, Glen Rock, NJ). Note the design features (grooves) aimed at maximizing implant–cement interface mechanics on both acetabular cup and femoral stem. (Courtesy of BioMedtrix and New Generation)

include roughening of the implant surface and precoating the implant with PMMA (Clayton et al. 2007). The juxta-articular portion of a stem is a common area for implant surface roughening because of the high interface shear stresses in this region. Sand or bead blasting can increase the shear strength of the cement–implant interface. This pattern of stem surface roughening is exhibited by the BioMedtrix CFX stem (BioMedtrix LLC, Boonton, NJ; Figure 5.1). In cemented systems the acetabular cup is made of UHMWPE, with multiple grooves on its outer side to increase the surface area of the implant–cement interface and improve resistance to torsion and pullout (Figure 5.1). CFX fixation is further described in Chapter 7.

Numerous factors affect the mechanical properties of PMMA and, subsequently, the mechanical factors of the cement–bone and cement–implant interfaces (Shields et al. 2002; Dearmin and Schulz 2004; Figure 5.2). First-generation hand-packed

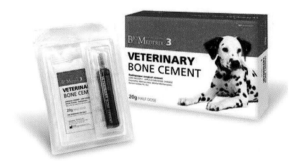

Figure 5.2 Commercially available veterinary PMMA product. (BioMedtrix, Boonton, NJ)

cementing techniques resulted in poor mechanical properties of the cement and inadequate interdigitation at the cement–bone interface. These problems have been implicated as important initiating factors in aseptic loosening (Ota et al. 2005). The second-generation cementing technique, using an intramedullary plug and cement gun, was introduced to achieve more uniform penetration and distribution of the cement (see Chapter 6). Human studies report significantly lower incidence of aseptic loosening using second-generation techniques compared with first-generation techniques. Third-generation cementing techniques include the use of centrifugation and vacuum mixing. The third-generation techniques further improved the strength of the cement mantle by minimizing air inclusion during cement preparation. Centrifugation and vacuum mixing improved tensile and fatigue properties of the cement in multiple *in vitro* mechanical studies (Davies et al. 1998). Modified third-generation cementing techniques (slow vacuum mixing) can be performed using commercially available instrumentation (Figure 5.3). The obvious disadvantage to this technique is the cost of the required equipment. Although it can diminish some mechanical properties, the benefits of mixing antibiotics with PMMA in primary total joint arthroplasty have been evaluated in several clinical studies (Weisman et al. 2000).

Because PMMA works as a cohesive, not as an adhesive, maximum strength of the cement–bone interface relies on the ability of the cement to penetrate irregularities in the bone surface (Schulz 2000). Drilling, reaming, and broaching results in filling of these irregularities with blood and bone fragments. Pulsatile lavage uses simultaneously pulsed lavage and suction to remove most of the blood and bone and has been shown, in combination with low-viscosity cement, to increase push-out strength (Askew et al. 1984). Pulsatile lavage is incapable of completely drying the femoral canal, and some additional bleeding is likely after cessation of lavage. Additional drying of the canal can be achieved with the use of femoral canal tampons or gauze sponges, further improving the strength of the cement–bone interface.

Similarly, the major goal of acetabular preparation in cemented systems is the maintenance of adequate cortical bone for structural support and the creation of appropriate surfaces for maximum cement cohesion. A number of techniques in acetabular bed preparation have been developed to maximize the strength and the longevity of the cement–bone interface. The strength of this interface is dependent on the bone surface area available for cement contact and filling. Techniques reported for use in cemented veterinary total hip systems include curette holes and connecting trough, three to five large drill holes, and multiple small drill holes (Schulz 2000).

Strength of the cement–bone interface may be further increased by pressurization of the cement within the femoral canal. Pressurization requires the use of a cement-restricting device to create a limited chamber into which the cement can flow. Cement restrictors were originally composed of PMMA plugs that were inserted into or formed within the femoral canal before insertion of the

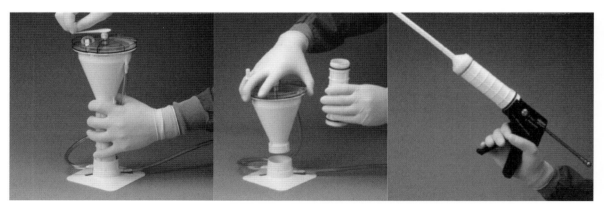

Figure 5.3 Modern "third-generation" cementing techniques can be performed with commercially available instrumentation (Advanced Cement Mixing System, Stryker Instruments, Kalamazoo, MI). Cement powder is poured into the bowl followed by the liquid monomer, the lid is secured, a 20–22 mmHg vacuum is applied, and the mixture is slowly mixed (*left*). The cement is transferred to the cartridge that is separated from the bowl (*middle*). The nozzle tip is applied, the cartridge is snapped into the cement injection gun, and cement is pressurized into the bone (*right*). (Image courtesy of Stryker Orthopedics, Mahwah, NJ)

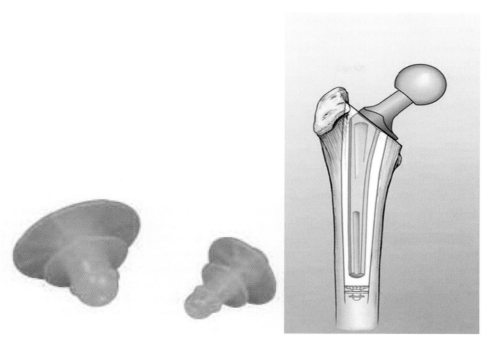

Figure 5.4   A cement restrictor plug (*left*) can be placed in the femur (*right*) to facilitate a better pressurization of cement. The implant is positioned to ensure maintenance of a cement mantle of 2 mm minimum surrounding the entire femoral stem (*right*). Substantial contact between the medial aspect of the ostectomy site and an implant collar also improves immediate implant stability (*right*). (Courtesy of BioMedtrix, Boonton, NJ)

remainder of the cement. Most current cement restrictors are pliable plastic plugs placed approximately 2 cm distal to the distal level of the tip of the femoral stem (Figure 5.4). The implant is positioned to ensure maintenance of a cement mantle of 2 mm minimum surrounding the entire femoral stem (Schulz 2000). Substantial contact between the medial aspect of the ostectomy site and an implant collar also improves immediate implant stability (Schulz 2000).

Postoperatively, the bone–cement interface may be immediately compromised due to cement polymerization, heat necrosis, the reaming process, or local monomer toxicity (Mann et al. 2008). As a consequence, a small layer of fibrous tissue can develop between the cement and the bone that creates a more compliant interface, reduces its strength, and leads to early implant migration. Under ideal conditions, the cement–bone interface can remain intact for years without an adverse biological response. However, conditions are often compromised, leading to progressive interface failure accompanied by clinical radiolucencies,

component migration, and pain. The exact mechanism for loosening is likely multifactorial with contributions from osteolysis and micromotion at the interface, bony changes due to stress adaptation and aging, and locally high fluid pressure. The reported incidence of loosening has been a major driving force toward the development of cementless implant systems (Mai et al. 2010; Khanuja et al. 2011).

Cementless systems

A variety of prostheses utilize cementless fixation as the means for initial implant stability. The types of cementless fixation used in veterinary prostheses are described below.

Cementless systems: Press-fit

"Osseointegration" (osteointegration) was first identified in the early 1950s by Per-Ingvar Brånemark as the attachment of lamellar bone to implants without intervening fibrous tissue (Brånemark 1983). It has been extensively studied (Albrektsson et al. 1981; Khanuja et al. 2011). Adequate osseous contact and firm fixation of the implant minimize micromotion. Micromotion of >150 μm leads to fibrous tissue formation, between 40 and 150 μm leads to a combination of bone and fibrous tissue formation, and <20 μm results in predominantly bone formation (Jasty et al. 1997). Initial fixation can be obtained by press-fitting a slightly oversized component. A number of factors influence the initial stability of primary fixation, including implant and bone geometry, roughness and coating of the implant, preparation technique, and bone quality.

Ingrowth occurs when bone grows inside a porous surface, and ongrowth occurs when bone grows onto a roughened surface (Khanuja et al. 2011). The surface characteristics of an implant determine which occurs. Ingrowth requires a pore size between 50 and 400 μm, and the percentage of voids within the coating should be between 30% and 40% to maintain mechanical strength (Albrektsson et al. 1981; Haddad et al. 1987).

Ingrowth surfaces include sintered beads, fiber mesh, and porous metals (Pilliar 2005). Ongrowth surfaces are created by grit blasting or plasma spraying. Osteoconductive materials such as hydroxyapatite can be applied to the surface of implants and may enhance the growth of mineralized bone onto the implant (see Chapter 3).

After the introduction of the canine cementless femoral stem and cup components in the 1980s, cementless implant design evolved in an effort to eliminate "cement-related" complications, such as aseptic loosening, progressive resorption of bone at the bone–cement interface, and loosening at the implant–cement interface. The canine uncemented porous-coated anatomic total hip prosthesis (PCA Canine Total Hip System, Howmedica, Mahway, NJ) has been extensively tested, but was never made commercially available (Marcellin-Little et al. 1999). Following the development of the PCA prosthesis, the Biologic Fixation (BFX) total hip system was introduced (BioMedtrix; Figure 5.5). The mechanical stability of this system initially relies on press-fit and, later, on bony ingrowth into both femoral stem and acetabular cup. The BFX system is made of cobalt-chromium or titanium

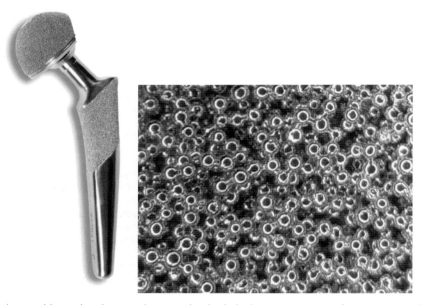

Figure 5.5   Cementless total hip arthroplasty implants, made of cobalt-chromium (stem) and titanium (cup) (*left*) with sintered beaded coatings (*right*; 250–300-μm bead diameter, pore size 150 μm, three layers, "stucco" application, 35% porosity). (BFX, courtesy of BioMedtrix, Boonton, NJ)

stem and the acetabular cup is made of titanium with sintered beaded coatings. Although it has not been critically evaluated, initial stability of this system appears to rely on multiple factors (Ganz et al. 2010; Lascelles et al. 2010). These factors include careful preoperative planning and case selection, and the precision of the surgical technique to prepare the bone surfaces for an ideal press-fit.

The TATE Elbow (BioMedtrix) also relies on a press-fit for initial stability. However, hollow posts are also utilized with the TATE prosthesis to maintain initial positioning of this cartridge component system. Fixation of the TATE Elbow is further described in Chapters 11 and 12.

The initial stability and femoral strain pattern during axial loading of BFX femoral implants were critically evaluated in an *in vitro* study.[1] The goal of cementless design is to create an initially stable press-fit that is conducive to bony ingrowth. The objective of the *in vitro* study was to determine whether osteotomy level or stem size affected initial implant stability of the BFX cementless stem and to assess femoral hoop strain under axial load. Axial load was applied to the potted femurs and cortical strain was measured with strain gauges. The study found that the more proximal osteotomy had a higher yield load, greater subsidence at failure, less canal fill, and less subsidence stiffness than did the more distal osteotomy. Larger implants had a higher yield load, greater subsidence stiffness, greater maximal load at failure, less subsidence at failure, and greater canal fill than did the undersized implants. Strain gauge data revealed nonuniform distributions of strain. Tensile strains were highest over fracture sites. The authors concluded that a proximal osteotomy and a large implant results in increased yield load prior to subsidence, likely due to increased stability resulting from a press-fit within the subtrochanteric cancellous bone block. Undersized implants and distal resection level results in lower subsidence stiffness and lower yield load, respectively.

The initial stability of the acetabular cup is thought to rely on press-fit at the cranial and caudal aspects of the acetabulum. The initial press-fit facilitates progressive osseointegration at the bone–implant interface. An *in vitro* study reported the biomechanical properties of the BFX acetabular cup impacted into a normal canine pelvis

(Margalit et al. 2010). Mean failure load was $3812 \pm 391\,N$, and the mode of failure was via bone fracture around the cup following minimal cup displacement in most cases (Figure 5.6). Mean failure load remained high ($2924 \pm 316\,N$), even when the medial wall of the acetabulum was intentionally penetrated with the reamer, in order to simulate a clinical situation where the dorsal rim of the acetabulum is absent and deep reaming becomes necessary. This study, using a normal pelvis, demonstrated that an appropriately positioned and seated BFX cementless cup is initially stable under physiological loading conditions. BFX fixation is further described in Chapter 7.

Cementless systems: Locking screws

The Zurich Cementless Hip Prosthesis (Kyon, Zurich, Switzerland) was the first cementless total hip arthroplasty system introduced to the veterinary market (Figure 5.7; Haney and Peck 2009).[2] Under the current design, immediate fixation of the acetabular cup is provided by a press-fit insertion, and long-term stability is achieved by bone ingrowth through the holes in the cup surface (Lauer et al. 2009). Locking screws are used for immediate fixation of the femoral stem, and ongrowth of bone along the rough titanium surface of the implant provides long-term stability (Guerrero and Montavon 2009). There are currently no data available regarding the immediate stability of this cementless total hip arthroplasty system (Hanson et al. 2006).

The outer shell of the acetabular cup is manufactured from perforated, highly compliant titanium, with an inner nonperforated shell, and a UHMWPE liner to receive the femoral head component. The double-shelled design is proposed to provide rapid and consistent osseointegration of the acetabular bone into the outer shell of the cup (Kyon).[3] The surface of the outer titanium shell is plasma titanium coated for additional microinterlock with the bone. For improved press-fit, the outer shell incorporates small protrusions, or "ribs," running circumferentially just below the equator. The pole of the shell is slightly flattened to prevent the cups from "bottoming out" at the pole without full engagement at the equator.[4]

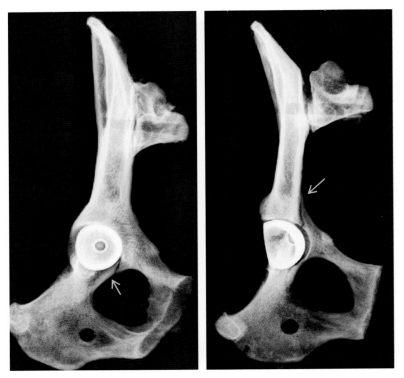

Figure 5.6 Radiograph of a cadaver pelvis made after implantation of a BFX cementless acetabular cup and mechanical testing. The cup–bone interface was immediately stable. Construct failure occurred after supraphysiological loading. The mode of failure was by ilial or ischial fractures (arrows) without major cup displacement.

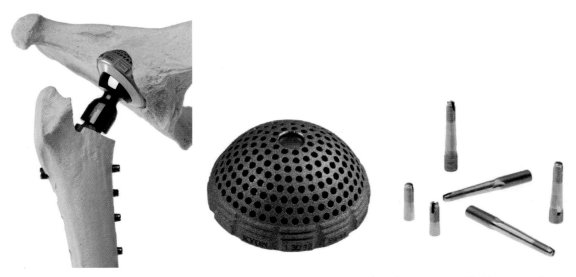

Figure 5.7 The Zurich Cementless Total Hip Replacement system (*left*). Immediate fixation is provided by a press-fit insertion for the acetabular cup (*center*) and by locking screws for the femoral stem (*right*). (Courtesy of Kyon, Zurich, Switzerland)

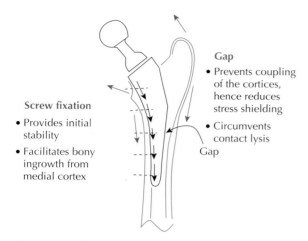

Screw fixation

- Provides initial stability
- Facilitates bony ingrowth from medial cortex

Gap

- Prevents coupling of the cortices, hence reduces stress shielding
- Circumvents contact lysis

Gap

Figure 5.8 Schematic representation of the hypothesis to support the concept of immediate and long-term stability of the Kyon cementless femoral implant. (Courtesy of Kyon, Zurich, Switzerland)

The cementless femoral stem of the Zurich Cementless Hip is designed to achieve permanent anchorage through bony ongrowth from the medial cortex without coupling to the lateral cortex. Immediate stability, required for ongrowth, is generated by locking screw fixation of the stem to the medial cortex of the femur (Figure 5.8). The mechanics of the femoral stem fixation are similar to the PC-Fix plating system of AO/ASIF (DePuy Synthes, West Chester, PA; Tepic et al. 1997). During normal cycling, the femur is subjected to compressive loading on the medial side and tensile forces on the lateral side. The femur is naturally more compliant than a solid canal-filling metal prosthesis. Physiological loading generates high interface shear stresses, which can initially be resisted by friction alone. It has been shown, by theoretical analysis, that canal-filling press-fitted metal stems cannot be stable at all contact areas with the femur under physiological-level loading. It has been hypothesized that if any motion occurs before the interface is secured by bone adaptation to the implant by ongrowth and/or ingrowth, true, solid anchorage of the prosthesis will fail.[4] Therefore, this cementless system was created based on a hypothesis for improved implant stability, as shown in Figure 5.8, where the medial and lateral cortices are "uncoupled." Fixation of the Zurich Cementless prosthesis is further described in Chapter 7.

Cementless systems: Screw-in implants

The Helica total hip prosthesis was developed in the 2000s in an attempt to reduce problems inherent with current conventional total hip replacement systems (Helica Canine Cementless Hip System, INNOPLANT Veterinary, Hannover, Germany; Figures 5.9 and 5.10). A helical orthopedic implant has been shown to be superior to conventional design in implant stability (Windolf et al. 2009; Wiebking et al. 2011). The authors hypothesized that the surrounding trabecular structure undergoes a volumetric compaction with the insertion of a helical implant, and this consolidation of the material in combination with the viscoelastic properties of cancellous bone enhances the implant anchorage; the increased implant surface projected orthogonally in the direction of the force may result in stress reduction at the bone–implant interface (Windolf et al. 2009).

The Helica acetabular and femoral implants screw into the acetabulum and femur, respectively, using self-cutting helical threads. The design allows a force-controlled implantation and firm anchorage in the bone. The roughened, titanium alloy, implant surfaces allow for bone apposition and ongrowth.

One suggested advantage of the Helica implant system is limited bone removal. The femoral implant replaces only the femoral head and preserves the neck. Consequently, bone resection is minimal, which, in theory, preserves more normal anatomical structure and original mechanical properties. Because the femoral neck is not excised, femoral neck version and inclination are maintained.

An *in vitro* mechanical study found that the Helica femoral prosthesis significantly alters strain distribution in the proximal aspect of the femur and exhibits initial micromotion (Kim et al. 2012). Failure strength in axial compression of the Helica-implanted femur is less than that of the normal femur, but much greater than expected *in vivo* loads associated with normal activity. This study also found that the Helica femoral prosthesis has shortcomings that are similar to other conventional femoral prostheses. Two recent clinical studies reported premature loosening of Helica implants (Hach and Delfs 2009; Andreoni et al.

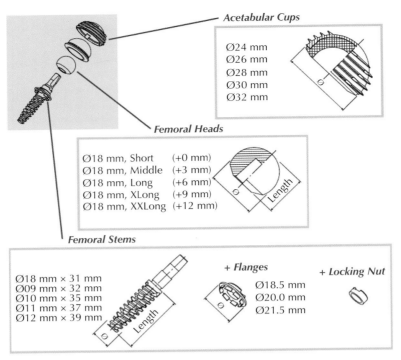

Acetabular Cups

Ø24 mm
Ø26 mm
Ø28 mm
Ø30 mm
Ø32 mm

Femoral Heads

Ø18 mm, Short   (+0 mm)
Ø18 mm, Middle   (+3 mm)
Ø18 mm, Long   (+6 mm)
Ø18 mm, XLong   (+9 mm)
Ø18 mm, XXLong   (+12 mm)

Length

Femoral Stems

Ø18 mm × 31 mm
Ø09 mm × 32 mm
Ø10 mm × 35 mm
Ø11 mm × 37 mm
Ø12 mm × 39 mm

Length

+ Flanges

Ø18.5 mm
Ø20.0 mm
Ø21.5 mm

+ Locking Nut

Figure 5.9 The Helica implant system (Helica TPS®). (Courtesy of INNOPLANT Veterinary, Hannover, Germany)

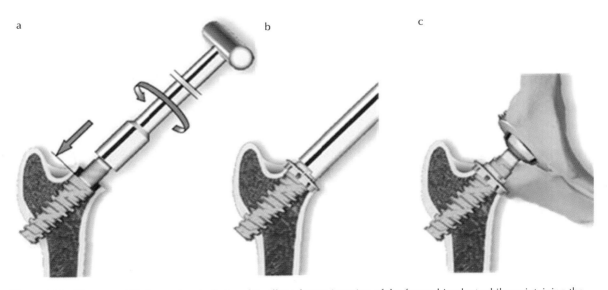

a   b   c

Figure 5.10 The current Helica system is designed to allow deeper insertion of the femoral implant while maintaining the integrity of femoral neck (a), and secured bone–implant interface by adjustable flanges (b). These modifications are proposed to result in stable construct in canine total hip replacement (THR) application (c). (Courtesy of INNOPLANT Veterinary, Hannover, Germany)

2010). Due to concerns associated with initial instability and subsequent implant loosening, a few modifications in implanting techniques have been suggested. Anecdotally, it is proposed that larger and longer femoral implants that engage in the lateral cortex appear to be more stable and to have a lower incidence of implant loosening.[5,6] To achieve secured engagement of femoral implant anchoring in the lateral cortex, a more distal neck ostectomy than originally proposed may be necessary, which may eliminate the proposed advantage of maintenance of femoral neck. Another proposed modification is the use of a steeper angle of femoral implant insertion than originally proposed. This modification was proposed in an attempt to reduce the force applied to the Helica femoral implant by shortening the lever arm length of femoral head and neck (Franklin et al. 2012). Clinical efficacy of these modifications has not been critically evaluated. However, these modifications have been incorporated in the second generation of the Helica implant (TPS®; Figures 5.9 and 5.10). The second-generation implant has also added an adjustable flange to increase surgical planning flexibility and improve resistance against shear forces at the interface between implant and femoral ostectomy site.

Combination: Hybrid fixation

As discussed above, the optimal method for implant fixation is a subject of considerable controversy in both human and veterinary total joint arthroplasty (Gemmill et al. 2011). The hybrid total hip arthroplasty (cementless acetabular component and cemented femoral component) has been proposed in human medicine (Harris 1996) and recently in veterinary medicine (Gemmill et al. 2011). The reverse hybrid method (i.e., cemented acetabular component and cementless femoral component) has also been evaluated (Lindalen et al. 2011). The current generation of the Iowa State University Elbow (ISU Elbow, BioMedtrix) utilizes a hybrid humeral component with a cemented humeral stem for immediate fixation, and a porous-coated humeral condyle for long-term fixation. Fixation of the ISU Elbow is further described in Chapters 11 and 12.

The rationale for this approach is well descried in a recent clinical study (Gemmill et al. 2011). A postmortem retrieval study reported that conventional canine total hip replacement fixation using PMMA was associated with a greater-than-50% incidence of implant loosening (Skurla et al. 2005), and complications relating to femoral components remain a problem in cementless canine total hip replacement (Ganz et al. 2010). The modern cementing techniques (described above) led to marked improvement in the survival of femoral components. However, only marginal improvements were noted in the performance of acetabular components, possibly because of the technical difficulties of achieving cement pressurization into a dry acetabular bone bed (Paul and Bargar 1987). These observations led many surgeons to adopt a hybrid approach to fixation, using a cementless acetabular cup and cemented femoral stem, and a recent clinical study reported a survival rate of the prostheses of 99% at a mean follow-up of 16 months (range: 6–40 months) (Gemmill et al. 2011).

Conclusion

To date, there is no consensus with regard to the optimal fixation method for total joint arthroplasty implants in human medicine (Clement et al. 2012, Khanuja et al. 2011; Ruben et al. 2012). Recent meta-analyses in human medicine could not support any single total joint arthroplasty system, and have generally concluded that an orthopedic surgeon should choose an established system based on patient characteristics, knowledge, experience, and surgeon preference (Corbett et al. 2010; Paxton et al. 2010; Huo et al. 2011; Pakvis et al. 2011) . Level of evidence of appropriate fixation method of total joint arthroplasty is low in veterinary medicine (Ganz et al. 2010; Margalit et al. 2010; Hayes et al. 2011). Randomized controlled trials are considered a standard for evaluating medical outcomes. However, such trials in total joint arthroplasty are impractical in evaluating long-term risks. A few studies in human medicine have demonstrated the effectiveness of national and regional registry systems in improving clinical practice, and such registries may be of benefit in the long-term evaluation of veterinary arthroplasty systems.

Endnotes

1. Townsend KL, Kowaleski MP, Johnson KA. Initial stability and femoral strain pattern during axial loading of canine cementless femoral prostheses: Effect of resection level and implant size. In: *Proceedings of the Veterinary Symposium, American College of Veterinary Surgeons*. 2007.
2. Vezzoni A. Revision of Kyon THR. In: *Proceedings of the 3rd World Veterinary Orthopedic Congress*. 2010, pp.464–467.
3. Tepic S. Development and mechanical basis for Kyon THR. In: *Proceedings of the Annual American College of Veterinary Surgeons Forum*. Denver, CO, 2004, pp. 289–291.
4. Tepic S. *Kyon Practicum Proceedings*. Las Vegas, NV, 2011.
5. Agnello K. Personal communication, January 2012.
6. Dosch M, Garcia TC, Hayashi K et al. Abstract: Biomechanical evaluation of the Helica femoral implant system using the traditional and a new modified technique. Veterinary Orthopedic Society, 2012.

References

Albrektsson T, Branenmark PI, Hansson HA et al. Osseointegrated titanium implants. Requirements for ensuring a long-lasting, direct bone to implant anchorage in man. Acta Orthop Scand 1981;52:155–170.

Andreoni AA, Guerrero TG, Hurter K, et al. Revision of an unstable HELICA endoprosthesis with a Zurich cementless total hip replacement. Vet Comp Orthop Traumatol 2010;23:177–181.

Askew MJ, Steege JW, Lewis JL, et al. Effect of cement pressure and bone strength on polymethylmethacrylate fixation. J Orthop Res 1984;1:412–420.

Beksac B, Taveras NA, Valle AG, et al. Surface finish mechanics explain different clinical survivorship of cemented femoral stems for total hip arthroplasty. J Long Term Eff Med Implants 2006;16:407–422.

Brånemark P. Osseointegration and its experimental background. J Prosthet Dent 1983;50:399–410.

Buechel FF, Pappas MJ. The design process. In: Principles of Human Joint Replacement: Design and Clinical Application. Berlin: Springer, 2011, pp. 77–90.

Charnley G, Judet T, Garreau de Loubresse C. Titanium femoral component fixation and experience with a cemented femoral prosthesis. In: Interfaces in Total Hip Arthroplasty, Learmonth ID (ed.). London: Springer, 2000, pp. 3–10.

Clayton R, Cravens R, Hupfer T, et al. Intermediate results of a cemented Femoral stem with a PMMA premantle. Orthopedics 2007;30:950.

Clement ND, Biant LC, Breusch SJ. Total hip arthroplasty: To cement or not to cement the acetabular socket? A critical review of the literature. Arch Orthop Trauma Surg 2012;132:411–427.

Corbett KL, Losina E, Nti AA, et al. Population-based rates of revision of primary total hip arthroplasty: A systematic review. PLoS One 2010;5:e13520.

Davies JP, Connor DO, Burke DW, et al. The effect of centrifugation on the fatigue life of bone cement in the presence of surface irregularities. Clin Orthop Rel Res 1998;229:156–161.

Dearmin MG, Schulz KS. The effect of stem length on femoral component positioning in canine total hip arthroplasty. Vet Surg 2004;33:272–278.

Eldridge JDJ, Learmonth ID. Component bone interface in cementless hip arthroplasty. In: Interfaces in Total Hip Arthroplasty, Learmonth ID (ed.). London: Springer, 2000, pp. 71–80.

Franklin SP, Franklin AL, Wilson H, et al. The relationship of the canine femoral head to the femoral neck: An anatomic study with relevance for hip arthroplasty implant design and implantation. Vet Surg 2012;41(1):86–93.

Ganz SM, Jackson J, VanEnkevort B. Risk factors for femoral fracture after canine press-fit cementless total hip arthroplasty. Vet Surg 2010;39:688–695.

Gemmill TJ, Pink J, Renwick A, et al. Hybrid cemented/cementless total hip replacement in dogs: Seventy-eight consecutive joint replacements. Vet Surg 2011;40:621–630.

Guerrero TG, Montavon PM. Zurich cementless total hip replacement: Retrospective evaluation of 2nd generation implants in 60 dogs. Vet Surg 2009;38:70–80.

Hach V, Delfs G. Initial experience with a newly developed cementless hip endoprosthesis. Vet Comp Orthop Traumatol 2009;22:153–158.

Haddad RJ, Cook SD, Thomas KA. Biological fixation of porous-coated implants. J Bone Joint Surg Am 1987;69:1459–1466.

Hallab NJ, Jacobs JJ, Katz JW. Application of materials in medicine, biology and artificial organs: Orthopedic applications. In: Biomaterials Science: An Introduction to Materials in Medicine, Ratner BD, Hoffman AS, Schoen FJ et al. (eds.), 2nd ed. Amsterdam: Elsevier Academic Press, 2004, pp. 527–555.

Haney DR, Peck JN. Influence of canal preparation depth on the incidence of femoral medullary infarction with Zurich Cementless Canine Total Hip arthroplasty. Vet Surg 2009;38:673–676.

Hanson SP, Peck JN, Berry CR, et al. Radiographic evaluation of the Zurich cementless total hip acetabular component. Vet Surg 2006;35:550–558.

Harris WH. Hybrid total hip replacement: Rationale and intermediate clinical results. Clin Orthop Relat Res 1996;333:155–164.

Hayes GM, Ramirez J, Langley Hobbs SJ. Does the degree of preoperative subluxation or soft tissue tension affect the incidence of postoperative luxation in dogs after total hip replacement? Vet Surg. 2011;40:6–13.

Huo MH, Dumont GD, Knight JR, Mont MA. What's new in total hip arthroplasty. J Bone Joint Surg Am 2011;19(93):1944–1950.

Jasty M, Bragdon C, Burke D, et al. *In vivo* skeletal responses to porous-surfaced implants subjected to small induced motions. J Bone Joint Surg Am 1997;79:707–714.

Khanuja HS, Vakil JJ, Goddard MS, et al. Cementless femoral fixation in total hip arthroplasty. J Bone Joint Surg Am 2011;93:500–509.

Kim JY, Hayashi K, Garcia TC, et al. Biomechanical evaluation of screw-in femoral implant in cementless total hip system. Vet Surg 2012;41:94–102.

Lascelles BD, Freire M, Roe SC, et al. Evaluation of functional outcome after BFX total hip replacement using a pressure sensitive walkway. Vet Surg 2010;39:71–77.

Lauer SK, Nieves MA, Peck J, et al. Descriptive histomorphometric ingrowth analysis of the Zurich cementless canine total hip acetabular component. Vet Surg 2009;38:59–69.

Lindalen E, Havelin LI, Nordsletten L, et al. Is reverse hybrid hip replacement the solution? Acta Orthopaedica 2011;82:639–645.

Mai KT, Verioti CA, Casey K, et al. Cementless femoral fixation in total hip arthroplasty. Am J Orthop 2010;39:126–130.

Mann KA, Miller MA, Cleary RJ, et al. Experimental micromechanics of the cement–bone interface. J Orthop Res 2008;26:872–879.

Marcellin-Little DJ, DeYoung BA, Doyens DH, et al. Canine uncemented porous-coated anatomic total hip arthroplasty: Results of a long-term prospective evaluation of 50 consecutive cases. Vet Surg 1999; 28:10–20.

Margalit KA, Hayashi K, Jackson J, et al. Biomechanical evaluation of acetabular cup implantation in cementless total hip arthroplasty. Vet Surg 2010;39:818–823.

Ota J, Cook JL, Lewis DD, et al. Short-term aseptic loosening of the femoral component in canine total hip replacement: Effects of cementing technique on cement mantle grade. Vet Surg 2005;34:345–352.

Pakvis D, van Hellemondt G, de Visser E, et al. Is there evidence for a superior method of socket fixation in hip arthroplasty? A systematic review. International Orthopaedics 2011;35:1109–1118.

Paul HA, Bargar WL. Histologic changes in the dog acetabulum following total hip replacement with current cementing techniques. J Arthroplasty 1987;2:71–76.

Paxton EW, Namba RS, Maletis GB, et al. A prospective study of 80,000 total joint and 5000 anterior cruciate ligament reconstruction procedures in a community-based registry in the United States. J Bone Joint Surg Am 2010;92:117–132.

Pérez MA, Seral-García B. A finite element analysis of the vibration behaviour of a cementless hip system. Comput Methods Biomech Biomed Engin 2012; [Epub]

Pilliar RM. Cementless implant fixation—Toward improved reliability. Orthop Clin North Am 2005;36:113–119.

Pruitt LA, Chakravartula AM. Orthopedics. In: Mechanics of Biomaterials: Fundamental Principles for Implant Design, Pruitt LA, Chakravartula AM (eds.). Cambridge, U.K.: Cambridge University Press, 2011, pp. 416–471.

Ruben RB, Fernandes PR, Folgado J. On the optimal shape of hip implants. J Biomech 2012;10(45): 239–246.

Schulz KS. Application of arthroplasty principles to canine cemented total hip replacement. Vet Surg 2000;29:578–593.

Shields SL, Schulz KS, Hagan CE, et al. The effects of acetabular cup temperature and duration of cement pressurization on cement porosity in a canine total hip replacement model. Vet Surg 2002;31:167–173.

Skurla CP, Pluhar GE, Frankel DJ, et al. Assessing the dog as model for human total hip replacement. Analysis of 38 canine cemented femoral components retrieved at post-mortem. J Bone Joint Surg Br 2005;87:120–127.

Tepic S, Remiger AR, Morikawa K, et al. Strength recovery in fractured sheep tibia treated with a plate or an internal fixator: An experimental study with a two-year follow-up. J Orthop Trauma 1997;11:14–23.

Weisman DL, Olmstead ML, Kowalski JJ. *In vitro* evaluation of antibiotic elution from polymethylmethacrylate (PMMA) and mechanical assessment of antibiotic-PMMA composites. Vet Surg 2000;29: 245–251.

Wiebking U, Birkenhauer B, Krettek C, et al. Initial stability of a new uncemented short-stem prosthesis, Spiron®, in dog bone. Technol Health Care 2011;19: 271–282.

Windolf M, Braunstein V, Dutoit C, et al. Is a helical shaped implant a superior alternative to the Dynamic Hip Screw for unstable femoral neck fractures? A biomechanical investigation. Clin Biomech (Bristol, Avon) 2009;24:59–64.

6 Biomechanical Considerations in Total Hip Replacement

Michael P. Kowaleski

Total hip replacement is a highly successful operation for the alleviation of discomfort secondary to debilitating conditions of the hip joint. Increasingly, patients and their owners are demanding more than just pain relief from replaced joints, challenging surgeons and implants to deliver highly athletic function as well as longevity. This challenge can be met by utilizing modern surgical techniques and implants to provide pain-free function and restore normal biomechanics and kinematics to the hip.

Functional anatomy of the hip joint

The femoral head comprises two-thirds of a sphere, and it is connected to the femoral metaphysis by the femoral neck. There are several anatomical aspects of the femoral head and neck that influence hip biomechanics. *Femoral neck anteversion* is the cranial (anterior) projection of the femoral head and neck relative to the anatomical axis of the femur. Anteversion of the femoral head and neck increases range of motion in flexion and extension that can occur prior to impingement of the femoral neck on the acetabular rim. *Femoral*

inclination angle is the angle formed between the anatomical axis of the femur and the long axis of the femoral head and neck (Figure 6.1). *Femoral offset* is the distance between the center of rotation of the femoral head and the anatomical axis of the femur (Figure 6.1). The offset distance is the lever arm for the abductor muscles of the hip (Figure 6.2). A decrease in the offset distance increases the force required by the abductor muscles to stabilize the pelvis during the stance phase of gait, while an increase in femoral offset decreases the force required. *Head–neck ratio* is the difference between the circumference of the femoral head and the femoral neck, which allows movements of the articulation to occur without impingement of the femoral neck on the acetabular rim (Sariali et al. 2008).

The acetabulum is a cotyloid (cup-shaped) cavity of the os coxae. In the normal hip, just under half of the femoral head is covered by the acetabulum. The less-than-hemispherical shape of the socket portends the Latin origin of the word, *acētum* (vinegar) and *–abulum* (container), from the Latin word for vinegar cup, a less-than-hemispherical vessel. The acetabular labrum is a fibrocartilaginous extension of the acetabular rim

Advances in Small Animal Total Joint Replacement, First Edition. Edited by Jeffrey N. Peck and Denis J. Marcellin-Little.
© 2013 John Wiley & Sons, Inc. Published 2013 by John Wiley & Sons, Inc.

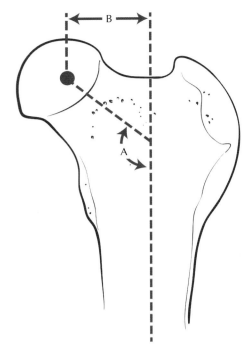

Figure 6.1   The femoral inclination angle (A) is the angle formed between the anatomical axis of the femur and the long axis of the femoral head and neck. Femoral offset (B) is the perpendicular distance between the center of rotation of the femoral head and the anatomical axis of the femur.

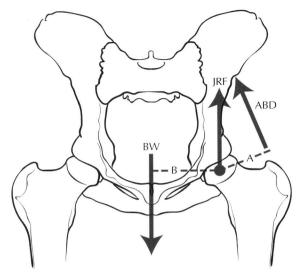

Figure 6.2   Schematic of the forces during the stance phase of gait. The abductor force (ABD) gains mechanical advantage due to the femoral offset (A). The force of body weight (BW) acts at a distance from centerline (B) to create the joint reaction force (JRF).

that effectively increases the depth of the acetabulum, resulting in coverage of the femoral head beyond its equator. The acetabular labrum extends across the acetabular notch as a free ligament, the transverse acetabular ligament (Evans 1993).

An understanding of normal and abnormal acetabular anatomy can be aided by evaluation of the orientation of prosthetic acetabular components. Acetabular component orientation can vary about three orthogonal axes, and is defined with reference to the angles of lateral opening, version, and inclination (Dyce et al. 2001). The angle of lateral opening is the angle between the dorsal plane and the open face of the cup (Figure 6.3A). The terms *closed* and *open* are used to describe acetabular components that have an angle of lateral opening of less than 45 degrees and greater than 45 degrees, respectively. The angle of version is the angle between the median plane and the open face of the cup (Figure 6.3B). Retroversion refers to a cup that faces caudally with respect to

the median plane, and anteversion refers to a cup that faces cranially with respect to the median plane. The angle of inclination is relevant only to acetabular components with a truncated open face, and is defined as the angle between the ilial-ischial axis and a line connecting the truncation points of the cup (Figure 6.3C). Radiographically, the truncation points of a metal-backed component are apparent; this is estimated by the long axis of the marker wire in an all-polyethylene component. Negative inclination (declined cup) refers to an inclination angle that is less than that of the ilial-ischial axis, and positive inclination (inclined cup) refers to an angle that is greater than that of the ilial-ischial axis (Dyce et al. 2001). Alternative nomenclature to describe the spatial orientation of cemented acetabular components has been reported (Cross et al. 2000). In this publication, the term inclination was used to describe the angle of lateral opening.

Many muscles cross, and therefore act upon the hip joint, not only producing motion but also increasing stability. The hip muscles can be grouped based on the direction in which they move the hip (Figure 6.4); flexion, extension, adduction, abduction, internal rotation, and

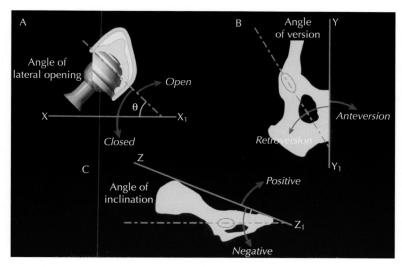

Figure 6.3 (A) Transverse plane cross section through an implanted acetabular component. The angle of lateral opening (θ) is the angle between the dorsal plane (X–X$_1$) and the plane of the nontruncated portion of the cup face. (B) Pelvis viewed from the ventral aspect, right hip. The angle of version is the angle between the median plane (Y–Y$_1$) and the long axis of the radiographic projection of the acetabular component. (C) Pelvis viewed from the lateral aspect, left hip. The angle of inclination is the angle between the ilial–ischial axis and the long axis of the marker wire or truncation points of a metal-backed component. (Reprinted with permission from Dyce et al. [2001]; Wiley-Blackwell).

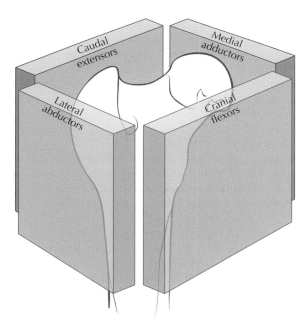

Figure 6.4 The hip muscles can be grouped based on their action on the joint; this is related to their anatomical location with respect to the femur.

external rotation are the major movements of the hip. All of these movements occur around a pivot point, or center of rotation, which is the center of the femoral head. The primary muscles that flex the hip are the iliopsoas, rectus femoris, and tensor fascia lata (Figure 6.5). The superficial, middle, and deep (*gluteus profundus*) gluteal muscles and the piriformis are the extensors of the hip (Figure 6.5). In order to rotate the femur toward the midline of the body (adduction), a series of muscles must contract, including the adductor (*adductor magnus et brevis* and *adductor longus*), gracilis, and pectineus (Figure 6.5). Abduction is achieved mainly through contraction of the superficial, middle, and deep gluteal muscles; these muscles extend from the lateral aspect of the ilium to the greater trochanter, except for the superficial gluteal that inserts on the third trochanter. Although these are relatively small muscles with short lever arms, it is likely that they are the most important muscle group for hip stability (Figure 6.2; Nevelos and Patel 2009); thus, is it critical to preserve these muscles during surgery of the hip. The torque created by these muscles is directly influenced by the femoral offset that defines the lever arm upon

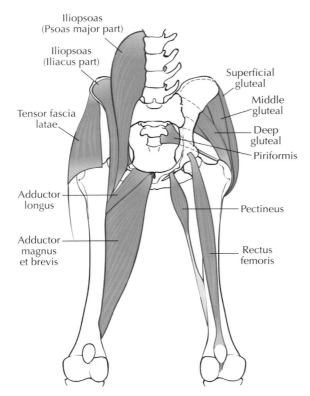

Iliopsoas
(Psoas major part)

Iliopsoas
(Iliacus part)

Superficial
gluteal

Middle
gluteal

Deep
gluteal

Piriformis

Tensor fascia
latae

Adductor
longus

Pectineus

Adductor
magnus
et brevis

Rectus
femoris

Figure 6.5   Flexor, extensor, adductor, and abductor
muscles of the hip joint.

which they act (Figures 6.1 and 6.2). Internal (or medial) rotation occurs with contraction of the superficial, middle, and deep gluteal muscles. External rotation is performed by a series of muscles that originate caudal to the acetabulum and insert within the trochanteric fossa, including the external obturator, internal obturator, gemelli, and quadratus femoris (Figure 6.6).

The range of motion of the hip joint in healthy Labrador retrievers, as determined by goniometry, was 50 ± 2 degrees of flexion to 162 ± 3 degrees of extension. The hip joint angle was measured at the intersection of the longitudinal axis of the femur and a line that joined the tuber sacrale and ischiadicum (Jaegger et al. 2002). A kinematic analysis using reflective markers attached to the skin on the dorsal iliac spine, greater trochanter, and stifle between the lateral epicondyle and fibular head was performed using motion capture to determine the sagittal plane joint motions in dogs and humans. During walking, the maximum flexion of the canine hip was 118 ± 3.6 degrees, and maximum extension was 147.9 ± 2.0 degrees (Richards et al. 2010). Note that in the later study, the angle measured and reported in the publication was the complementary angle to that measured by Jaegger; for simplicity, the data was transformed to the analogous angle reported by

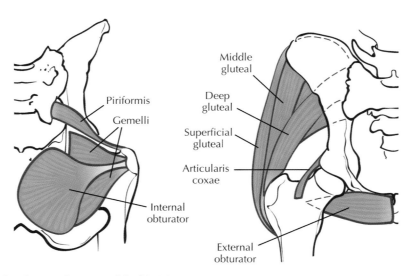

Piriformis

Gemelli

Internal
obturator

Middle
gluteal

Deep
gluteal

Superficial
gluteal

Articularis
coxae

External
obturator

Figure 6.6   Internal and external rotators of the hip joint.

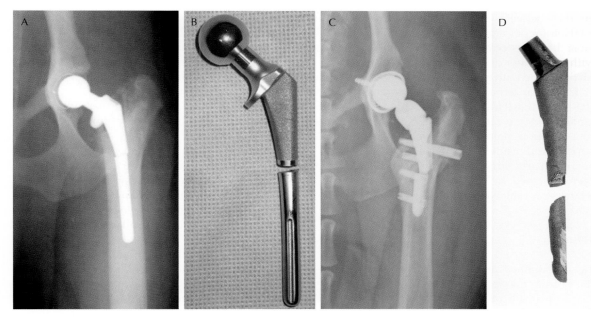

Figure 6.7 Fatigue failure of a cemented (A and B) and a cementless (C and D) femoral component. Images A and B courtesy of Dr. Jonathan Dyce.

Jaegger by subtracting the original values from 180 degrees.

Mechanics of total hip replacement

Basic concepts of mechanics are important in understanding the performance and limits to longevity of total joint replacements. *Stress* is defined at force/unit area, and *strain* is a dimensionless measure of deformation, defined as change in length/original length. *Stiffness* is a measure of how much deformation a material will undergo with a given applied force. *Ultimate strength* is the amount of stress necessary to reach the failure point of a material or construct with a single application of load. Modes of failure include fracture or plastic deformation.

Devices or constructs may fracture following the serial application of loads below their ultimate strength. This type of failure is known as *fatigue failure*. Fatigue failure occurs because all materials contain imperfections or flaws, which may be propagated as cracks under conditions of high stress, a large numbers of cycles, or both. As cycling continues, these cracks coalesce, causing

complete structural failure (Figure 6.7). The fatigue behavior of a material can be determined experimentally and expressed as stress versus log (number of cycles) to failure, referred to as an S–N curve. The lower limit of stress below which the material can be cycled infinitely without fatigue failure is termed the *endurance limit* (Hollister 1995).

A primary function of total hip replacement is to bear and transfer load (Hollister 1995). The primary point of load transfer is the contact between the head of the femoral component and the socket of the acetabular component. In contrast to the viscoelastic nature of hyaline cartilage, the articulating components in a total hip replacement are simple solids that do not exhibit the time-dependent viscoelastic properties of cartilage. The elastic modulus, as determined by the stress–strain curve, of cartilage ranges from less than 1 MPa to 3 MPa, while that of polyethylene is 1400 MPa (Hollister 1995).

The secondary region of load transfer occurs at the interface between the implants and the surrounding bone (Hollister 1995). In a normal joint, no such interface exists, as there is a continuous transition from trabecular to cortical bone. The

between either a cemented or cementless
replacement is not as seamless. The load
transferred from the metallic implant
a stiffness of 100,000–200,000 MPa to either
cortical bone with a stiffness of 15,000–20,000 MPa
or trabecular bone with a stiffness ranging from
100–1000 MPa (Hollister 1995). This mismatch in
modulus may create large shear stresses or stress
concentration points at the material interfaces,
which could result in fatigue failure or the generation of wear debris. Low-modulus implants have
been designed to decrease bone surface strains
(Harrysson et al. 2008; Marcellin-Little et al. 2010).

Wear

Wear is defined as the progressive loss of sub-
stance from the operating surface of a body occurring as a result of relative motion at the surface
(Jin et al. 2006). The moving contact between a
metal head and ultrahigh-molecular-weight polyethylene (UHMWPE) bearing surface is the first
point of load transfer in total hip replacement.
This moving contact between these two apposing
surfaces generates wear debris that result in the
cytokine-mediated osteolysis and bone resorption
that has been implicated as the primary long-term
failure mode in total joint replacement.

Five types of wear have been described. *Adhesive* wear is the transfer of material from one
surface to another during relative motion by the
process of solid-phase welding. Adhesion occurs
during contact of the opposing bearing surfaces.
Sliding breaks these contacts; however, if the
strength of the adhesion exceeds the strength of
the material, particles (wear debris) are pulled
from the material. These adhesive wear debris are
typically generated from the polyethylene acetabular component because polyethylene is the
weaker of the two bearing surfaces.

Abrasive wear is the displacement of materials
by hard particles. Two-body abrasive wear occurs
when a hard projection on one surface cuts into
the opposing surface. Abrasive wear is also typically observed in polyethylene components. Abrasive wear also occurs when freely moving, hard
particles are trapped between adjacent surfaces
causing damage; this is known as *third-body* wear.
For example, particles of polymethylmethacrylate

(PMMA) bone cement, bone, metal, or polyethylene trapped between the femoral head and
acetabular cup may result in third-body wear.
Scratching of the metallic femoral heads is commonly observed during revision surgery, and this
is likely caused by third-body wear.

Adhesive wear and *fatigue* wear may work
together, with the surface asperities of the two
surfaces momentarily sticking together, causing
shear stresses that, over time, lead to eventual
fatigue of the asperity (Stewart 2010). In addition,
surface fatigue, occurs because contact forces
produce subsurface stresses in both the polyethylene and metal as they undergo cyclic compression
and tension. In a process similar to fatigue failure,
these cyclic stresses propagate cracks from subsurface imperfections that eventually cause pitting of
the surface and generation of large free fragments
or shards.[1]

Erosive wear is the loss of material from a solid
surface due to relative motion in contact with a
fluid that contains particles. This is often subdivided into impingement erosion and abrasive
erosion. If no solid particles are present, erosion
can still take place, such as erosion caused by rain
or by cavitation (Jin et al. 2006). *Corrosive* wear is
a process in which chemical or electrochemical
reactions with the environment dominate, such as
oxidative wear (Jin et al. 2006). To avoid corrosive
wear, it is important to avoid placing metals with
different nobility in contact with each other in the
body. Metal nobility is described in the galvanic
series.

Not all wear debris are generated from the
bearing surfaces. Wear debris can be produced
from any modular junction at which there is relative motion between the components, for example,
backside wear between the inside of the metallic
outer shell and the outside of the inner polyethylene liner in a metal-backed acetabular component.
Unintended contact, such as impingement of the
femoral neck on the acetabular component will
generate debris. These wear mechanisms apply
equally to both hard-on-soft (e.g., metal or ceramic
on polyethylene) and hard-on-hard (e.g., ceramic
on ceramic, metal on metal, and ceramic on metal)
bearing surfaces.

Of the five types of wear, abrasive wear, adhesive wear, and surface fatigue are the most relevant in total joint polyethylene wear. It should be

Sliding Distance = $r\alpha$, where $\alpha = 2(160 - 50)\pi/180$
Sliding Velocity = sliding distance/Time

Diameter	Distance	Velocity
14 mm	27 mm	34 mm/s
19 mm	36 mm	45 mm/s

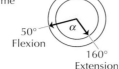

50°
Flexion

160°
Extension

Figure 6.8 Sliding distance and velocity as a function of bearing diameter during a single step at a walking gait with a stride frequency of 1.25 strides per second.

noted that the various wear types might occur simultaneously or sequentially. For example, wear particles produced as a result of adhesive wear can then act as third bodies causing abrasive wear (Jin et al. 2006). Once particles come between adjacent bearing surfaces, the amount of wear debris generated through abrasive wear depends on the hardness of the material, the magnitude of the contact force, and the sliding distance. Sliding distance is related to the diameter of the femoral head. For a given range of motion, a small femoral head will have a shorter sliding distance than a large femoral head; thus, the small femoral head will generate less wear in abrasion and fatigue (Figure 6.8). Mechanical factors affecting surface fatigue include material hardness, material fatigue resistance, contact stress magnitude, and the amount of cycling between tensile and compressive subsurface stresses. The magnitude of both contact and subsurface stresses depends on joint reaction forces, surface friction, material stiffness, the thickness of surface materials, and the conformity of bearing surfaces (Hollister 1995). Utilizing finite element analysis of human acetabular cups, Bartel demonstrated that higher conformity, that is, a better fit between surfaces, reduced contact stresses, and polyethylene thickness of less than 6–8 mm greatly increased subsurface stresses (Bartel et al. 1985, 1986). Metal backing appears to slightly elevate the contact stresses, although this effect is greater on thinner polyethylene than on thicker polyethylene. Thicker polyethylene reduces cement stresses (Hollister 1995). To reduce contact stress, the surgeon can choose hip replacements with highly conforming articular surfaces, ensure proper alignment at implantation, and use the thickest polyethylene liner that is practical, balanced with the available bone stock (Hollister 1995).

The volumetric wear rate of UHMWPE in post-mortem retrievals of human acetabular components has been reported to be 35.0 mm³/year (Jasty et al. 1997), and that of dogs has been reported to be 6.9 mm³/year for implants produced by BioMedtrix (Boonton, NJ) and 8.3 mm³/year for implants produced by Richards (Memphis, TN) (Skurla and James 2001). Analysis of periprosthetic tissues from patients with failed cemented total hip replacement has revealed a total mass of polyethylene debris of 216–518 μg/g of tissue for human patients and 200–400 μg/g of tissue for canine patients.[1] It appears that the osteolytic process responsible for aseptic loosening in man has a threshold of $1–10 \times 10^9$ polyethylene particles per gram of tissue, and in the dog it has been estimated to be $4.1–8.2 \times 10^8$ particles per gram of tissue.[1] The total mass of metallic particles in the periprosthetic tissues of failed cemented total hip replacements is reported to be 6000–25,000 μg/g of tissue in human patients and was found to be 1333–20,000 μg/g of tissue in a cohort of canine patients.[1]

In summary, there are three laws of wear that should be considered in the context of total joint replacement:

1. Wear volume increases as the normal load increases.
2. Wear increases as the sliding distance increases.
3. Wear decreases as the hardness of the softer sliding component increases.

Cemented implant interfaces

The implant–bone interface is the second major site of load transfer; thus, it represents the other potential site for mechanical failure of total joints. The implant interface of a cemented component can be subdivided into three regions including the cement–implant interface, the inner cement mantle, and the cement–bone interface. Defects or voids within these regions result in stress concentration at the edge of the defect, increasing the likelihood that the cement will mechanically fail locally. Local failure propagates the defect, limiting the mechanical performance of the implant system and increasing the likelihood of implant failure. The material properties of the components of the implant interface of a cemented component vary widely. A metallic femoral stem can be made from titanium alloy with a stiffness of 114,000 MPa, endurance limit of 400 MPa, and ultimate strength of 850 MPa, or cobalt-chromium with a stiffness of 200,000 MPa, endurance limit of 350 MPa, and ultimate strength of 900 MPa. The bony portion is a combination of trabecular bone with an average stiffness of 500 MPa and an ultimate strength of 20 MPa or cortical bone with an average stiffness of 15,000 MPa and ultimate strength of approximately 150 MPa. The PMMA bone cement is the weak link of this interface, as it has a stiffness of 2200 MPa and an ultimate strength of 8–10 MPa (Hollister 1995). Thus, the high endurance limit of metal, and the bone's ability to repair itself, relatively protect these elements, leaving the cement as the most susceptible to fatigue failure. Mechanical loosening or debonding at the cement–implant interface appears to be the initial failure event in both cemented acetabular and femoral components in dogs (Skurla and James 2005; Skurla et al. 2005).

Cortical area and cortical porosity are significantly increased in the femurs of dogs with stable, long-term cemented femoral implants compared with nonimplanted femurs (Bergh et al. 2004a). Net bone loss proximally and increased bone mass distally support stress shielding as an important mechanical factor associated with this bone adaptation (Bergh et al. 2004a). Interface loosening occurs due to direct mechanical failure, or due to bone resorption secondary to wear debris. The histomorphometric changes of femurs with unstable cemented implants include periosteal bone formation and endosteal bone resorption, supporting mechanisms of stress shielding and wear debris-mediated osteolysis as factors that may contribute to femoral adaptation and implant loosening (Bergh et al. 2004b).

The mechanical performance of PMMA bone cement can be enhanced by refinement of the cementing technique, thereby increasing cement intrusion into trabecular bone and decreasing voids and porosity of the cement. Bone cement is a viscoelastic material that can undergo creep. It is much stronger in compression than tension, and is weakest in shear (Santavirta et al. 1998). Decreased porosity has been shown to increase tensile strength and fatigue strength of cement,

Table 6.1   Evolution of contemporary cementing techniques

Technique	First-generation	Second-generation	Third-generation
Filling	Antegrade	Retrograde	Retrograde
Cement gun	No	Yes	Yes
Distal femoral restriction	No	Yes	Yes
Proximal femoral restriction	No	No	Yes
Hand mixing cement	Yes	Yes	No
Vacuum mixing/ centrifugation cement	No	No	Yes
Canal brushing	No	Yes	Yes
Pulsed lavage	No	No	Yes
Distal centralization	No	Yes	Yes
Proximal centralization	No	No	Yes/No

theoretically increasing the cement's longevity (Davies et al. 1988, 1989). Contemporary cementing techniques have followed an evolutionary process (Table 6.1). First-generation cement technique included hand mixing with manual insertion (finger packing). This technique allowed for cement lamination, creation of voids within the cement, inadequate or incomplete cement mantles, and poor penetration of cement into cancellous bone. In spite of these limitations, many authors reported good long-term survivorship (Nercessian et al. 2005).

Since PMMA bone cement has no adhesive characteristics, it functions as a grout, and not as glue. Pressurization increases the penetration of cement into the interstices of cancellous bone; it is this intrusion of cement into the bone that is responsible for the shear strength of the interface. Pressurized cement has better tensile and shear strengths at the bone–cement interface than finger-packed cement in adult mongrel dogs (MacDonald et al. 1993). Bone preparation by removing fat, blood, and debris promotes better cement penetration, improving mechanical interlock and interface shear strength (Breusch et al. 2000). Based on these findings, second-generation cement techniques, involving canal preparation with brushing, retrograde liquid-phase injection of cement using a cement gun, a distal canal plug (cement restrictor), and stem centralizer, were introduced in the 1980s (Table 6.1). These advances in cementing technique resulted in a marked reduction in the incidence of femoral component loosening in people (Savory et al. 2006).

Contemporary or third-generation techniques introduced the concept of maintaining pressurization of the cement before and during cement insertion by adding proximal restriction to distal femoral occlusion (Table 6.1). Retrograde filling, proximal restrictions, and liquid-phase injection with the cement gun allow increased pressurization of the cement, and thus greater cement intrusion into the interstices of the cancellous bone. In addition, centrifugation and vacuum mixing have been advocated to decrease porosity and to remove the noxious fumes of the monomer. The amount of reduction in porosity that is achieved remains somewhat controversial. In addition, although voids can act as crack initiators, they can also be crack terminators (Savory et al. 2006). Nonporous cement can exhibit excessive contraction after polymerization, and this contraction can compromise fixation by diminishing microinterlock.

Cementless implant interfaces

Unlike cemented implants that rely on mechanical interlock for stability, cementless ingrowth and ongrowth implants rely on the interaction between the biological healing process and mechanical stimuli to achieve long-term fixation. In addition, the initial stability of these implants achieved by frictional forces or screw fixation is often inferior to that of the long-term stability that occurs in the weeks following implantation. The processes of bone ingrowth and ongrowth are thought to occur in two stages. The initial stage is similar to indirect or secondary bony union, in which the initial hematoma differentiates into either fibrous tissue, if the implant is unstable, or woven bone, if the implant is stable. The threshold of stability necessary to achieve bony ingrowth has generally been defined as 100 μm of motion at the bone–implant interface (Hollister 1995). The second stage of bone ingrowth is remodeling of the interface tissue. Fibrous tissue at the interface generally remains at the interface wherever it was initially deposited, and bony tissue remodels in response to the implant-imposed strains. In order to create and maintain bone ingrowth or ongrowth, osseointegration, or synthesis of mineralized tissue within the interface, during the initial phase of healing must occur, and the subsequent implant-imposed strains must be large enough to maintain the initially deposited bone.

It is not certain how much bone ingrowth or ongrowth is necessary for implant stability; however, it has been demonstrated that the mechanics of the implant–bone interface depend substantially on the amount and type of tissue that grows into or onto the implant surface. In a model of bone ingrowth, Ko evaluated the effect of the percentage of bone ingrowth on interface stiffness. In the case of 65% bone ingrowth, the stiffness parallel to the interface was 25,094 MPa and that perpendicular to the interface was 1644 MPa. With 50% ingrowth the parallel stiffness was 24,850 MPa, and perpendicular was 996 MPa. If ingrowth is reduced to 15%, the parallel stiffness was reduced by only 1%, while the perpendicular stiffness was reduced by 40%. Based on these results, it appears that the amount of bone tissue ingrowth will dramatically affect load transfer perpendicular to the interface, while it has a much lower effect on load transfer parallel to the interface.[2] Schiller et al. (1993) reported that the mean percentage of bone ingrowth, expressed as mean percent of ingrowth surface volume, into the porous-coated beaded surface of the acetabular component of the PCA Canine Total Hip System (Howmedica, Mahwah, NJ) was 12% at 6 months, 24% at 12 months, and 24% at 24 months. Lauer et al. (2009) reported that the median bone ingrowth, expressed as percent of ingrowth surface area, into the cup perforations of the Zurich Cementless Total Hip (Kyon, Zurich, Switzerland) acetabular component was 50%, 20%, and 44% at 2, 6, and 12 months, respectively.

Center of rotation

The center of rotation of the hip joint is the geometrical center of the femoral head. Careful preoperative planning and intraoperative execution should ensure that, after total hip replacement, the center of rotation is restored to its predisease position. Utilization of modern, highly modular hip prostheses allows selection of appropriate neck length to reestablish femoral offset and soft tissue tension, once the center of rotation has been established.

In the dysplastic patient, it is common for the center of rotation to be displaced dorsally. Restoration of the hip center to the center of the true acetabulum during arthroplasty confers both anatomical and biomechanical advantages (Sariali et al. 2008). The best acetabular bone stock is generally found in the true acetabulum; thus, positioning the acetabular component within the true acetabulum optimizes dorsal coverage and medialization of the component. Returning the center of rotation to the true acetabulum in these cases also increases the lever arm for the abductor muscles, restoring biomechanics (Sariali et al. 2008). "High hip center" and cup lateralization have both been implicated in early failure in people (Stans et al. 1998; Sariali et al. 2008).

Version

The complementary retroversion of the acetabular component and anteversion of the neck of the femoral component should reflect normal patient anatomy, thus restoring range of motion to normal or near-normal levels prior to impingement. Relative, or absolute, anteversion of the cup, for instance, reduces impingement-free range of motion in external rotation, predisposing to craniodorsal luxation. While anteversion of the stem improves range of motion, it reduces femoral offset.

Offset

Cup position, cup size and center of rotation, femoral head size, stem size, neck length, stem version, and stem position within the medullary canal all influence offset, which is defined as the distance between the center of the femoral head and the center of the medullary canal, or anatomical axis of the femur (Figure 6.1). Medialization or lateralization of the acetabular component alters the offset by changing the center of the femoral head. Although offset can be corrected by making a reciprocal adjustment to the neck length, the incorrect center of the hip will remain. Reduced offset results in abductor muscle dysfunction owing to a diminished lever arm. Therefore, the abductor muscles must generate a larger force to balance body weight. The increased force creates a larger joint reaction force and increases wear (Sariali et al. 2008). In addition, reduced offset results in soft tissue laxity that predisposes to luxation. Subluxation during the stance or swing phase also likely results in increased wear by causing microseparation edge loading (Stewart et al. 2001).

Bearing diameter

In order for dislocation to occur, the femoral head has to displace a distance "AB" within the cup (Figure 6.9). This distance, referred to as the *jumping distance*, is the translation of the center of

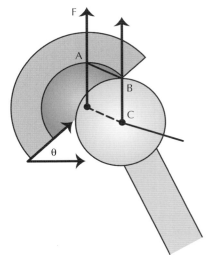

Figure 6.9 The jumping distance is the lateral translation (AB) of the center of the femoral head (C) that must occur before dislocation occurs. F is the joint reaction force and Θ is the angle of lateral opening measured in the transverse plane.

the femoral head that precedes luxation. The jumping distance increases proportionally as the diameter of the femoral head increases, and is inversely related to angle of lateral opening; that is, as the angle of lateral opening increases, jumping distance decreases. Bearing diameter also affects wear rate, since sliding distance increases as diameter increases, as discussed above. Therefore, selection of femoral head diameter must take resistance to luxation and wear into consideration. The jumping distance is also related to the geometry of the cup, and if the design is not a complete hemisphere, the distance is reduced. Considering an acetabular component with a perfect hemispherical shape and a 45-degree angle of lateral opening, distance "AB" is equal to 0.77 times the bearing radius (Figure 6.9). The distance is reduced to 0.43 times the bearing radius if the cup is positioned with a 65-degree angle of lateral opening (Sariali et al. 2008).

Bearing type

Bearings can be broadly divided into hard-on-soft (e.g., metal or ceramic on polyethylene) and hard-on-hard (e.g., ceramic on ceramic, metal on metal, and ceramic on metal). Hard-on-soft bearings operate with boundary lubrication (also known as border lubrication), a condition in which a complete fluid film does not develop between apposing surfaces. Thus, there is momentary dry contact between wear surface high points or asperities; in this case, friction and wear are significant, and wear is proportional to sliding distance; a function of bearing diameter, as illustrated in Figure 6.8. Hard-on-hard bearings operate with mixed lubrication, a mixture of characteristics between boundary, or thin film, and fluid film lubrication, in which there is complete separation of elements by fluid. Mixed lubrication can lead to lower wear; thus hard-on-hard bearings are ideal for use in larger bearings, since these lubrication mechanisms may improve with higher sliding velocities (Fisher et al. 2006).

Femoral head materials

The metallic alloys that have been used with the UHMWPE bearing surfaces are stainless steel,

cobalt-chromium alloy, and titanium alloy. Laboratory and clinical studies in man have shown that wear rates of UHMWPE coupled with either stainless steel or cobalt-chromium are comparable (Manley and Dumbleton 2006). Historically, cobalt-chromium was chosen over the 316L stainless steel available at the time because the cobalt-chromium alloy was more resistant to corrosion. Newer more corrosion-resistant stainless steel alloys are now available, and the use of these newer alloys is increasing. Titanium alloys are more vulnerable to abrasion than cobalt-based alloys; therefore, they are not commonly used as bearings in people. Hardening of the surface of titanium alloy heads using techniques such as gas nitriding, solution nitriding, ion implantation, and diamond-like carbon coating may improve performance, but wear can still occur if the hardened layer is penetrated (Manley and Dumbleton 2006).

In man, cast or forged cobalt-chromium alloy predominates as the choice of femoral head material for articulation against UHMWPE. For this reason, the wear of cobalt-chromium alloy against UHMWPE bearing combination is the standard against which all other bearing combinations are measured (Barrack et al. 2004).

Polyethylene

UHMWPE is manufactured from powder that is converted into solid form by ram extrusion of rods, or compression molding of blocks. The component is then machined from the solid UHMWPE. Sometimes a near net shape component is molded from powder prior to final machining. The final step in the manufacturing process is sterilization, which can be performed by ethylene oxide, gas-plasma, or gamma irradiation in air. Sterilization of UHMWPE by gamma radiation introduces cross-linking of the polyethylene molecules from the interaction of the free radicals formed during irradiation. Laboratory and clinical studies in man have demonstrated improved wear resistance of gamma-sterilized UHMWPE compared with UHMWPE sterilized by nonionizing means (ethylene oxide or gas-plasma) (Manley and Dumbleton 2006). Sterilization by gamma radiation in air creates the potential for oxidation of UHMWPE because of the existence of free radicals that are not cross-linked. Oxidation reduced the mechanical properties of these components. For this reason, some manufacturers have changed the sterilization process to gamma irradiation in an inert atmosphere such as nitrogen, argon, or vacuum; the lack of oxygen in these environments prevents initiation of the oxidative process (Manley and Dumbleton 2006).

Since cross-linking was shown to reduce UHMWPE wear, it was theorized that increasing cross-linking further would result in an even more wear-resistant UHMWPE. *Highly cross-linked* UHMWPE can be produced by using higher doses of radiation followed by or combined with heat to enhance the cross-linking process and the removal of free radicals. Among the many variables that can be manipulated in the production of highly cross-linked UHMWPE, the key variables are radiation dose and the temperature of heating (Manley and Dumbleton 2006). Manufacturers of UHMWPE components for people have introduced different highly cross-linked polyethylenes by different choices in the radiation dose and heating temperature. These efforts have been largely successful, and studies on highly cross-linked UHMWPE liners have consistently showed lower femoral head penetration and an 87% lower risk of osteolysis (Kurtz et al. 2011). However, cases of *in vivo* oxidation at the rim and rim delamination in annealed polyethylene, and rim fracture in remelted polyethylene have provided motivation for ongoing research on the long-term stability and mechanical performance of this first generation of highly cross-linked UHMWPE (Kurtz et al. 2011).

Design considerations of cemented femoral components

The durability of a cemented femoral stem is highly dependent on both the quality of the cementing technique and the design of the implant. Two separate design philosophies have emerged from the last four decades of total hip arthroplasty experience: the tapered slip and the composite beam models of femoral design.

The taper slip design is thought to take advantage of the viscoelastic behavior of cement (creep). Under loading conditions, the cement deforms, resulting in slight subsidence of the stem. The axial migration of the stem results in tighter wedging of the loaded, tapered stem within the cement mantle, creating compressive stresses within the cement and reduced shear at the cement–bone interface (Savory et al. 2006).

According to the composite beam model, the mechanical bond between the cement–implant interface can be strengthened by features on the stem surface. These features include roughened stem surfaces or precoating the stem with PMMA. Collars on the stem are thought to strengthen the cement-stem bond by pressurizing the cement, reducing subsidence, and transferring load to the proximal portion of the femur (Savory et al. 2006).

Implant material, cross-sectional geometry, and length of cemented stems affect cement stresses (Schulz 2000). Stiff materials, such as cobalt-chromium alloys and stainless steel, create less cement stresses. In addition, since these materials are harder, they are more resistant to abrasion than softer, less stiff materials. Sharp corners concentrate stresses, thus they should be avoided. Broad medial borders reduce proximal cement strain, and broad lateral borders increase component strength (Estok et al. 1997). In a canine cemented total hip replacement model, shorter implants had higher cement strains medial and lateral to the stem tip; however, changes in neck length did not significantly affect cement strain (Dassler et al. 2003). In canine total hip replacement, implant positioning, including fit and geometry of reconstruction, has been shown to vary depending on the implant design and manufacturer (Schulz et al. 2000). Longer femoral stems result in decreased compressive stresses in the cement; however, long straight implants have been shown to be difficult to accurately position in the curved canine femur (Schulz et al. 1998, 1999). Increasing the cross-sectional area of the stem also reduces compressive stresses in the cement, and increases the ratio of compressive to tensile forces, which is preferable, since PMMA is more resistant to compressive loads than tensile loads.

Design considerations of cementless acetabular components

Cementless acetabular components were introduced in the early 1980s in an attempt to improve the long-term results of acetabular fixation. Although cemented acetabular components provided reliable early results in people, long-term studies noted increased rates of radiographic and clinical loosening. In addition, an increased understanding of the factors affecting the quality of cement technique revealed the demanding nature of implanting a cemented all-polyethylene cup. Specifically, difficulties were noted in routinely obtaining a bloodless surgical field and providing for optimal cement pressurization.

A variety of strategies for obtaining initial stability were explored including dome screws, peripheral screws, peripheral threads, dome spikes, peripheral fins, and insertion with a press-fit technique in which the component is oversized relative to the diameter of the acetabular preparation (Savory et al. 2006). These cementless components rapidly became the most popular type of acetabular implant in both human and veterinary total hip replacement surgery because the surgical technique is more versatile and reproducible than acetabular fixation with cement.

The geometry of cementless acetabular components varies widely, from hemispheric, oblong, or threaded designs to dual geometry designs. Most threaded acetabular components do not have a biological surface for bone ingrowth or ongrowth and rely on a mechanical interlock with the acetabular bone bed. These components have been shown to have poorer mechanical stability than hemispherical components and a smaller amount of surface area in contact with the acetabular bone bed. Few of the threaded designs have demonstrated acceptable survivorship in humans (Savory et al. 2006). Threaded implants with biological surfaces for bony ingrowth have been associated with acceptable results; however, the preparation of the acetabular bed and the reproducible insertion of these components is generally more challenging than those with a press-fit hemispherical design (Savory et al. 2006).

Some dual geometry designs are characterized by a larger radius of the component at the periphery than at the dome, while others feature a cylindrical locking zone at the face of the hemispherical cup. The dual geometry design is intended to maximize the contact of the biological surface at the rim of the acetabulum with the use of a press-fit technique. These designs were developed for use in people in response to concerns over the use of screws for fixation and in an attempt to maximize initial component stability without the use of adjunctive forms of fixation (Savory et al. 2006). Although the intermediate results with components of this design in people have been acceptable, there is a concern that this design may decrease total contact between the dome of the component acetabular bone bed, resulting in a decreased amount of bone ingrowth compared with components with a simple hemispherical design.

Threaded screws have been shown to be the strongest method to provide or augment the initial stability of cementless acetabular components. Screw holes can be placed in the dome of the component, or at the periphery; however, since placement of peripheral screws often requires a wider exposure, most modern primary acetabular components for people utilize dome screws. Concerns with the use of screws include the potential for neurovascular injury during drilling or screw insertion, concerns that screw holes may act as access channels for polyethylene wear debris to access the implant–bone interface, the potential for fretting corrosion and material loss between the screw head and the metal shell, and direct contact and subsequent abrasive wear of the screw head against the femoral head as the polyethylene liner thins (Savory et al. 2006; Figure 6.10).

Design considerations of cementless femoral components

Cementless femoral components were first introduced in the 1970s in an attempt to improve the long-term survivorship experienced with cemented femoral stems. A variety of design and material factors should be considered when evaluating the performance of a femoral component since these factors may influence the initial and long-term stability, durability, and ease of implantation. These factors include stem material, stem shape, extent and type of surface coating, and the modularity of the system.

Cobalt-chromium and titanium are the two most common materials used to produce femoral components, and comparable long-term results have been obtained using both. Implants made of

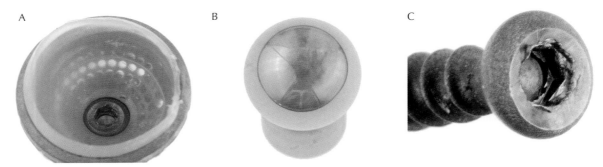

Figure 6.10   Abrasive wear of the dome screw of an acetabular component. Note the extensive polyethylene wear (thinning) (A) that occurred prior to contact of the femoral head (note gray discolored area) (B) and the screw head (note concavity in screw head due to wear) (C).

titanium have a lower modulus of elasticity that more closely approximates that of cortical bone. This provides the theoretical advantages of more predictable and physiological patterns of bone modeling, remodeling, and less stress shielding, which should yield better long-term stability. Bone density studies using dual-energy X-ray absorptiometry in people have corroborated this, demonstrating less overall stress shielding and better maintenance of proximal bone density with stems made of titanium with proximal ingrowth compared with stems made of cobalt-chromium, or those with distal ingrowth (Gibbons et al. 2001). Despite these theoretical benefits and the observed differences in bone density, superiority of one stem design over another has not been demonstrated in long-term clinical studies with revision for stem loosening as the outcome measure (Khanuja et al. 2011).

Femoral components have been designed with a variety of shapes including tapered, cylindrical, and anatomical, depending on the intended method of fixation. In addition, varying degrees of craniocaudal and mediolateral taper can be designed into these stems.

Tapered stems, those with a pronounced proximal to distal taper, are designed to interlock into the metaphyseal region with little or no diaphyseal fixation. These stems are usually a collarless design to allow wedging of the prosthesis into the metaphyseal region. The proximal fixation surface is typically a porous coating, plasma spray macrotexturing, or fiber mesh pads, designed to create adequate initial stability to achieve bony ingrowth.

The tapered geometry of the stem takes advantage of the viscoelastic nature of bone, allowing the stem to subside to a position of tightest fit, enhancing proximal load sharing of the device.

Cylindrical stems usually have a circumferential porous coating over most or all of the surface area of the stem. Both proximal and distal coating of these stems is intended to maximize the region of potential bone ingrowth and enhance the long-term stability of the implant. Initial stability can be achieved by obtaining a tight diaphyseal fit by machining the tubular femoral diaphysis in people, or by utilizing screw fixation in dogs. Monocortical, locking screw fixation to the medial cortex theoretically allows independent motion of the medial (compression) and lateral (tension) surfaces of the proximal femur. This motion may be mitigated as bony ongrowth or ingrowth occurs.

Anatomical stems, designed to fit the anatomy of the proximal femur, have been associated with significant rates of thigh pain and osteolysis in people (Knight et al. 1998). Factors that appear crucial to their long-term success and to avoid thigh pain are adequate fill of the metaphyseal region in both the coronal and sagittal planes. A prospective analysis of 50 consecutive cases using a similar stem design in dogs revealed long-term stability and excellent clinical function (Marcellin-Little et al. 1999).

Modularity of the head and neck is common to most implant designs, and allows customization of the implants to individual patients. Intraoperative flexibility allows more accurate adjustment of the prosthetic articulation that may reduce the risk of postoperative luxation (Schulz 2000). The greatest concern for modularity is corrosion at the junction between the modular parts, particularly between dissimilar metals such as cobalt-chromium head and a titanium trunion. The generation and release of particulate debris can lead to local tissue hypersensitivity and cause third-body wear at the bearing surface. Wear products from corrosion at the head-neck junction have been identified in periprosthetic tissue from human patients in as little as 8 months following surgery (Urban et al. 1994).

An understanding of hip biomechanics including the range of motion and kinematics of normal gait, the static and dynamic loads applied to the articulation, the transmission of mechanical stress within and across the joint, and the mechanical interplay of various tissues and structures that cross the joint are fundamental to treating a wide range of disorders with total hip replacement. Characteristics of implant materials and implant design play a large role in the function and longevity of a total hip replacement. Precise manipulation of these factors can optimize implant design, long-term patient outcome, and function.

Endnotes

1. Wood I. Particulate debris and implant failure in cemented canine total hip replacements. MS thesis, The Ohio State University, Columbus, OH, 2004.
2. Ko CC. Mechanical characteristics of implant/tissue interphases. PhD dissertation, The University of Michigan, Ann Arbor, MI, 1994.

References

Barrack RL, Burak C, Skinner HB. Concerns about ceramics in THA. Clin Orthop Relat Res 2004;429:73–79.

Bartel DL, Burstein AH, Toda MD et al. The effect of conformity and plastic thickness on contact stresses in metal-backed plastic implants. J Biomech Eng 1985;107:193–199.

Bartel DL, Bicknell VL, Wright TM. The effect of conformity, thickness and material on stresses in ultra-high molecular weight components for total joint replacement. J Bone Joint Surg Am 1986;68:1041–1051.

Bergh MS, Muir P, Markel MD et al. Femoral bone adaptation to stable long-term cemented total hip arthroplasty in dogs. Vet Surg 2004a;33:214–220.

Bergh MS, Muir P, Markel MD et al. Femoral bone adaptation to unstable long-term cemented total hip arthroplasty in dogs. Vet Surg 2004b;33:238–245.

Breusch SJ, Norman TL, Schneider U et al. Lavage technique in total hip arthroplasty: Jet lavage produces better cement penetration than syringe lavage in the proximal femur. J Arthroplasty 2000;15:921–927.

Cross AR, Newell SM, Chambers JN, et al. Acetabular component orientation as an indicator of implant luxation in cemented total hip arthroplasty. Vet Surg 2000;29:517–523.

Dassler CL, Schulz KS, Kass P et al. The effects of femoral stem and neck length on cement strains in a canine total hip replacement model. Vet Surg 2003;32:37–45.

Davies JP, O'Connor DO, Burke DW et al. The effect of centrifugation on the fatigue life of bone cement in the presence of surface irregularities. Clin Orthop Relat Res 1988;229:156–161.

Davies JP, Jasty M, O'Connor DO et al. The effect of centrifuging bone cement. J Bone Joint Surg Br 1989;71:39–42.

Dyce J, Wisner ER, Schrader SC et al. Radiographic evaluation of acetabular component position in dogs. Vet Surg 2001;30:28–39.

Estok DM, Orr TE, Harris WH. Factors affecting cement strains near the tip of a cemented femoral component. J Arthroplasty 1997;12:40–48.

Evans HE. The skeleton, arthrology, the muscular system. In: Miller's Anatomy of the Dog, Evans HE (ed.), 3rd ed. Philadelphia: WB Saunders, 1993, p. 245.

Fisher J, Zin J, Tipper J et al. Tribology of alternative bearings. Clin Orthop Relat Res 2006;453:25–34.

Gibbons CE, Davies AJ, Amis AA et al. Periprosthetic bone mineral density changes with femoral components of differing design philosophy. Int Orthop 2001;25:89–92.

Harrysson OLA, Cansizoglu O, Marcellin-Little DJ et al. Direct metal fabrication of titanium implant components with tailored materials and mechanical properties using electron beam melting technology. Mat Sci Eng C 2008;28:366–373.

Hollister SJ. Mechanical factors influencing the outcome of total joint replacement. Curr Orthop 1995;9:2–8.

Jaegger G, Marcellin-Little DJ, Levine D. Reliability of goniometry in Labrador retrievers. Am J Vet Res 2002;63:979–986.

Jasty M, Goetz DD, Bragdon CR et al. Wear of polyethylene acetabular components in total hip arthroplasty: An analysis of one hundred and twenty-eight components retrieved at autopsy or revision operations. J Bone Joint Surg Am 1997;79:349–358.

Jin ZM, Stone M, Ingham E et al. Biotribology. Curr Orthop 2006;20:32–40.

Khanuja HS, Vakil JJ, Goddard MS et al. Cementless femoral fixation in total hip arthroplasty. J Bone Joint Surg Am 2011;93:500–509.

Knight JL, Atwater RD, Guo J. Clinical results of the midstem porous-coated anatomic uncemented femoral stem in primary total hip arthroplasty: A five to nine-year prospective study. J Arthroplasty 1998;13:535–545.

Kurtz SM, Gawel HA, Patel JD. History and systematic review of wear and osteolysis outcomes for first-generation highly crosslinked polyethylene. Clin Orthop Relat Res 2011;469:2262–2277.

Lauer SK, Nieves MA, Peck J et al. Descriptive histomorphometric ingrowth analysis of the Zurich cementless canine total hip acetabular component. Vet Surg 2009;38:59–69.

MacDonald W, Swarts E, Beaver R. Penetration and shear strength of cement-bone interfaces *in vivo*. Clin Orthop Relat Res 1993;286:283–288.

Manley MT, Dumbleton J. Bearing surfaces. In: *Orthopaedic Knowledge Update. Hip and Knee Reconstruction*, Barrack RL, Booth RE, Lonner JH et al (eds.), 3rd ed. Rosemont, IL: American Academy of Orthopaedic Surgeons, 2006.

Marcellin-Little DJ, DeYoung BA, Doyens DH et al. Canine uncemented porous-coated anatomic total hip arthroplasty: Results of a long-term prospective evaluation of 50 consecutive cases. Vet Surg 1999;28:10–20.

Marcellin-Little DJ, Cansizoglu O, Harrysson OLA et al. *In vitro* testing of a low modulus mesh canine prosthetic hip stem. Am J Vet Res 2010;71:1089–1095.

Nercessian OA, Martin G, Joshi RP et al. A 15- to 25-year follow-up study of primary Charnley low-friction arthroplasty: A single surgeon series. J Arthroplasty 2005;20:162–167.

Nevelos J, Patel A. *Hip Biomechanics and the Implications of Total Hip Replacement*, 1st ed. Mahwah, NJ: HSC Press, 2009.

Richards J, Holler R, Bockstahler B et al. A comparison of human and canine kinematics during level walking, stair ascent, and stair descent. Vet Med Austria 2010;97:92–100.

Santavirta S, Xu JW, Hietanen J et al. Activation of periprosthetic connective tissue in aseptic loosening of total hip implants. Clin Orthop Relat Res 1998;352:16–24.

Sariali E, Veysi V, Stewart T. Biomechanics of the human hip—Consequences for total hip replacement. Curr Orthop 2008;22:371–375.

Savory CG, Hamilton WG, Engh CA et al. Hip designs. In: *Orthopaedic Knowledge Update. Hip and Knee Reconstruction*, Barrack RL, Booth RE, Lonner JH et al (eds.), 3rd ed. Rosemont, IL: American Academy of Orthopaedic Surgeons, 2006.

Schiller TD, DeYoung DJ, Schiller RA et al. Quantitative ingrowth analysis of a porous-coated acetabular component in a canine model. Vet Surg 1993;22:276–280.

Schulz KS. Application of arthroplasty principles to canine cemented total hip replacement. Vet Surg 2000;29:578–593.

Schulz KS, Vasseur P, Stover SM et al. Transverse plane evaluation of the effects of surgical technique on stem positioning and geometry of reconstruction in canine total hip replacement. Am J Vet Res 1998;59:1071–1079.

Schulz KS, Vasseur P, Stover SM et al. Effect of surgical technique and use of a rigid centralizing device on stem positioning and geometric reconstruction in the sagittal plane during total hip replacement in canine cadavers. Am J Vet Res 1999;60:1126–1135.

Schulz KS, Nielsen C, Stover SM et al. Comparison of the fit and geometry of reconstruction of femoral components of four cemented canine total hip replacement implants. Am J Vet Res 2000;61:1113–1121.

Skurla CT, James SP. A comparison of canine and human UHMWPE acetabular component wear. Biomed Sci Instrum 2001;37:245–250.

Skurla CP, James SP. Assessing the dog as a model for human total hip replacement: Analysis of 38 postmortem retrieved canine cemented acetabular components. J Biomed Mater Res B Appl Biomater 2005;73:260–270.

Skurla CP, Pluhar GE, Frankel DJ et al. Assessing the dog as a model for human total hip replacement. Analysis of 38 canine cemented femoral components retrieved at post-mortem. J Bone Joint Surg Br 2005;87:120–127.

Stans AA, Pagnano MW, Shaughnessy WJ et al. Results of total hip arthroplasty for Crowe Type III developmental hip dysplasia. Clin Orthop Relat Res 1998;348:149–157.

Stewart T, Tipper J, Streicher R et al. Long-term wear of HIPed alumina on alumina bearings for THR under microseparation conditions. J Mater Sci Mater Med 2001;12:1053–1056.

Stewart TD. Tribology of artificial joints. Orthop Trauma 2010;24:435–440.

Urban RM, Jacobs JJ, Gilbert JL et al. Migration of corrosion products from modular hip prostheses. Particle microanalysis and histopathological findings. J Bone Joint Surg Am 1994;76:1345–1359.

7 Clinical Application of Total Hip Replacement

Jeffrey N. Peck, William D. Liska, David J. DeYoung, and Denis J. Marcellin-Little

Introduction and background

Documentation of joint pathology dates to prehistoric times. For millennia, little could be done to treat joint pain or dysfunction. Remedies were likely discovered on a trial and error basis and relied in part on rest and placebo effect. Nonsteroidal anti-inflammatory drugs were discovered and modified over time to increase their safety and efficacy. These drugs have made a great contribution to the quality of life of humans and animals.

Prearthroplasty era surgical attempts to alleviate pain included amputation, joint debridement (Magnuson 1946), corrective osteotomies, excision arthroplasty, denervation, and arthrodesis. The flourishing era of joint replacement was ushered in by John Charnley's pioneering development of a human total hip replacement (THR) in the 1960s using metal, plastic, and bone cement (Charnley 1960, 1970).

The first report of THR in dogs was published in 1957 (Gorman 1957). Widespread clinical interest in canine THR grew from the need to treat dogs with hip pain and the success of THR in humans. The initial clinical reports were published by Olmstead in the 1980s using a cemented fixed-head femoral component and an all-polyethylene acetabular cup prosthesis (Olmstead et al. 1983; Olmstead 1987), and later using the modular prosthesis in 1995 (Olmstead 1995a).

Ingrowth cementless THR was developed in the early 1980s to address the issue of component loosening that was identified in cemented implants. Several cementless THR systems were developed and used in experimental studies or in short case series (Chen et al. 1983; Paul et al. 1992). The stems were made of titanium alloy, and fiber metal was present on surfaces intended for bone ingrowth. The canine porous-coated anatomical hip (Canine PCA, Howmedica, Mahway, NJ) was developed by DeYoung and was used for a nonrandomized long-term prospective clinical trial that lasted approximately 10 years at North Carolina State University (NCSU; DeYoung et al. 1992; Marcellin-Little et al. 1999a). The system was also used at several other colleges of veterinary medicine (Montgomery et al. 1992). Through a series of clinical studies, information on radiographic criteria for evaluation, short- and long-term radiographic assessment, bone ingrowth

Advances in Small Animal Total Joint Replacement, First Edition. Edited by Jeffrey N. Peck and Denis J. Marcellin-Little.
© 2013 John Wiley & Sons, Inc. Published 2013 by John Wiley & Sons, Inc.

assessment, and long-term clinical assessment, the NCSU clinical program formed the scientific foundation of our current clinical knowledge in ingrowth cementless THR (DeYoung and Schiller 1992; DeYoung et al. 1992, 1993; Schiller et al. 1993; Marcellin-Little et al. 1999a).

The BioMedtrix press-fit cementless Biological Fixation (BFX) system (BioMedtrix LLC, Boonton, NJ) was designed in the early 2000s. The system addressed many of the shortcomings of the Canine PCA system, including its lack of commercial availability; the relative lack of modularity with regard to stem size, cup size, and prosthetic neck length; the risk of luxation because of a relatively small (15-mm diameter) prosthetic head; and the need to stock left and right anatomical stems. The BFX system became commercially available in 2003. In 2007, the BFX and the Modular Total Hip systems were combined into the Universal Total Hip system with a common instrument set and surgical technique.

The Zurich Cementless Total Hip system (Kyon, Zurich, Switzerland) with screw fixation was developed in the late 1990s. Guerrero reported its clinical outcome in 2009 (Guerrero and Montavon 2009). Stability of this prosthesis is provided by bone ingrowth into the cup and locking-screw fixation of the femoral stem to the medial femoral cortex. The histomorphometric analysis of bone ingrowth into the acetabular component was reported in 2009 (Lauer et al. 2009). Other concepts in canine THR have been explored. A screw-in femoral implant that replaces the femoral head is in the early phase of commercialization and clinical assessment (Hach and Delfs 2009; Kim et al. 2012).

The size range of hip prostheses was initially limited so only large- (>20 kg) and giant-breed dogs were candidates for THR. More recently, smaller prostheses have become available. A miniature prosthesis for use in dogs less than 25 kg was reported by Warnock in 2003 (Warnock et al. 2003) and Matis in 2008.[1] In 2010, Liska reported on the use of an even smaller cemented prosthesis used in cats and small dogs with a mean weight of 7.2 kg (Liska 2010).

In 1996, Budsberg documented significant improvement of loading function following hip replacement in dogs using gait analysis (Budsberg et al. 1996). Radiographic assessment standards of

the uncemented prosthesis were established by DeYoung in 1992 (DeYoung and Schiller 1992; DeYoung et al. 1993) and Marcellin-Little in 1999 (Marcellin-Little et al. 1999a). These radiographic studies described the radiographic changes following cementless THR in the dog and standardized the nomenclature. The studies detailed the short- and the long-term clinical and radiographic results, and set the standards for other surgeons to aspire to achieve.

The increased interest in canine and feline hip replacement encourages continued biomaterials research. Function and long-term survivorship of implants can be increased through improved materials, implant design, and methods of fixation.

Equally important, surgeons must be trained to maximize results and to minimize risks and complications (Hayes et al. 2011b). It is paramount that surgeons be able to recognize potential risks and be capable of and willing to manage complications when they arise. The profession must demand unbiased prospective research reporting patient outcomes and implant survivorship as the primary agent of change in arthroplasty.

Tremendous advancements in canine and feline THR have been made in the past 30 years. Joint replacement in animals will no doubt continue to evolve and expand as clients expect the elimination of hip pain and the return to normal function for their pets. However, it is important to bear in mind that total joint arthroplasty is a salvage procedure resulting from the failure to adequately treat or eliminate the underlying disease condition. Genetic engineering and cell biology offer the promise for future medical treatment options for osteoarthritis (OA). However, until such time, research and development must continue to improve total joint arthroplasty.

Indications and contraindications

THR in dogs is most often performed to alleviate the pain resulting from OA secondary to hip dysplasia (Figure 7.1; Olmstead et al. 1983; Marcellin-Little et al. 1999a; Guerrero and Montavon 2009). However, any cause of nonseptic OA may be an indication, whether its cause is traumatic, developmental, acquired, or idiopathic. In one report,

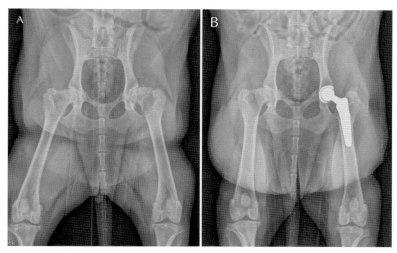

Figure 7.1   Ventrodorsal radiographs of a 7-year-old Labrador retriever. The dog had severe bilateral hip dysplasia (A) and a total hip replacement was performed. Fifteen months later, the prosthesis is stable (B) and the dog is free of clinical signs.

12 large-breed dogs with traumatic hip luxation were treated successfully with cemented THR (Pozzi et al. 2004).

Not all animals presenting with hip pain have sufficient indications that justify imminent THR. Animals with coxofemoral OA, with or without clinical signs or previous attempts to alleviate pain nonsurgically, are potential THR candidates. In some scenarios, surgery can be delayed until pain management is only partially effective and/or clinical signs worsen. Additionally, if pain management combined with attaining an ideal body condition score of 4 or 5 out of 9 (Mawby et al. 2004) plus exercise resolves symptoms, surgery can be delayed (Marcellin-Little 2008). Conversely, in the presence of uncomplicated unrelenting hip pain, a THR recommendation should be made to improve the quality of life of the pet.

THR is becoming more common in cats and small-breed dogs (Figure 7.2). Just as in large-breed dogs, OA secondary to hip dysplasia is the predominant indication for THR in cats and small dogs. Other problems, including coxofemoral luxation, avascular necrosis, or physeal fractures, are common indications for THR in small dogs and cats. In one report, hip luxation, avascular necrosis, and capital physeal fractures were the respective indications for 15 (23%), 17 (26%), and 11 (17%) of 66 small-breed THRs (Liska 2010). Other

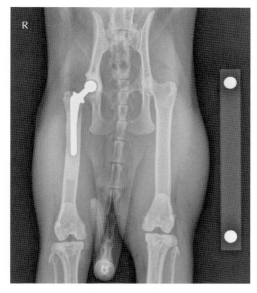

Figure 7.2   Ventrodorsal radiograph of the pelvis of a 4-year-old cat made 26 months after THR. The THR was done to revise a femoral head ostectomy that had led to disuse of the limb. The femoral head ostectomy was performed to manage a nonunion of the capital femoral physis. The implants are stable and no radiolucent lines at the bone–cement interface are visible in the acetabulum or femur.

recent case series have also reported the use of THR for the treatment of capital femoral physeal fractures and for avascular necrosis of the femoral head (Jankovits et al. 2012; Kalis et al. 2012). THR has also been performed to manage unsuccessful femoral head ostectomy (Liska et al. 2010; Fitzpatrick et al. 2012).

Patient age is an important consideration both physiologically and from the perspective of the stage of hip dysplasia. Surgery should be delayed in immature animals until the acetabular growth plates are closed, while surgery prior to closure of the capital physeal plate is inconsequential. Surgery may be performed if the physeal plate at the base of the greater trochanter is only partially closed. However, this growth plate could separate during surgery and require reduction and stabilization. The status of the distal femoral physeal plate is also inconsequential since it is not disrupted during preparation of the femoral canal.

The stage of hip dysplasia seen in dogs presenting between 5 and 12 months of age is important in the timing of surgery. A favorable window of opportunity may exist in young dogs with severe coxofemoral subluxation or developmental luxation (Figure 7.3). For these patients, it is generally advantageous to recommend surgery early rather than waiting until the animal and the disease are mature. Chronic hip dysplasia may result in severe morphological changes, making surgery more technically challenging. The adverse changes include luxation, acetabular hypoplasia, dorsal acetabular rim wear, lateral drift of the proximal-medial femoral cortex, medialization of the greater trochanter, sclerosis of the proximal aspect of the femoral medullary canal, narrowing of the femoral isthmus, lateralization of the proximal aspect of the femur, and muscle atrophy including contracture of the hip musculature muscles resulting from hip luxation (Figure 7.4). The muscle atrophy and contracture make rearticulation of the prosthetic joint more difficult and increase the risk of luxation after surgery (Hayes et al. 2011a).

Concurrent orthopedic and neurological disease is often present in patients presenting for THR surgery. These conditions may exacerbate the clinical signs of hip dysplasia or may lead one to incorrectly attribute the severity of the clinical signs to the hip joint. Degenerative myelopathy and lumbosacral disease may produce symptoms similar to severe bilateral hip dysplasia.

A thorough physical examination including neurological evaluation must be undertaken to rule out or to identify concurrent disease conditions during the planning process. Concurrent neurological or orthopedic disease must be carefully assessed and may necessitate postponement of THR until these conditions are resolved or evaluated in light of the patient's overall condition or function.

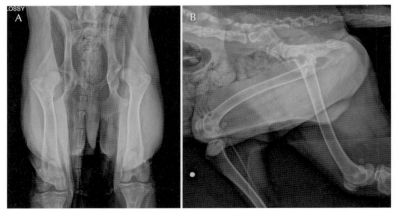

Figure 7.3   Ventrodorsal (A) and lateral (B) radiographs of the pelvis of a 9-month-old golden retriever with severe developmental hip subluxation. Valgus angulation of the femoral shaft is present. The left acetabulum is poorly developed and the left femoral head is cranially and dorsally displaced, compared with the right femoral head. This type of hip joint presents challenges during total hip replacement because of the shallow acetabulum, abnormal femoral shape, and tissue tension after reduction of the prosthetic components.

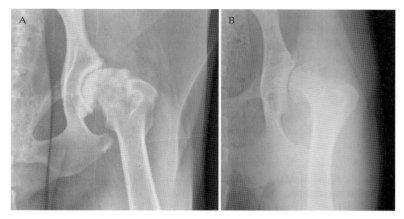

Figure 7.4 Ventrodorsal radiographs of the hip joint of an older Labrador retriever (A) and German shepherd (B). The dogs were referred for total hip replacement because of clinical signs resulting from severe osteoarthritis of the hips. Osteophytes or enthesophytes surround the femoral neck. The acetabula are shallow due to filling with new bone. Subchondral sclerosis of the acetabulum is evident. The German shepherd's acetabulum is nearly flat, resembling a saucer.

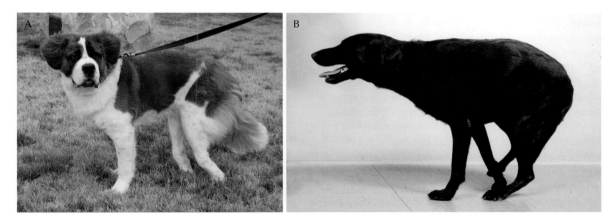

Figure 7.5 (A) An 11-month-old Saint Bernard is shifting weight forward because of severe hip pain resulting from hip subluxation. Bilateral talocrural joint hyperextension is present and is most likely the consequence of his weight shift and reluctance to extend his hip joints. The dog was managed with a THR. (B) A 3-year-old Labrador retriever is shifting most of his weight to his forelimbs because of partial tears to his cranial cruciate ligaments. Weight shifts from cranial cruciate ligament disease and hip dysplasia may resemble each other.

Ipsilateral or contralateral orthopedic pathology, such as medial patella luxation (MPL) or cranial cruciate ligament (CrCL) injury, are frequently present concurrent with hip pathology (Figure 7.5). Hip dysplasia and MPL appear to be significantly correlated in cats (Smith et al. 1999). When concurrent hip and knee problems are suspected, it must be determined whether symptoms (lameness and/or pain) originate at the hip, the knee, or both. If both joints are responsible for clinical signs, the hip and knee procedures are in most cases staged, with the knee problem usually given a higher priority.

Serious and often life-threatening medical conditions must also be considered. Patients with concurrent systemic disease must be treated with caution. Examples include uncontrollable bacterial dermatitis, neoplasia, coagulopathy, and compensated heart, liver, or renal failure. Likewise, the systemic effects of immunosuppression, diabetes mellitus, Cushing's disease, and generalized immune-mediated polyarthropathy may pose a significant risk to the THR patient. Thoughtful preoperative assessment and owner counseling is recommended if THR surgery is contemplated, even after successful treatment of these or similar diseases. Consideration should be given to testing for von Willebrand factor deficiency in predisposed breeds.

Septic arthritis is an absolute contraindication for THR. The presence of ipsilateral hindquarter or generalized dermatitis, otitis externa, urinary tract infection, and periodontal disease should be resolved prior to surgery.

Even though neoplasia with or without metastatic disease may be a relative contraindication, neoplasia localized to the hip region may not be. It is feasible to implant a custom-made prosthesis in selected cases (see Chapter 14). The prosthesis fixation is typically cemented and shielded if immediate postoperative radiation therapy is anticipated. Osseointegration fixation of porous-coated implants is adversely affected by radiation at 2 weeks, but not at 4 or 8 weeks. The porous-coated area of the prosthesis should also be shielded from radiation until ingrowth has ceased (Sumner et al. 1990).

When financial constraints preempt THR surgery, a femoral head and neck ostectomy (FHO) may be an option in selected cases. An FHO carries the risk of not achieving acceptable pain relief and restoration of function in all breed sizes (Off and Matis 2010). An FHO disrupts the normal hip biomechanics, results in limb leg length discrepancy and unpredictable pain relief, and may require prolonged rehabilitation (Liska et al. 2009). In some cases, it is possible to revise a painful FHO to a THR, but an FHO should never be advised as an interim procedure.

Preoperative planning

Preoperative planning starts with critical assessment of the anatomical and pathological changes in the hip joint. Failure to recognize all changes will increase the risk of complications. Regardless of the THR system, the approximate size of the acetabular cup and femoral stem are determined preoperatively using acetate template overlays on radiograph film or digital templates for digital radiographs. Accurate magnification-calibrated radiographic images of the acetabulum and of the femur are essential for correct implant size selection.

The ventral-dorsal radiographic view of the pelvis is positioned primarily for assessment of the pelvis and acetabulum, including acetabular cup size and dorsal rim wear (Figure 7.6). When making the radiograph, preference is given to provide square alignment of the pelvis rather than the accurate positioning of the femurs. The lateral radiographic view of the pelvis is made with the hemipelves superimposed (Figure 7.7). An accurate representation of the femur is best obtained from a cranial-caudal radiographic view of the affected femur (Figure 7.8). The dog is positioned in lateral recumbency with the affected limb up with the radiographic cassette placed caudal and parallel to the femur. The X-ray beam is directed horizontally from cranial to caudal. This view provides an accurate and reproducible representation of the femur. An open-leg lateral radiographic view of the femur is obtained with the dog positioned in lateral recumbency with the affected limb down (Figure 7.9). The contralateral limb is abducted and flexed to expose the groin area and proximal aspect of the femur being examined. This positioning provides an oblique view of the acetabulum and a view of the proximal aspect of the femur without superimposition of the opposite femur. The implant–bone and cement–bone interfaces can be clearly assessed using these positions. The same radiographic protocol is followed for postoperative and serial radiographic follow-up.

Once the radiographic magnification is determined, the appropriate templates are superimposed over the radiograph of the femur in the cranial-caudal and lateral views to determine the likely femoral implant size (Figure 7.10). Fit and fill of the stem in the canal at the appropriate level are the key indicators for selection of stem size. When determining the implant size for a cementless press-fit stem, the surgeon should plan to place the largest implant that fills the confines of the endosteal margins of the metaphysis and diaphysis. In narrow, "champagne fluted" femurs, the diaphysis, rather than the metaphysis, may be the size-limiting point.

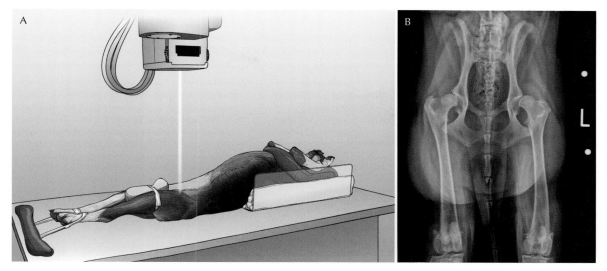

Figure 7.6   (A) The preoperative assessment of patients evaluated for THR includes a ventrodorsal (VD) radiograph made with the patient in dorsal recumbency with the pelvic limbs extended. (B) The size of the VD radiograph is calibrated using a magnification marker. The acetabular size and shape, degree of hip subluxation, and femoral size and shape are assessed.

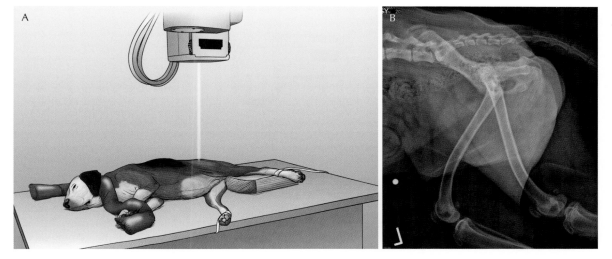

Figure 7.7   (A) The lateral radiograph is made with the dog in lateral recumbency. (B) The shape of the pelvis and amount of dorsal displacement of the femur in relation to the pelvis is assessed radiographically using this position.

When determining the size for a screw fixation stem, the same radiographic views are used. Femoral stem size is initially evaluated on the cranial-caudal view of the femur (Figure 7.11). The proximal-medial aspect of the "shoulder" of the template is placed against the endosteal medial cortex of the femur, just proximal to the lesser trochanter. The medial aspect of the template is aligned against the endosteal surface of the medial cortex. Adequate space within the medullary canal should be present. Space medial to the greater trochanter should be present. On the medial-lateral

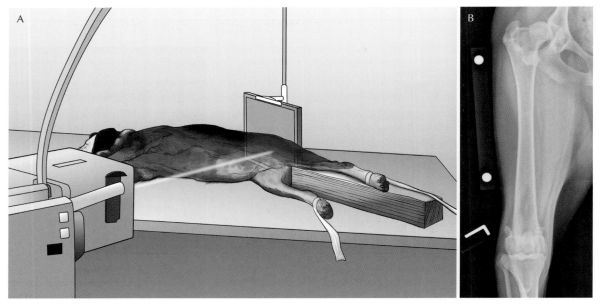

Figure 7.8 (A) The cranial-caudal horizontal beam radiograph is made with the patient in lateral recumbency with the leg of interest up and extended. (B) This view provides the most accurate craniocaudal projection of the femur.

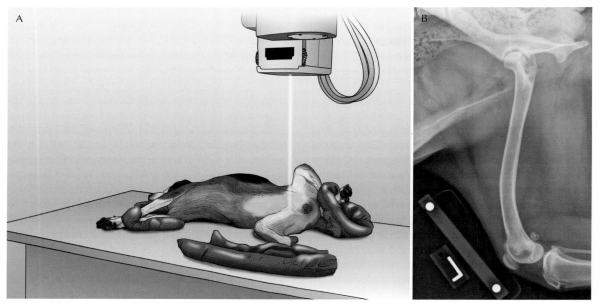

Figure 7.9 (A) The open-leg lateral radiograph is made with the dog in lateral recumbency with the leg of interest down and held in a neutral position. (B) This view provides the most accurate lateral projection of the femur. The size of the acetabulum can be assessed on this view.

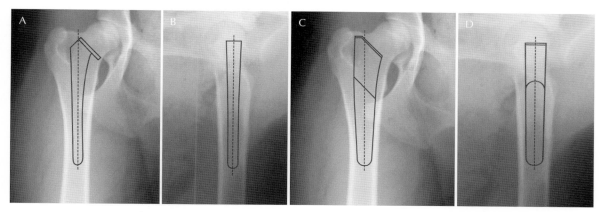

Figure 7.10 The size of the CFX femoral component is determined by superimposing the templates over the craniocaudal (A) and the lateral (B) radiographic views. The largest CFX stem is selected that allows space for an adequate cement mantle in the medullary canal of the femoral diaphysis. A BFX stem is selected that fills the confines of the endosteal space of the metaphysis and diaphysis on both the craniocaudal (C) and lateral (D) radiographic views.

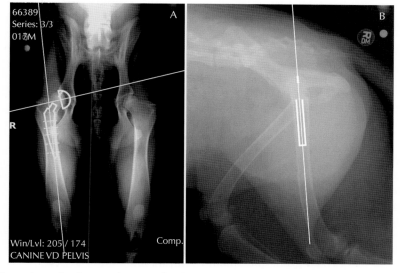

Figure 7.11 Digital templating for the Zurich Cementless hip using the Orthoview software (Orthoview LLC, Southampton, UK). On the ventrodorsal hip-extended view (A), the appropriately sized acetabular cup template should extend, both cranially and caudally, just beyond the sclerotic subchondral bone. On the same view, the appropriately sized femoral component will clear both the greater trochanter and lateral cortex when seated just proximal to the lesser trochanter and apposed to the endosteal surface of the medial cortex. The lateral radiographic view (B) is evaluated to ensure that the femoral component will also fit in the cranial-caudal plane.

radiographic projection of the femur, the template is used to evaluate adequate cranial-caudal fit for the femoral stem (Figure 7.11).

The proper size of the acetabular component is determined by choosing a template that fills the cranial and caudal dimensions of the acetabular bed (Figures 7.11 and 7.12). In most instances, the medial aspect of the cup template will contact the medial cortical wall of the acetabulum. If the template does not contact the medial wall, it may indicate that the cup is too small. The next size template should be superimposed over the acetabulum. A

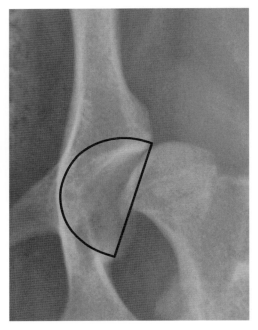

Figure 7.12 The appropriate-size acetabular cup is determined by selecting a template that fills the acetabulum in the cranial-caudal direction. It is not necessary, however, that the cup contacts the medial wall. The rim of the cup should not protrude out beyond the acetabular cranial and caudal margins.

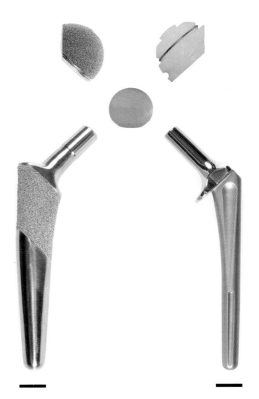

Figure 7.13 The Universal Total Hip system consists of the BFX press-fit cup and stem (*left*) and the CFX cemented cup and stem (*right*). Both fixation options use the same-size femoral head giving surgeons the option of combining both cemented and cementless components in the same joint. Multiple femoral head sizes and neck lengths are available that provide a variety of options. The horizontal bars measure 10 mm.

size cup should be selected that fills the cranial-caudal dimension of the acetabulum and is flush with the bone cranially and caudally. Too small a cup may be placed medially and too large a cup may not seat deep enough to provide press-fit fixation of a cementless press-fit cup. Likewise, with a cemented cup, the bone cement may not be supported by bone of the dorsal acetabular rim. While templating should be performed accurately, final implant size selection is determined during surgery.

Surgical overview

The most common THR systems in use and with outcomes reported in the literature are the Universal Total Hip (BioMedtrix), the Micro Total Hip (BioMedtrix), and the Zurich Cementless Total Hip (Kyon). The BioMedtrix Universal Canine Hip System consists of Biological Fixation (BFX™) and Cement Fixation (CFX™) implants (Figure

7.13). A common surgical technique allows surgeons the option to change the fixation method intraoperatively. The two applications in the same modular total hip system increase the surgeon's options during both primary joint replacement and revision surgeries. Both applications use the same femoral head, allowing the use of cemented and cementless components in the same patient. The cementless cup and stem achieve their initial stability using the interference press-fit concept.

The Micro Total Hip system components and instrumentation share their design with the Universal CFX system (Figure 7.14). The system consists of cemented components only and the implant sizes are appropriate for small-breed dogs and cats. Micro THR may be performed in small-breed

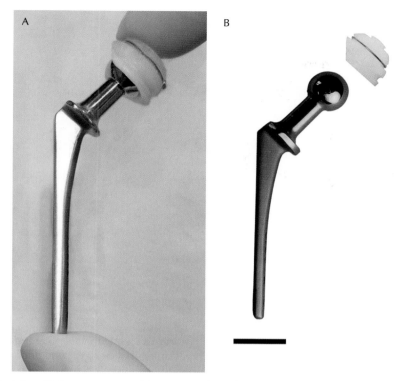

Figure 7.14   (A) The Micro THR system is a modular cemented prosthesis. The outside diameter of the cups is 12, 14, or 16 mm. The femoral stems are #2 or #3, with 2- or 3-mm-diameter stem tips, respectively. The 8-mm femoral heads have two neck lengths of +0 and +2 mm. (B) The Nano THR system is also a cemented system. The outside diameter of the cup is 10 mm. The femoral stem and head components are fixed, with neck lengths of 0, +2, or +4 mm. The femoral head diameter is 6 mm. The horizontal bar measures 10 mm.

dogs weighing less than 12 kg, and as small as 2.5 kg, and in cats. The Nano THR is the smallest implant available and the prosthesis has a fixed head (Ireifej et al. 2012).

The femoral stem of the Zurich Cementless Total Hip system achieves both immediate and long-term fixation with bone screws, while the cup is press-fit (Figure 7.15). Perforations in the metal backing of the cup allow bone ingrowth in addition to a plasma-sprayed surface. The most novel approach of the system is the departure from achieving stability of the femoral component by press-fit fixation. The stem achieves primary fixation to the endosteal surface of the medial femoral cortex using locking-screw fixation. The primary screw fixation of the stem is augmented in time by bone ingrowth to a plasma-sprayed surface. The rationale of anchoring the stem to the cortex is to ensure immediate fixation and minimize stress

shielding of the femur that can occur with conventional canal filling femoral components.

These systems and the broad range of implants offer the surgeon a variety of options for fixation and cover a wide range of patient sizes. The choice of implant depends on surgeon training and experience with a particular system, as well as the needs of the patient. Generally, the indications for hip replacement are the same regardless of the method of implant fixation or the choice of hip system. Currently available total hip systems should be able to accommodate almost all of the needs of the diverse canine and feline breeds and sizes presented to the veterinary surgeon.

Cement fixation requires less precision in femoral canal fit and final positioning of the femoral stem. Therefore, in some patients, a cemented stem may be the preferred choice because of the large size or "stovepipe" shape of

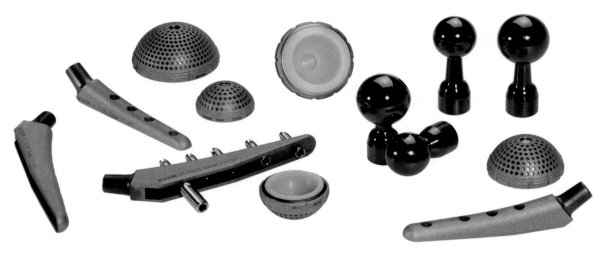

Figure 7.15 The Zurich Cementless system consists of a variety of size stems, cups, and heads with different neck lengths. The polyethylene-lined acetabular component is assembled into a perforated metal shell. The femoral stem is fixed using conical screws that wedge into the implant. The proximal screw is bicortical and the remaining screws are monocortical. (Image courtesy of Kyon, Zurich, Switzerland)

the femur, poor bone quality, or advanced age. Likewise, in very small dogs and cats, cement fixation of the cup and stem allows the surgeon flexibility of implant sizes. In younger patients with a flared proximal metaphyseal region of the femur, a press-fit cementless stem may be preferred.

Because its initial stability relies on intimate contact with bone, the conventional press-fit stem may offer less flexibility in patient selection than a cemented stem or a cementless screw fixation stem. In all but the smallest patients, a press-fit cup is preferred over a cemented cup regardless of the type stem fixation used. During revision of a failed cemented stem, a cementless stem may offer the surgeon a better option for revision than recementing a femoral component. The decision to use cemented or cementless implants is preferably made prior to surgery and varies with surgeon experience, preference, and the bone morphology.

The specific surgical techniques for the Universal and the Zurich Cementless total hip systems are described in detail in the "Addendum" section. Although there are differences in technique dictated by the implant design and fixation, the procedures have many common and similar steps. In general terms, the surgical procedure starts by positioning the dog with the hemipelvi

superimposed in the sagittal plane and held securely in position using a positioning device. The positioning device stabilizes the pelvis and prevents movement during retraction, reaming, and impaction of the implants. This is especially important during placement and alignment of the acetabular component.

The hip joint is exposed using the modified cranial-lateral approach to the hip joint (Piermattei and Johnson 2004). An L-shaped tenotomy of the deep gluteal tendon of insertion and muscle is performed, leaving the proximal one-third to one-half of the tendon intact. A T-shaped capsulotomy is performed. If the ligament of the femoral head is intact, it can be transected with a sharp Hatt spoon or other narrow sharp instrument that will enter the joint space. The hip is luxated, externally rotated 90 degrees and the femoral neck is osteotomized. The dissection is further developed to provide clear and unobstructed access the acetabulum and unhindered access to the central axis of the femoral canal. If a press-fit cementless cup and stem are to be used, the acetabular bone bed is prepared first and the cup implanted, followed by preparation and implantation of the femoral component. The Zurich Cementless system prepares the femur first, followed by acetabular preparation and implantation. If both components are cemented, the femur is prepared first, followed by the acetabulum. The cup is then cemented, followed by cementing of the femoral stem. This places the cementing procedures in sequence. In cemented hip replacement, the bone is prepared to allow the surgeon to accurately position the implant within the cement mantle. In cementless hip replacement, the preparation of the bone determines the exact positioning and stability of press-fit implants. Also, the absence of a cement mantle necessitates that bone preparation be precise to result in initial press-fit stability and eventual stable fixation by bone ingrowth.

Following implantation of both components, a prosthetic femoral head with the appropriate neck length is assembled onto the femoral stem. The range of motion of the reduced joint is evaluated. If the range of motion and stability of the joint are satisfactory, the joint and the wound are lavaged copiously with pulsatile irrigation in preparation for closure. If bone cement was used, the joint and adjacent tissues are carefully inspected and any remnants of bone cement are removed. The wound is closed in layers, beginning with the joint capsule. The transected tendon of the deep gluteal muscle is reattached securely to its insertion. The reflected vastus lateralis muscle is sutured to its origin or, if necessary, to the ventral edge of the tendon of the deep gluteal muscle. The overlying tissues are closed in layers.

Postoperative care and physical rehabilitation

The postoperative management of patients following THR is basically identical, regardless of the hip system or method of fixation. Dogs are discharged to their owners once they can independently get up and lie down and can walk outside for short distances. This occurs after a day or two in most instances, but very large or overweight dogs may need prolonged hospitalization. Activity should be restricted to surfaces with good traction, indoors, for 6 weeks postoperatively with no running, jumping, playing, or stair climbing. Outdoor activity during this time should always occur under supervision and should be controlled with a leash. Walking must be limited to a few minutes, several times per day. Leash walks of

progressively longer duration and distance can begin 6 weeks after surgery. Patients are reevaluated after 3 months and their activity is unrestricted afterward. Specific rehabilitation plans are rarely necessary after THR. They may be considered in patients with limited hip joint motion because of tissue tightness. For example, some patients whose femur is dorsally displaced for extended periods of time before surgery have tight periarticular muscles after surgery, including external rotators, gluteal muscles, and rectus femoris. These tight muscles interfere with comfortable locomotion. A controlled stretching and exercise program may be considered for these patients. The rehabilitation of THR patients that are amputees on their opposite hind limb may include specific assisted stance and locomotion exercises (Figure 7.16). Rehabilitation may also be necessary in patients that had traumatic luxation of a dysplastic hip and have other concomitant orthopedic injuries.

The aftercare of small dogs and cats after Micro THR is often simplified compared with that of larger dogs because small animals can be carried from place to place during rehabilitation. Cats require confinement to a space that does not permit jumping. Cats are allowed free activity starting 6 weeks after surgery.

Clinical outcomes and postoperative complications

The outcome of Howmedica's Canine PCA ingrowth cementless prostheses has been reported (DeYoung et al. 1992; Marcellin-Little et al. 1999a). A long-term (>5 years) assessment of 50 consecutive patients was included. All patients had bone ingrowth in their prosthetic cups and stems. The complications included six luxations. Five of these luxations occurred in the short term and one in the long term, after trauma. One dog developed an osteosarcoma at the site of medullary bone infarction, distal to the prosthetic stem (Marcellin-Little et al. 1999b).

The short-term clinical outcome of the BioMedtrix BFX cementless prostheses has been reported.[2] In a consecutive case series studied from 2003 to 2009, 204 primary BFX THR were performed. The patients ranged in weight from 18 to 72 kg (mean:

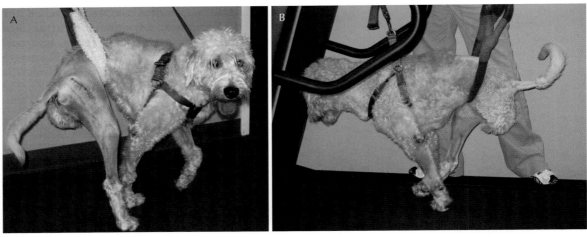

Figure 7.16   A young mixed-breed dog with a previous left pelvic limb amputation underwent a right THR. The dog was not able to walk without assistance after surgery and was uncoordinated. (A) In this picture made 4 days after surgery, the dog is assisted and protected from falls with a chest harness and a sling. (B) Rehabilitation includes trotting on a treadmill while controlled and supported by the chest harness and a soft sling.

36 ± 10 kg). The implants used most often were 24- and 26-mm cups (n = 78 and 76, respectively); #7, #8, and #9 stems (n = 53, 59, and 40); and 0- and +3-mm prosthetic heads (n = 78 and 67). Forty-eight percent of patients were free of complications. Minor complications requiring no additional surgery occurred in 25% of patients. They included stem subsidence without fissure with (n = 1) or without rotation (n = 13) and stem rotation without fissure (n = 3). Intraoperative and postoperative femoral fissures were also seen (n = 19). Of these, some occurred without subsidence (n = 11), some with subsidence and rotation (n = 3), and some with subsidence only (n = 4) or rotation only (n = 1). Three dogs had intraoperative fractures of the greater trochanter and one had an acetabular fracture managed conservatively. The fissure rate decreased over time, from 30% for the first group of 50 patients, to 14% for the second group of 50, 12% for the third group of 50, and 4% for the fourth group of 50. Major complications requiring a surgical revision occurred in 11% of patients. Luxation was the most common major complication (n = 17; 8.4% of patients). The causes of luxation included subsidence and rotation, impingement, and lack of tissue tension. Closed reduction was done in one patient. Open reduction was done in all other patients. The prosthetic neck length was increased in most patients.

Iliofemoral sutures were placed in 10 patients. One patient underwent a triple pelvic osteotomy. Femoral fractures occurred in nine patients (4.4%). Five of these were propagations of fissures that occurred at the time of implantation. All fractures but one were managed successfully with surgical reduction and internal fixation and placement of a BFX stem (n = 6) or a cemented stem (n = 3). Five of nine fractures occurred in dogs older than 6 years of age. One dog had sciatic neurapraxia. Lack or loss of bone ingrowth was identified with two cups. These cups were successfully revised with larger BFX cups. One of the patients with a loose cup had an infection due to a *Staphylococcus* sp. that was diagnosed based on a bacterial culture made at the time of revision. That *Staphylococcus* sp. also had been cultured from the dog's skin after an episode of pyoderma that preceded the occurrence of lameness. No other infection was identified. Loss of bone ingrowth in the stem was not identified. This is similar to the long-term results of the Canine PCA THR.

The functional outcome after BFX THR was evaluated prospectively using a pressure-sensitive walkway in 35 dogs (Lascelles et al. 2010). Weight distribution to the operated limb was normal 3 months after surgery. Large canal fill in the proximal portion of the femur and the presence of a large flare of the proximal portion of the femur negatively impacted the normalization of weight distribution.

Overall, the BFX procedure has been a successful method for primary THR. Bone ingrowth into the cup and the stem is consistent. The most common complications, fissures, and luxations appear to be technique-related. The fissure rate in this series of cases decreased dramatically with improved broaching technique. The BFX system has also been used for the revision of failed cemented THR. One report described the successful use of BFX stems to revise three failed cemented stems (Torres and Budsberg 2009). Our group has successfully revised two failed cemented stems and one failed screw prosthesis stem (Helica, INNOPLANT, Hannover, Germany) with BFX stems. One report documented the successful revision of experimental carbon composite stems in two dogs. Septic loosening of the experimental stem developed in one dog, and aseptic (polyethylene wear debris-induced) loosening in the other dog. The single-stage revisions were performed using the Canine PCA cementless hip (Massat et al. 1998).

The clinical outcome of cemented THR has been reported in several clinical case series (Olmstead et al. 1983; Massat and Vasseur 1994; Edwards et al. 1997). A cumulative complication rate of 18% and a cumulative satisfactory outcome of 90.7%, extrapolated from six clinical reports, were reported after 506 Richards Canine II prostheses (Smith & Nephew Richards, Memphis, TN) (Montgomery et al. 1992). Complications included aseptic loosening (5.7%), luxation (5.1%), infection (4.7%), sciatic nerve palsy (1.6%), and fractures (1.6%). The outcome of the BioMedtrix CFX procedure was reported in a prospective clinical study that included 51 dogs (Olmstead 1995b). The complication rate was 7%.

In a retrospective study including 284 canine cemented THR, the cementing methods did not influence the short-term complication rate (Ota et al. 2005). In a retrospective study of 97 CFX hips, a revision rate of 12.1% was reported for the first side THR (Bergh et al. 2006). Not all cases with major complications in this series underwent revision surgery. The authors discussed several potential reasons for this relatively high complication rate, including a low case load, eccentrically placed femoral stems, and the presence of radiolucent lines at the bone–polymethylmethacrylate (PMMA) interfaces. The overall luxation rate in that study was 11.8%.

Factors predisposing to luxation after CFX were evaluated in several studies. Cup orientation (increased angle of lateral opening [ALO]) was identified as a predisposing factor for dorsal luxation in one report (Dyce et al. 2000). Another report concluded that the ALO and cup retroversion were poor predictors for THR luxation (Cross et al. 2000). Body size and conformation (e.g., Saint Bernard type), a short femoral neck, and cup orientation were identified as factors predisposing to ventral hip luxation in a report (Nelson et al. 2007). Preexisting hip subluxation was identified as a factor predisposing to luxation of CFX THR in one study (Hayes et al. 2011a). A femoral fracture rate of 2.9% was reported to occur in a consecutive case series of 684 CFX THR performed by a single surgeon (Liska 2004).

The outcome of micro and nano cemented THR has been reported in several case series (Warnock et al. 2003; Liska 2010; Ireifej et al. 2012). The overall success rate in the largest series was 91% and complications included luxation and cup loosening (Liska 2010).

The outcome of cemented THR has also been assessed through several histological studies (Paul and Bargar 1986, 1987; Skurla and James 2004, 2005; Skurla et al. 2005). In one report analyzing 38 cemented acetabular components retrieved from client-owned dogs postmortem, 53% of acetabular cups were loose, when tested on a materials testing machine. The apparent source of loosening was a mechanical failure of the bone–cement interface. In another report assessing the cemented stems collected from the same patient series, 63% of the stems were loose (Skurla et al. 2005). Debonding (loosening of the implant–cement interface) was identified as the primary mode of failure. Debonding was also identified as a mode of failure after cemented THR in a group of 10 dogs (Edwards et al. 1997). These various studies identified or suggested that the metal used for stem fabrication, stem handling during surgery, and stem orientation within the femoral canal as factors predisposing to debonding.

The clinical outcomes and complications for Micro THR in cats and small dogs are comparable with those seen in medium or large dogs treated with cemented THR. Sciatic neurapraxia (Andrews et al. 2008), infection, femoral fractures, femoral fissures, pulmonary embolism, and aseptic loosening are all potential complications following Micro THR. These complications had a very low frequency or did not occur in a series of 66 consecutive Micro THR (Liska 2010). There are no reported complications that are specific to Micro THR. In one report of seven dogs that underwent THR for unilateral avascular necrosis, ground reaction forces did not differ between normal hips and hips receiving the Micro THR (Jankovits et al. 2012). Luxation is the most common Micro THR complication. Luxation occurred in 9 of 66 consecutive cases in one study (Liska 2010). Five luxations were managed with revision. Four dogs had dorsal and ventral luxations for reasons not well understood. Explantation (6%) was the end result. There was no detectable correlation between luxation and the angle of lateral cup opening. Oversizing as well as undersizing the components can predispose to luxation in dogs or cats weighing <2.5 kg. Smaller implants (Nano THR, BioMedtrix LLC) are now manufactured to eliminate the risk of oversizing in small cats and dogs weighing 2-to 4 kg.

Complications reported for the Zurich Cementless hip are common to all THR systems and include luxation, aseptic loosening, femur fracture, septic loosening, implant failure, neurapraxia, and patellar luxation. Of published reports, two retrospective studies evaluated complications of both the femoral and acetabular components (Guerrero and Montavon 2009; Hummel et al. 2010), and one study evaluated only the acetabular component (Hanson et al. 2006). Even with this limited number of reports, the complication rates have varied widely. Hummel et al. reported an intraoperative femur fracture rate of 7.4% (Hummel et al. 2010). Interestingly, these fractures were reported as diaphyseal, but were described as occurring in the calcar region, which is metaphyseal. The overall femoral fracture rate ranges from 1.5% to 7.9% (Guerrero and Montavon 2009; Hummel et al. 2010). Fractures of the greater trochanter and acetabulum, as well as transient sciatic neurapraxia, are also occasionally reported. Luxation rates in two reports were 10% and 17% (Guerrero and Montavon 2009; Hummel et al. 2010). Aseptic loosening rates ranged from 0% to 11% (Hanson et al.

2006; Guerrero and Montavon 2009;Hummel et al. 2010). Implant-associated infection or septic loosening has been reported in 0%–3.7% of patients (Hanson et al. 2006; Guerrero and Montavon 2009; Hummel et al. 2010). Other than rates of aseptic loosening, Hummel et al. reported a substantially higher overall complication and failure rate than had been previously published or described. The authors of that study commented that technical errors and surgeon inexperience were the cause of a large portion of their complications. Cases of failure of stem fixation and cup dislodgement have also been described anecdotally, but have not been reported in peer-reviewed literature. In an unpublished retrospective study of 623 consecutive cases operated between 2001 and 2008, Vezzoni reported an overall complication rate of 10.4%. Of the 65 cases with complications, 59 were successfully revised and 6 were explanted.[3]

Femoral medullary infarction (FMI) and pulmonary embolism are two additional potential sequelae to THR (Sebestyen et al. 2000; Liska and Poteet 2003). FMI is identified on radiographs made several months after surgery as sclerotic linear opacities within the medullary canal distal to the femoral stem tip. These opacities are typically described as cigarette smoke or "serpigenous," meaning creeping or spreading. The incidence of FMI associated with the Zurich system was investigated in two studies. The first study (Marsolais et al. 2009) reported a 19.5% incidence of FMI, comparable with the 14% rate of FMI in a previous report that included a combination of cemented and press-fit femoral stems (Sebestyen et al. 2000). An increased incidence of FMI in young dogs was identified in both studies. A follow-up study by Haney et al. in which reaming for Zurich femoral stems was carefully controlled to not exceed the depth of reamer flutes or rasp teeth reported a decrease in incidence of FMI to 2.9% (Haney and Peck 2009). While the specific cause of FMI remains unknown, the Haney study strongly suggests that FMI is caused by excessive reaming depth and damage to endosteal blood supply during femoral preparation. The clinical consequences of FMI are not well known. However, a femoral osteosarcoma that developed at the site of a medullary infarct following cementless press-fit THR was reported in one patient (Marcellin-Little et al. 1999b).

Pulmonary embolism associated with THR was initially reported after cemented THR (Otto and Matis 1994; Liska and Poteet 2003). The incidence of pulmonary embolism associated with the Zurich THR was evaluated by Tidwell et al. A combination of computed tomography (CT) pulmonary angiography and nuclear scintigraphy were used to detect pulmonary embolism in 11 dogs. No cases of pulmonary embolism were detected. However, intraoperative transesophageal ultrasound, a modality that may be used to detect emboli in real time, was not used in that study (Tidwell et al. 2007). Sudden intraoperative death was reported in one patient due to pulmonary embolism associated with cemented THR (Liska and Poteet 2003).

Addendum: surgical procedures

Universal hip system

The general philosophy of this surgical technique is regardless of whether a BFX cementless or a CFX cemented implantation is intended, the bone bed of the acetabulum and the femoral canal are always prepared using the precision technique required for the BFX implants. If it is desired to cement a CFX implant, the preparation is modified at the end of the BFX preparation. This approach allows the surgeon to develop one consistent surgical technique and have the intraoperative flexibility to change implants. In the femur, the mantle for bone cement is created by simply downsizing the CFX stem from the BFX preparation. On the acetabular side, the CFX cup is 1 mm smaller than the BFX preparation, allowing space for a cement mantle.

The BFX technique will be described first, followed by modifications for the CFX technique. The Micro Hip technique is similar to the CFX with a few differences in instrumentation related to the small size of patients.

Neck resection

The femur is rotated externally 90 degrees to expose the femoral head and neck. The neck resection guide is held aligned with the central axis of the femur as in the radiographic templating process. The femoral neck resection is made parallel to the neck cutting guide using the medial edge of the greater trochanter as the point of reference. The neck resection is identical for both the collared CFX and the collarless BFX stems. A high osteotomy is made to preserve proximal cancellous and cortical bone and to enhance stability and torsional resistance of the implanted stem. The angle of the neck cut is most important when using a collared CFX stem. When the collar is seated against the neck cut, it sets the axial alignment of the stem in the femoral canal.

Acetabular preparation

An unobstructed view of the acetabulum is necessary for proper preparation of the bone bed and press-fit of the cup. In patients with chronic dysplastic changes, the junction of the joint capsule and the bony acetabular rim must be identified and the joint capsule undermined 2–3 mm with a scalpel blade around the circumference of the acetabulum. Meyerding retractors are placed under the reflected joint capsule cranial, dorsal, and caudal to the acetabulum. The caudal retractor can simultaneously retract the femur.

In severe cases of hip dysplasia, identification and isolation of the acetabular rim helps to ensure a stable interference fit and seating the cup against bone without an interposed thick fibrous joint capsule. Likewise, it is crucial to ream the true acetabulum and not a dorsally migrated pseudo-acetabulum resulting from hip dysplasia. Before reaming, reliable reference landmarks must be located. The ventral aspect of the true acetabulum can be determined by locating the transverse acetabular ligament (Figure 7.17). The ventral edge of the acetabular reamer is maintained just dorsal to this landmark. Any large osteophytes are removed, especially ventrally and caudally, to facilitate positioning of the reamer and insertion of the cup and to improve the range of motion of the prosthetic joint. The acetabulum is reamed to create a hemispherical bone bed, free of cartilage, eburnated bone, or fibrous tissue.

To minimize removal of the dorsal rim and prevent dorsal migration of the reamer, reaming is started with the reamer shaft directed at an angle of approximately 15–20 degrees ventral to perpendicular (Figure 7.18), rather than at the 45-degree

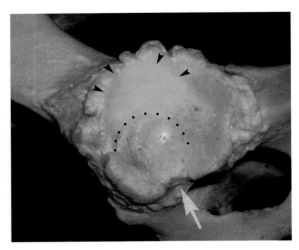

Figure 7.17 An acetabulum from a dog with advanced osteoarthritis secondary to hip dysplasia. The location of the true (original) acetabulum is delineated by black dots forming a semicircle. The articular surface migrated over time to the white circular area delineated by black arrowheads. The true acetabulum must be identified and reamed to place the cup in the original location. Locating the ventral acetabular ligament original location (white arrow) helps identify the correct location of the acetabulum. A large osteophyte is visible cranial and caudal to the transverse acetabular ligament. The ventral rim of protruding osteophytes should be removed. A cup with a relatively large diameter should be implanted to lateralize the cup in relation to the bone cranial and caudal to prevent impingement resulting in dislocation. Other osteophytes causing impingement should be removed.

anatomical central axis of the acetabulum. To minimize deviation of the reamer or wobbling, the surgeon must hold the reamer without a wobble and directed at the correct angle. This requires the surgeon to hold the power reamer in one hand and the reamer shaft close to the reamer head with the other hand. The reamer handle and shaft are held stationary as the depth and diameter of the bone bed are expanded. Acetabular reaming must be deliberate and accurate to ensure proper positioning and press-fit.

Preparation of an accurate acetabular bone bed is accomplished using a two-stage reaming technique. First, a starter reamer ("cheese grater" style), 1 mm smaller than the intended BFX cup, is used to establish the depth of the bone bed. Second, a solid core finishing reamer the same size as the BFX cup is used to expand the diameter of

the bone bed to achieve an accurate preparation within the required tolerance for a press-fit. The starter reamer is used initially to create the depth because of its ability to remove cartilage and penetrate hard subchondral bone. The hollow reamer head also collects cancellous bone that can be used later in the procedure for a bone graft. The finishing reamer is designed to expand the bone bed in diameter only. It does not add additional depth to the reamed bone bed. Once the acetabular bone bed has been prepared, if the surgeon decides to use the next largest BFX or CFX cup, the bone bed must be prepared first with the next-size starter reamer and completed with the appropriate-size finishing reamer. If the starter reamer is not used to increase the depth of the preparation, the rim of the BFX cup will not seat nor achieve press-fit stability and the bed will not be deep enough for the CFX cup. The starter reamers are odd-numbered (19, 21, 23, 25, 27, 29, 31, 33 mm) and the finishing reamers are even-numbered sizes (20, 22, 24, 26, 28, 30, 32, 34 mm). The surgeon should select CFX cups that are the same size as the starter reamers and BFX cups the same size as the finishing reamer. The CFX cup is 1 mm smaller than the finishing reamer. A finishing reamer can be used when implanting a CFX cup to create cement mantle space. For example, if a 26-mm BFX cup is to be implanted, the reaming is started with a 25-mm starter reamer (or with a smaller reamer followed by incrementally larger reamers to 25 mm) then completed with the 26-mm finishing reamer. Both the starter and finishing reamer heads are the same depth as the corresponding CFX and BFX cup and are used to determine the depth of the reamed bed. The best anatomical indicators for depth are the cranial and caudal aspects of the acetabulum. Because the reamer is a full circle and the cup is truncated, it is not possible to judge the depth of the ream dorsally. Also, the dorsal rim is frequently partially worn away, providing a poor anatomical reference. In general, reaming is to the depth of the medial cortical wall of the acetabulum, but occasionally, adequate depth is achieved before reaching the medial wall. In such cases, care should be taken to avoid placing the cup too deep, or medialized, as this can reduce joint reduction tension and result in impingement during external rotation of the prosthetic joint. Both decreased joint reduction tension and

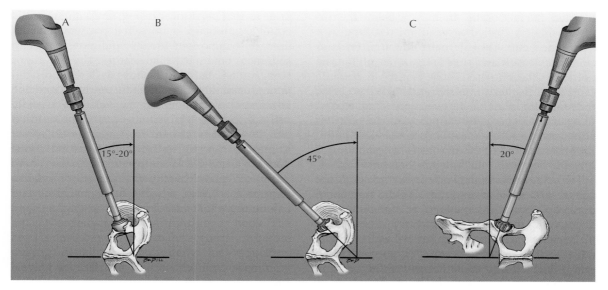

Figure 7.18 Acetabular reaming is initiated using the starter reamer positioned approximately 15–20 degrees ventral to perpendicular to minimize dorsal migration and minimize removal of the acetabular rim (A). Once the depth of the hemispherical bone bed has been established, the finishing reamer is used to create a press-fit and set the orientation of the cup. The finishing reamer is aligned with the anatomical axis of the acetabulum at approximately 45 degrees ventral to perpendicular (B) and in 20 degrees of retroversion (C).

impingement increase the risk of luxation. Impingement also increases the production of wear debris, thus increasing the likelihood of future aseptic loosening.

Once the initial bed is established, the reamer shaft must be positioned in the correct anatomical axis of the final cup position (Figure 7.18). The BFX cup is a hemisphere to within 3 mm of the rim. Beyond that depth, it becomes a cylinder and sets the axis or orientation of the cup. This necessitates the last 3–4 mm of reaming depth be done at an angle of 45 degrees ventral to perpendicular and in 20 degrees of acetabular retroversion. All reaming with the finishing reamer should be done in the anatomical axis of the acetabulum. This angle is determined by placing the acetabular alignment guide on the two dorsal columns of the pelvic positioning device and holding the reamer shaft parallel to the guide. Alternatively, the acetabular alignment assembly is attached to the reamer sleeve and the horizontal retroversion alignment rod is inserted into the appropriate hole labeled "right" or "left". When properly oriented, this guide will align the reamer 45 degrees ventral to perpendicular, with the appropriate degree of retroversion.

The cementless cup is metal backed; therefore, it is not as imperative that its entire dorsal aspect be covered by bone as it is with a cemented polyethylene cup. The perceived advantage of dorsal coverage must be weighed against the pitfalls of a deep, or medialized, cup. To place a cup deeper to provide better dorsal coverage, the surgeon can carefully penetrate the medial wall with the reamer. The size of the opening must remain small to prevent the cup from migrating through the medial wall. The periosteum should be left intact to promote bone ingrowth. This step is not recommended except in special situations, that is, small pelvis, poor acetabular development, or extreme dorsal rim loss. Reaming through the medial wall must be done with caution; and once done precludes the use of bone cement or it will require sealing the opening with a layer of bone cement prior to cementing a CFX cup.

In advanced stages of hip dysplasia, the acetabulum may be shaped like a large flat, or shallow, saucer and consist of hard cortical bone (Figure 7.17). In these instances, the bone bed should be expanded to the outer rim of the acetabulum by using sequentially larger reamers and a large-diameter cup implanted. If an undersized cup is inserted, the face of the cup may be below the rim of the shallow dished acetabulum resulting in a medialized cup. On external rotation, a fulcrum effect may result and predispose to luxation. The presence of eburnated bone in these patients causes the reamer to chatter and makes accurate reaming difficult. The starter reamers are used to sequentially expand the diameter of the acetabular bone bed. Once the desired diameter and depth has been established, the final preparation is accomplished with the finishing reamer.

The trial acetabular cup is used to assess the reamed bone bed and provide an indication of the final cup position, orientation, and dorsal coverage, and to help identify the location of any osteophytes or soft tissues that may require removal. Large ventral osteophytes should be removed so that they do not displace the cup dorsally during insertion.

Once the acetabular bone bed has been prepared, the acetabulum is irrigated and any remnants of the round ligament, redundant joint capsule, and osteophytes are removed with the aid of a scalpel blade or rongeur before placement of the cup. With BFX implants, it is not necessary to stop all hemorrhage in the bone bed as it is with a cemented application. In fact, the formation of a blood clot is the first step toward fibrous tissue ingrowth and eventual bone formation.

Cup insertion

BFX cup

The cup positioner handle is fitted with the appropriately sized central cup positioner head. When handling the cup, avoid excessive manipulation in order to minimize contamination. The cup is started into the prepared bone bed parallel to the axis in which the reaming was carried out. It is often helpful to place the cup into the prepared bone bed from a ventral aspect taking care to retract the ventral soft tissues. If tissue is pulled into the acetabular bone bed as the cup is seated, it may prevent seating and press-fit of the cup. The angle is determined by aligning the positioner handle with the acetabular alignment guide positioned on the two dorsal columns of the pelvic positioning device, or alternatively using the acetabular alignment assembly attached to the positioner handle. The angle of cup insertion is the same as that used for reaming. Once alignment is achieved, the cup is impacted partway. At this time, it is important to stop and assess the cup alignment before the final seating. The cup alignment can be altered by using the offset cup positioner head. Any adjustments are made and the alignment assessed using the positioner handle and appropriate alignment guide. Once satisfied that the alignment is correct, the cup is seated the remaining distance using the central cup positioner head by briskly impacting with the mallet until fully seated. Following seating, the alignment of the cup is verified using the positioner handle and the acetabular alignment guide. It is difficult to reposition the cup at this point. The offset cup positioner head can be used to attempt small changes in cup orientation. If the cup is grossly malaligned and its orientation cannot be altered, it is best to drive the cup from its bed, reposition it, and impact it at a correct orientation. The cup can be removed by impacting the dorsal aspect of the metal shell at midtruncation at the 12 o'clock position. The tip of the impactor handle is placed on the metal shell and impacted with the mallet to "rotate" the cup out of its bone bed around its cranial-caudal axis. If appropriate care is taken in removing the cup, it can usually be replaced into the same bone bed without loss of press-fit.

A properly placed cup should be flush with the acetabulum cranially and caudally. Having the cup elevated above the acetabulum caudally (anteversion) may result in reduced range of motion in external rotation and could result in luxation due to neck impingement. The offset cup positioner head can be used to impact the cup into retroversion. If the cup is not seated flush with the cranial and caudal columns of bone (i.e., the cup is "proud"), this may indicate that the cup is not seated deep enough in the acetabulum. In this case, the cup should be removed and the bone preparation reamed deeper.

CFX cup

If a CFX cup is to be placed, two to three keyholes may be made in the cancellous bone dorsally using a high-speed bur, small curette, or drill bit (Figure 7.19). The acetabular bone bed is flushed to clean the cancellous bone of debris and packed

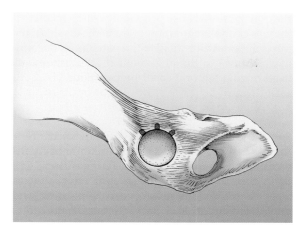

Figure 7.19 If a cemented polyethylene cup is to be implanted, three or more keyholes are made into the dorsal acetabular cancellous bone to allow cement intrusion and aid the mechanical stability of the cement–bone interface. (Image courtesy of BioMedtrix, Boonton, NJ)

until all hemorrhage is stopped. The acetabulum is filled with bone cement and a CFX cup 1 mm smaller than the finishing reamer is selected and mounted on the cup positioner. As with the BFX cup, the CFX cup is fitted onto the cup positioner handle with the central cup positioner head. The cup is inserted into the cement-filled bone bed using the same alignment instrumentation described for the BFX cup. The CFX cup is seated by hand rather than impacted with the mallet. Once seated and positioned, excess bone cement is removed, being careful not to disturb the cup orientation. Bone cement particles are removed from the joint and adjacent soft tissues. If a femoral stem (sizes 5–9) centralizer is being used, the appropriate femoral stem is placed into a warm centralizer mold (flash sterilized just prior to use). Prior to injecting cement into the acetabulum, a portion of the cement batch is injected into the mold until cement emerges from the top of the mold around the stem. The mold is set aside to cure while the acetabular cup is cemented.

Femoral canal preparation

The limb is rotated 90 degrees and the proximal portion of the femur is elevated from the wound using a large blunt-tipped Hohmann retractor. The proximal aspect of the femur must be elevated enough to allow unimpeded passage of the femoral

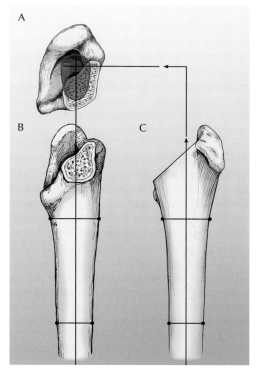

Figure 7.20 The initial opening into the femur (A, red dot) is made over the central axis of the femur as viewed from orthogonal planes, medial-lateral (B), and cranial-caudal (C). The central axis (red dot) lies in the trochanteric fossa adjacent to the greater trochanter, not in the femoral neck osteotomy site. The initial opening is made with a Steinmann pin or drill bit and a fluted reamer and then expanded to the appropriate implant size (A, blue oval) using a series of broaches with increasing sizes. (Image courtesy of BioMedtrix, Boonton, NJ)

instrumentation down the central axis of the canal. Femoral canal preparation consists of two basic steps: initial opening and final canal preparation.

Initial opening

The initial opening is made into the femoral canal over the central axis of the femur. The central axis is located in the trochanteric fossa medial to the greater trochanter (Figure 7.20). Proper identification of this point is crucial for canal preparation and positioning of both the BFX and the CFX stems. The point of entry is difficult to visualize because of the presence of soft tissue, and potentially osteophytes, in the trochanteric fossa. The femoral canal must not be entered through the neck osteotomy site. Accurate placement of the opening is facilitated by creating a pilot hole in the trochanteric fossa with a sharp 3.2-mm intramedullary pin. The pin will penetrate soft tissues and osteophytes and engage the sloping surface of the trochanteric fossa. This step can be done prior to or after resection of the femoral head and neck. Presence of the head and neck may provide better orientation during pin placement. This is the same technique used to place an intramedullary pin or interlocking nail during fracture repair. Once the appropriate point is identified, the pin is driven into the femoral canal, parallel to the long axis of the femur. The alignment of the pin must be carefully assessed prior to entering the proximal femur. Valgus-varus deviation is avoided by directing the pin toward the center of the patella. Cranial-caudal tipping is avoided by ensuring that the pin is aligned with the long axis of the proximal aspect of the femur as determined during templating on the lateral radiographic view. Intraoperative review of the orientation of the long axis relative to the patella is helpful in obtaining the correct alignment. With normal femoral anatomy,

the pin is aimed just proximal to the patella. If there is caudal angulation of the femoral shaft, the pin is aimed well cranial to the patella. These landmarks apply to the alignment of all instruments used during femoral canal preparation.

Final canal preparation

After the opening is made in the trochanteric fossa, the preparation is expanded through the remaining caudal wall of the femoral neck. The hard cortical bone of the caudal femoral neck offers considerable resistance to broaching and makes it difficult to expand the preparation into the osteotomy site. This cortical bone may cause the broach to rotate into retroversion rather than penetrate the neck wall and enter the osteotomy site. An opening through the caudal femoral neck wall is created using a rongeur followed by a side-cutting tapered reamer. Using a rongeur first to remove the caudal neck facilitates the reaming process. The location of this opening or pathway through the caudal neck is important as it sets the version of the broach and the stem (Figure 7.21).

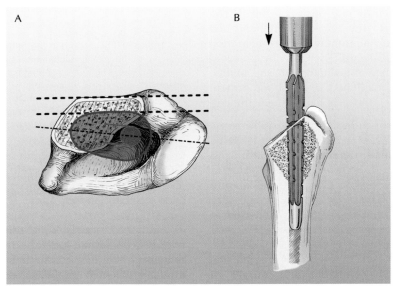

Figure 7.21 Once the initial opening into the femoral canal is made, removing the remaining femoral neck (A, between the parallel red lines) with a rongeur facilitates the reaming and broaching process. The power reamer is held axially and directed or forced against the surface of the cortical wall medially (B). During the insertion of the broaches, the cranial face of the broach is held parallel to the cranial face of the femoral neck. This sets the version of the stem (dot-dash line through implant center) to match the original version of the femoral neck (A, heavy dotted parallel lines). (Image courtesy of BioMedtrix, Boonton, NJ)

The stem version can be determined by placing the tip of the #4 broach into the 3.2-mm pinhole opening and aligning the cranial surface of the broach with the cranial surface of the femoral cortex at the level of the osteotomy. The point at which the broach contacts the remnants of the caudal femoral neck is noted and that portion of the neck wall is removed using a rongeur, followed by a power-driven, side-cutting, tapered reamer. The #2–3 or the #5 tapered reamer is inserted axially into the opening (Figure 7.21). During power insertion, the reamer is initially positioned axially and held firmly against the neck wall as it is inserted. After partial insertion, the reamer is migrated through the caudal neck wall into the osteotomy site at the point previously identified. Care must be taken not to violate the envelope of the stem shape and only remove enough bone to facilitate the initiation of the broaching process. The opening through the caudal neck must be made in the location that will direct the broach into the canal in neutral rotation, not in excessive anteversion or retroversion. If a larger size stem is to be implanted, the initial opening made with the 3.2-mm pin can be expanded using a 5-mm drill bit followed by the #5 reamer. If a #4 or #5 stem is to be used, the #2–3 reamer should be used following the 3.2-mm pin. To ensure press-fit stability when implanting a smaller stem, use the least amount of power reaming to remove the neck wall and never insert the reamer to a depth beyond the notch on the reamer fins.

To continue the preparation, the cylindrical tip of the #4 broach is introduced into the opening made with the reamer. The handle of the broach is held parallel to the long axis of the femur as viewed from two planes. To avoid placing the stem in excessive anteversion or retroversion, the cranial surface of the broach is aligned parallel to the cranial cortex of the femoral neck as it is impacted. This will place the stem in a near-neutral position or similar to the original degree of femoral neck anteversion. The stem should be placed neutral or in slight anteversion. The stem should never be placed in retroversion. Care must simultaneously be taken to ensure proper axial alignment of the broach as it is impacted. If the broach becomes malaligned in varus or if the tip is directed caudally, it should not be forcibly redirected or straightened in the canal. The broach should be retracted until it can be correctly aligned and the impaction process resumed with the shaft of the broach held parallel to the long axis of the femur. The surgeon must resist letting the broach slide back into malalignment during reinsertion. Holding the broach using a golfer's grip, with the thumb extended on the shaft rather than like a fist, helps stabilize the shaft axially. If the malalignment is severe, the broach may be partially extracted and the tip used as a rasp to remove bone medial to the trochanter or caudally until the broach can be aligned axially. Once aligned, the broach is advanced with the mallet until the proximal-lateral "shoulder" of the broach is seated 2–3 mm below the junction of the femoral neck with the greater trochanter (Figure 7.22). In surgery, this anatomical reference point is palpable as a bony ridge at the level of the origin of the vastus lateralis muscle on the cranial surface of the femur. This is the reference point for seating the broach in the canal. The slotted slap hammer is used to extract the broach in the same direction in which it was inserted. The next larger size broach is inserted and impacted to the appropriate level.

Femoral preparation is continued with sequentially larger broaches until press-fit stability is achieved. Like the acetabular reamer, the broach serves as the trial component. When the appropriate broach size is seated, it should offer "considerable" resistance to further advancement. The final size selection is influenced by preoperative radiographic templating, but is determined intraoperatively by the change in resistance during sequential broaching. For that reason, sequential broaching is recommended so the surgeon learns to "feel" the sequential change in resistance to subsidence of the broach as the canal is prepared and to "hear" the mallet handle "tuning fork" sound emission change when the broach impact is resisted by cortical bone contact. As a general rule, provided the broach is properly aligned in both planes, the last 5 mm of seating the broach should be significantly more difficult than the previous advancement. In addition, the surgeon should note the amount of cancellous bone between the teeth of the broach and the medial and cranial cortical walls when the broach is seated. If there is 4 mm or more of cancellous bone cranial and medial, the next broach size

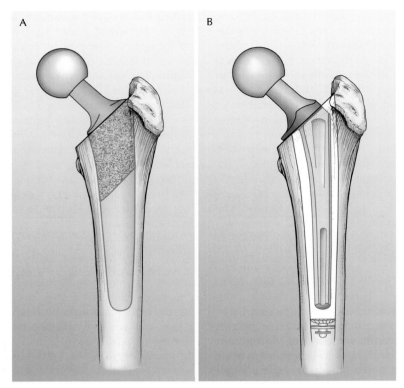

Figure 7.22   (A) BFX stem press-fit into the femoral canal following preparation using the broaches. (B) A CFX stem surrounded by bone cement. The distal flow of bone cement is limited by a cement restrictor placed distal to the stem tip. To allow space for the cement mantle, a CFX stem is selected one size smaller than the final broach. If the femur was prepared only using reamers, then the stem size matches the final reamer size. The stem is inserted until the collar contacts the femoral neck cranial and medial. (Image courtesy of BioMedtrix, Boonton, NJ)

may be indicated. However, it is desirable that, whenever possible, a margin of cancellous bone be preserved between the implant and the cortex, especially when cementing an implant.

When making the decision to increase the size of the stem, the surgeon must always keep in mind the largest stem tip that will fit in the femoral diaphysis as determined during preoperative templating. In "champagne fluted" femurs, the diaphysis may be the size-limiting point, not the metaphysis. If the surgeon is not comfortable impacting a broach the remaining distance because it does not advance with "reasonable" impaction force, the broach should be removed and not forced further into the canal. When this occurs, the technique of inserting, impacting, removing, and cleaning the broach multiple times until seated may be utilized. Alternatively, a smaller broach can be reinserted into the femoral canal and used

as a rasp to selectively remove bone caudally and laterally along the greater trochanter. Caution must be exercised not to rasp away too much bone when this technique is used to seat the final broach size. The broach must be custom fit slowly; one or two strokes or rasping motions with the broach may be sufficient. The finishing file should only be used very judiciously for this procedure.

Forces resulting from impaction of the broach are distributed uniformly outward. These forces are unlikely to result in a fissure fracture, provided the broach is aligned parallel with the long axis of the femur and enters the canal over the central axis. Situations predisposing to femoral fissure or fracture include starting the femoral broach into the canal from the femoral neck osteotomy site, varus and/or caudal alignment of the broach, and excessive bending or rotation of the broach in the femur or during extraction. Also, inadequate elevation of the proximal aspect of the femur, or the femur slipping off the retractor used for elevation, may tempt the surgeon to use the broach as a lever to elevate the femur from the surgical site. The resulting bending force can cause a fracture. Twisting the broach around its long axis or placing the broach in excessive anteversion can wedge the cortical walls apart resulting in a fracture. It is recommended that the mallet with a slotted handle be used to impact the broach. Fissure fractures are technique related and most often result from varus or caudal alignment of the broach. Attention to proper elevation of the proximal aspect of the femur and appropriate use and alignment of the broaches, combined with selective rasping, reduces or eliminates the incidence of fissure fractures. Also, during femoral canal preparation, an assistant should provide resistance at the stifle joint to counteract the impact of the mallet on the broach in order to minimize the chance of the proximal aspect of the femur slipping off the retractor.

The craniomedial region of the femoral neck should be closely observed during broaching and stem insertion for the development of a fissure. If a fissure does occur, canal preparation or stem insertion should be stopped and the broach or stem removed. A double-loop cerclage wire is placed around the femur at the level just distal to the greater trochanter and proximal to the lesser trochanter. Broaching or stem insertion is then resumed. If the fissure extends more than 2 cm distally or the patient's bone appears brittle and/ or thin, double-loop cerclage wires may be placed every centimeter, continuing beyond the most distal extent of the fissure (McCulloch et al. 2012). In the event that the broaching process or stem implantation cannot proceed without the fissure widening, despite the application of cerclage wire, conversion to a CFX stem may be necessary.

Femoral stem insertion

BFX stem

The femur is maintained in the same position as during the broaching procedure. The appropriate BFX femoral component is held by the femoral neck and inserted by hand into the prepared femoral canal in the same plane and degree of anteversion as the broach. When resistance to hand seating is met, the component is seated the

remaining "drive" distance with the femoral component impactor and a mallet. The proximal-lateral "shoulder" of the femoral stem is seated approximately 2–3 mm below the most proximal aspect of the junction of the femoral neck with the greater trochanter (Figure 7.22). In reality, the level of final seating may be anywhere from 2 to 3 mm above or below this ideal insertion point, based on the degree of resistance to impaction. If the component was easily advanced beyond the desired seating point, subsidence is likely to occur when the implant is loaded. In that case, the femoral component should be extracted and the medullary canal expanded with the next broach size to accommodate a larger implant.

Following hand seating the stem, the surgeon must assess the remaining drive distance prior to impaction with the mallet. The drive distance should be approximately two-thirds to one-half of the length of the beaded portion of the stem. If the drive distance is greater than this, the preparation is cautiously expanded using the next larger broach. This must be done in a manner to avoid oversizing the preparation resulting in loss of press-fit. The stem should be removed from the canal and the next largest broach size hand inserted until it stops. The broach is advanced approximately two teeth, removed, and the desired stem reinserted. The drive distance is reassessed. This sequence is continued until the stem has a drive distance equal to two-thirds to one-half of the beaded section. Leaving the extractor attached to the stem facilitates its insertion and removal during this custom fitting process.

In the event that a stem must be extracted during surgery, the stem extractor is attached firmly to the stem and the stem is removed using the slotted mallet against the impaction block. If the stem resists removal with the extractor, the femoral neck is firmly gripped using a large Vise-Grip and the implant extracted by impacting the Vise-Grip.

CFX stem

If a CFX stem is to be implanted, the femoral canal is prepared as described above. A CFX trial stem, one size smaller than the broach used for the preparation, is inserted into the prepared bone bed until the collar contacts the cranial and medial cortex (Figure 7.22). If the collar contacts the caudal neck cortex first, preventing seating on the cranial cortex, a rasp or rongeur can be used to remove a portion of the caudal neck. If necessary, the angle of the osteotomy can be altered using the finishing file to optimize the axial alignment of the stem.

Alternatively, if the surgeon intends to implant a CFX implant from the beginning, the femur can be prepared using sequential power reamers inserted axially into the original opening in the trochanteric fossa. The final power reamer used is the same size as the intended stem size. The opening can then be finished by impacting a broach one size larger than the CFX stem or hand rasping using a smaller broach as a rasp to remove bone until the stem can be axially aligned.

With cement fixation, the trial cup and stem, rather than the components to be implanted, are always used to determine the adequacy of the bone bed preparation. Fat and marrow cannot be adequately washed off the implant surface during surgery. Studies have shown that the bonding strength of a stem with the cement is decreased by more than 80% if wet or contaminated with fat or marrow (Stone et al. 1989). This can predispose to debonding at the implant–cement interface.

Once the canal preparation has been completed, a polyethylene cement restrictor is inserted into the diaphysis below the level of the stem tip to restrict the flow of cement down the distal femoral canal. The small restrictor is generally used in canals prepared for stem sizes #5 or #6, and the large restrictor for sizes #7 to #10, although this may vary based on canal preparation. Following placement of the cement restrictor, the canal is flushed using pressure to remove any debris, blood, and loose cancellous bone from the canal. The canal is dried and injected with bone cement in the low-viscosity stage, starting from the cement restrictor out. Once the canal is filled with cement, thumb pressure over the neck resection area can be helpful to pressurize the cement into the cleaned and dried cancellous bone. The CFX stem is inserted into the cement-filled canal until the collar of the prosthesis contacts the femoral neck cut. If a centralizer was used on the stem tip, and resistance is encountered during seating, the mallet is used to tap the stem impactor handle and seat the stem the remaining distance into the canal.

The stem is firmly held in place while the excess cement is removed from the surrounding tissues, especially in the area of the joint and acetabular cup. It is recommended that a centralizer and cement restrictor be used whenever the bone size allows. The centralizer has 1-mm flanges that keep the stem tip away from the cortical wall and allows bone cement to remain or flow between the centralizer and the cortical wall.

In summary, the integrity and survival of a cemented stem may be influenced by the preparation of the bone bed, the amount of cancellous bone left proximally, elimination of hemorrhage, cleaning and drying the bone, avoiding stem tip contact with the cortical wall with a centralizer, restricting the cement flow distally, injecting a homogeneous mass of cement that is free of blood, pressurizing the cement into the bone, inserting a clean and dry implant in axial alignment, and holding the implant motionless until the cement has cured. Bone cement should always be mixed following the manufacturer's recommendations. It is highly recommended to fill the canal with cement from distal to proximal whether or not a cement restrictor was used. If a cement restrictor is not used, care must be taken that the cement is not pumped distally and inadequate cement remains in the syringe to fill the proximal canal. Also, it is important to recognize that operating room temperature significantly influences setting time of the cement. A cooler atmosphere slows down the setting time and a warmer atmosphere (>22°C/72°F) accelerates it.

Trial reduction

Trial reduction is performed with trial heads to determine the reduction tension of the joint. The reduction tension should not be excessively tight or loose. Proper alignment of the cup and range of motion are more important in maintaining reduction than joint tension. Trial reduction generally begins with the +3-mm trial head and is adjusted up or down based on the reduction tension. During trial reduction, the correct alignment of the acetabular component can be verified by holding the limb in a normal walking position in relation to the body. With the limb in this position, the flat surface on the back of the femoral head

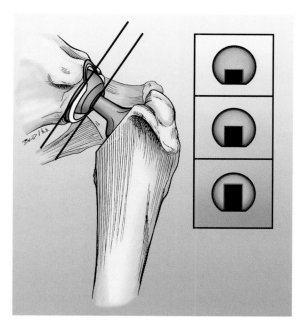

Figure 7.23 Trial reduction of the joint is done using trial femoral head components to determine the correct neck length and joint tension. The orientation of the cup is assessed by holding the limb in a normal standing position to verify that the face of the cup is parallel to the back of the femoral head (parallel lines). (Image courtesy of BioMedtrix, Boonton, NJ)

component should be parallel with the plane of the nontruncated aspect of the cup (Figure 7.23). This is the best indication the surgeon will get of the cup positioning, especially with the BFX cup. It is difficult to assess the position of a metal-backed cup on postoperative radiographs. Cup position should be ascertained during trial reduction and should be corrected at that point, if deemed necessary.

The range of motion should be checked during trial reduction, particularly external rotation. If external rotation is limited, the caudal area of the cup and acetabular bone bed should be checked for interference or impingement with the femoral neck. Correction of impingement is more easily performed before final head assembly, with the joint luxated. If large osteophytes or bone on the rim of the acetabulum limit range of motion or appear to act as a fulcrum resulting in luxation, they are removed with a rongeur. Similarly, large osteophytes present on the caudal aspect

of the greater trochanter should be removed. Lengthening the femoral neck may also increase the range of motion on external rotation. When removing the trial head from the trunion, the head should be firmly grasped with the fingers to prevent loss in the wound.

Head assembly

The trunion is first wiped free of blood and fat and dried before attachment of the head. The head, with the appropriate neck length, is placed onto the trunion and impacted with a mallet using the head impactor. Caution must be taken to prevent contact of the head component with any metal instruments or the rim of the metal acetabular shell during placement or during reduction to avoid scratching the head surface. It is recommended that cotton gauze be placed between the impactor head and the bearing surface to prevent scratching.

Reduction and closure

The femoral head is reduced into the acetabular cup. The range of motion of the reduced joint is again evaluated. The joint and the wound are lavaged copiously with pulsatile irrigation. The joint and adjacent tissues are carefully inspected and any remnants of bone cement are removed. The wound is closed in layers, beginning with the joint capsule. The transected tendon of the deep gluteal muscle is reattached securely to its insertion. The reflected vastus lateralis muscle is sutured to its origin or, if necessary, to the ventral edge of the tendon of the deep gluteal muscle. The overlying tissues are closed in layers. Postoperative radiographs are made using the same technique as described for the preoperative assessment and templating (Figures 7.24 and 7.25).

Zurich hip system technique

The Zurich Cementless THR has been commercially available since the late 1990s. Several changes have been made since its introduction, in response to challenges faced over the past 12 years. This section will primarily discuss the prosthesis in its current form, with a discussion of prior versions, where appropriate.

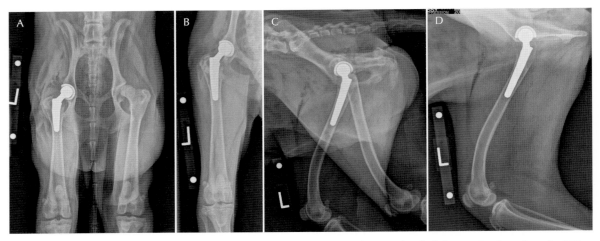

Figure 7.24 Ventrodorsal (A) and craniocaudal (B) radiographic views made immediately following implantation of a BFX press-fit stem in a young dog with hip dysplasia. The femoral component is oriented parallel to the long axis of the femur and fills the metaphysis. On the lateral (C) and open-leg lateral (D) radiographic views, the stem is positioned in the neutral axis of the femur and fills the canal adequately. On the open-leg lateral view, the acetabular component is fully seated against the bone bed and is flush with the cranial and caudal poles of the acetabulum.

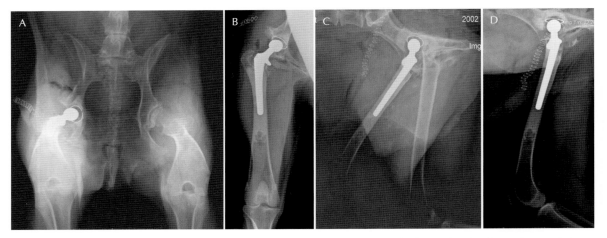

Figure 7.25 Postoperative radiographs of a CFX total hip replacement in a dog with chronic hip dysplasia. The metal ring around the radiolucent polyethylene cup is used to assess the cup position on the ventrodorsal and lateral radiographic views (A and C). The femoral component cannot be assessed on the ventrodorsal view because the chronic changes in the joint prevent full extension of the limb. The femoral component is best assessed on the craniocaudal radiographic view (B) and the lateral and open-leg radiographic views (D). The stem is centrally oriented parallel to the femoral axis in both planes and there is adequate and uniform cement mantle. A cement restrictor outline is visible, distal to the stem tip.

The Zurich hip is a modular total hip system with three components: acetabular cup, head/neck, and femoral stem. The acetabular component is a press-fit component with a double titanium shell and an ultrahigh-molecular-weight polyethylene (UHMWPE) liner. The outer shell is perforated, and plasma sprayed with commercially pure titanium. The inner shell is solid. There is a 1-mm space between the outer and inner shells to allow for "open convection." The open convection reportedly permits free fluid and cellular flow into and out of the perforations in the outer shell during weight bearing to allow improved bone ingrowth, compared with blind-ended channels.[4] Bone ongrowth and ingrowth into the Zurich acetabular cup was assessed using histomorphometric analysis (Lauer et al. 2009). Bone apposition with the outer shell of the cup was 75% and bone ingrowth into the perforations was 44%, 12 months after implantation. The outer shell, as a result of its perforations, has a lower elastic modulus that more closely resembles that of bone (Bragdon et al. 2004). The acetabular polyethylene liner is not spherical. Rather, there is a fossa at the apex of the cup. That fossa decreases the stress on the polyethylene liner by a factor of 2.5 and reduces the coefficient of friction by a factor of 2 compared with a spherical control, based on finite element analysis (Bishop et al. 2008).[5] The acetabular cups are available in five sizes (21.5, 23.5, 26.5, 29.5, and 32.5 mm). The 29.5- and 32.5-mm cups accept 19-mm-diameter femoral heads, while other sizes accept 16-mm-diameter femoral heads. The femoral stem is also made of titanium and has a plasma-sprayed, commercially pure titanium coating. Five stem sizes are available. The stems are fixed to the medial cortex of the femur with conically shaped screws that are wedged into the implant itself. The smaller two stem sizes (extra-small and small) are fixed with four screws, and the others (medium, large, and extra-large) are fixed with five screws. In the original version of the stems, all screws were monocortical and obtained purchase only in the medial cortex. The rationale for monocortical, rather than bicortical, screws was that the medial and lateral cortices cycle at slightly differing rates during loading. Since screw fixation was initially expected to be load bearing ad infinitum in THR patients, this design was thought to decrease the likelihood of screw loosening or screw failure.[4] Additionally, based on a three-dimensional finite element analysis study, stress shielding of the proximomedial femoral cortex is significantly lower with the Zurich prosthesis than with a cemented prosthesis (Shahar et al. 2003). This advantage, primarily attributed to the method of fixation, suggests a lower risk of proximal femoral bone loss. Manufacturer recommendations now include placing a bicortical screw in the most proximal hole. That screw is thought to decrease the likelihood of avulsion of the stem from the medial cortex prior to its

osseointegration, particularly in giant breeds. Since the prosthesis is not press-fit, several millimeters of open medullary cavity are often present lateral to the prosthesis. The femoral head/neck component is titanium alloy with a diamond-like carbon coating. The head/neck component is affixed to the stem trunion with a Morse taper. The angle of inclination of the head/neck with the femoral stem is 135 degrees. Twelve millimeters of neck length modularity are available in five 3-mm increments (extra-short, short, medium, long, and extra-long necks). Each neck length is available for both 16- and 19-mm-diameter heads.

Surgical procedure

Neck resection

The femoral head and neck excision is performed via a biplanar osteotomy (Figure 7.26). The vertical portion of the osteotomy is made just medial to the greater trochanter, as lateral as possible to ensure access to the central axis of the femur. The

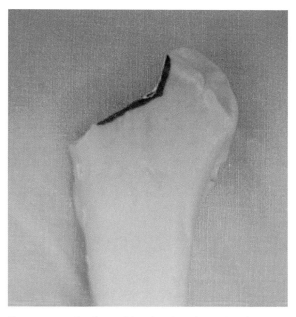

Figure 7.26 The femoral head and neck excision for a Zurich Cementless hip is performed in a biplanar fashion. The vertical portion of the osteotomy extends distally to the level of the distal extent of the femoral head. The transverse portion of the osteotomy exits the medial cortex just proximal to the lesser trochanter.

vertical portion of the osteotomy terminates at the level of the distal aspect of the femoral head. The transverse portion of the osteotomy originates at the proximal extent of the lesser trochanter medially and angles proximally to meet the distal end of the vertical osteotomy.

Femoral canal preparation

During femoral canal preparation, the leg is held in 90 degrees of external rotation and at approximately 90 degrees of extension. To improve access to the medullary canal, the femur is lateralized using a modified Hohmann retractor placed just distal to the osteotomy. Initial entry into the femoral canal should be made as caudolateral as possible and visualization of the tendon of insertion of the internal obturator muscle is a useful landmark within the trochanteric fossa. A teardrop-shaped proximal portion of the femur rather than an oval or elliptical shape suggests that the neck cut is too proximal. This complicates the entry into the central axis of the femur and predisposes to stem tipping into a varus and caudal orientation. Perforation into the medullary canal can be performed using a rongeur, a high-speed bur, or the 6-mm drill bit that is used for initial femoral canal preparation. Femoral canal preparation is performed by hand, using two drill bits (6 and 8 mm) and two files. The drill bits are manually rotated approximately 180 degrees in both clockwise and counterclockwise directions. Each bit needs only be inserted to the point where proximal extent of the flutes of the bit is at the level of the osteotomy (Figure 7.27). As the bit is removed from the medullary canal, its T-handle should be gradually brought cranially while continuing handle rotation to remove the medullary bone associated with the medial cortex to create appropriate stem contact with that cortex. The small and large files are used sequentially (Figure 7.28). All file cutting is lateral (Figure 7.29). The large file is not necessary for the extra-small or small stems. In order to file for appropriate stem anteversion, the file may be externally rotated by approximately 20 degrees or the limb may be internally rotated (from the 90-degree position) to approximately 70 degrees of external rotation.

Filing should be done in short strokes and wedging or jamming the file should be avoided.

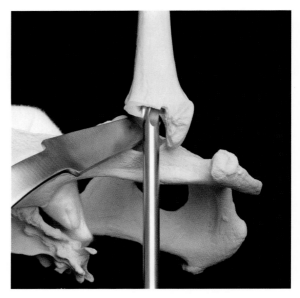

Figure 7.27   Femoral canal preparation for a Zurich Cementless hip is initiated by hand-drilling with a 6-mm and then an 8-mm T-handle mounted bit. Note the presence of the Hohmann retractor used to lateralize the femur during femoral canal preparation. (Image courtesy of Kyon, Zurich, Switzerland)

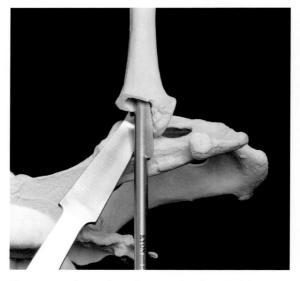

Figure 7.28   Femoral canal preparation for a Zurich Cementless hip is completed with the small file (pictured) for small stems or large file for medium or large stems. The teeth of the file cut laterally only and the file is oriented at approximately 20 degrees of femoral anteversion. (Image courtesy of Kyon, Zurich, Switzerland)

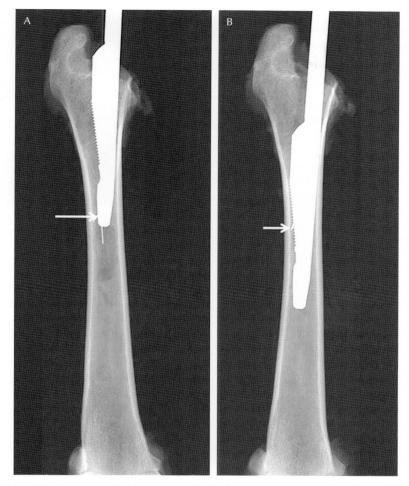

Figure 7.29 Cranial-caudal radiographs of cadaver bone with the femoral preparation file in the medullary canal at appropriate final depth (A) and at excessive depth (B). The arrows indicate the level of the nutrient foramen. Excessively distal femoral canal preparation is associated with an increased incidence of femoral medullary infarction.

If the file becomes jammed in the femoral canal, careful, small amplitude rotations will generally free the file. Careful filing will result in the formation of a central ridge laterally, with space between the two columns of the file. This ridge can be removed, if desired, by refiling at +5 and −5 degrees from the original angles, or by using a high-speed bur. The most proximal portion of the ridge can also prevent full seating of the femoral stem. Removal of the ridge allows greater freedom to adjust femoral anteversion at the time of implantation, but requires greater care between drilling of holes and screw placement. As with

the drill bits, filing should not proceed distally beyond the end of the cutting portion of the file. After filing is complete, a trial fit should be evaluated for contact with the medial cortex and ability to seat the stem roughly to the level of the shoulder of the prosthesis. The Zurich stem is not a collared prosthesis and does not require full seating. In fact, it may be advantageous to have the stem placed 4 or 5 mm "proud" to further lateralize the femur. The stem must, however, be inserted far enough so that the proximal screw hole is at least one screw hole diameter distal to the osteotomy.

Acetabular preparation

Acetabular bed preparation follows femoral canal preparation. The femur is retracted caudodistally using an Army-Navy retractor or can be levered using a small Hohmann retractor hooked on the ischium just caudal to the caudal acetabular rim. Care must be taken to avoid damage to the sciatic nerve. In poorly muscled dogs, transient sciatic neurapraxia can occur with even moderate retraction. Gelpi retractors are placed perpendicular to the capsular incision. The joint capsule is undercut circumferentially at its attachment to allow clear visualization of the dorsal rim, as well as the cranial and caudal poles. At this point, the dorsomedial aspect of the dorsal rim is palpated to evaluate bone support and dorsal migration. In patients with more advanced degenerative changes, the acetabular fossa may not be visible, as it is hidden behind a false medial wall and does not appear until after reaming has progressed several millimeters. The ventral (transverse) acetabular ligament is a useful landmark at this point in the procedure, as it identifies the true ventral limit of the acetabulum. It is often hidden behind a ventral rim of osteophytes that must be removed. The surgeon should not confuse the tendon of insertion of the iliopsoas muscle with the transverse ligament. If desired, if the acetabular fossa is not visible, a small-diameter pilot hole can be drilled in the cranioventral one-third of the acetabulum for monitoring of medial wall thickness during acetabular reaming. Reaming should begin fairly central and ventral, based on previously discussed landmarks, and should start with a reamer that is at least one size smaller than the final cup size. The final reamer size can be used to complete the acetabular bed preparation. In order to ensure complete spherical bone preparation, pivoting or wobbling of the reamer is necessary during reaming. However, the surgeon should be careful not to allow the reamer to drift or shift, otherwise the ability to achieve a press-fit will be lost. It is not necessary, and it is frequently undesirable, to ream the acetabulum entirely to the medial wall. Doing so can decrease lateralization of the femur, resulting in impingement or the requirement of a longer neck than would otherwise be necessary. The depth of preparation should allow the rim of the final reamer to be covered at the cranial and

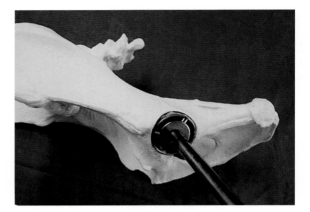

Figure 7.30 Acetabular reaming for a Zurich Cementless cup. Adequate acetabular reaming depth is reached when the rim of the reamer is just below the bone surface cranially and caudally.

caudal poles, based on planned cup orientation (Figure 7.30). Osteophytes that might interfere with cup impaction should be removed. Some surgeons will drill vascular ingrowth channels in prepared areas that do not have exposed cancellous bone. Reamers have a diameter that is 0.5 mm smaller than the corresponding cup in order to achieve press-fit.

Cup insertion

Appropriate patient positioning is confirmed before cup insertion. A marker (skin staple or hemostatic forceps) is placed over the ischiatic tuberosity and another halfway between the tuber coxae and tuber sacrale. The horizontal bar of the cup positioner is the central hole and should be parallel to floor and aligned with the long axis of the femur to create an ALO of 45 degrees. The craniocaudal bar (upper hole for right hip) should be parallel to the line connecting the previously placed markers. This bar sets the anteversion / retroversion angle of the cup (Figure 7.31). The surgeon should also check for anatomical alignment based on equal cranial and caudal pole depth of the cup. The ALO is evaluated prior to complete seating of the cup.

Using the spherical impactor, when the impactor shaft is at 90 degrees to the table, it should just contact the plastic liner (for 29.5- and 32.5-mm cups, the shaft should be approximately 0.5 mm from the liner). When the cup is fully seated, the

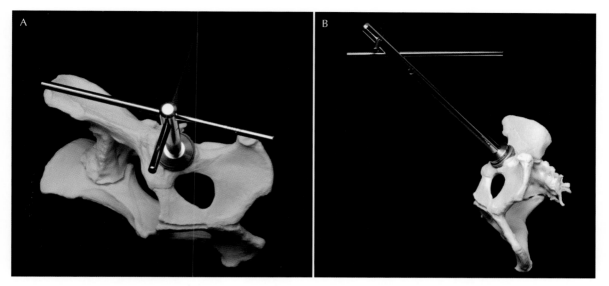

Figure 7.31   Acetabular cup impactor/positioning guide. The sagittal bar is parallel to a line connecting the center of the wing of the ilium to the center of the ischiatic tuberosity (A). This bar sets the retroversion angle of the acetabular component. The transverse bar is set parallel to the floor to achieve an angle of lateral opening of 45 degrees. (Image courtesy of Kyon, Zurich, Switzerland)

cranial and caudal rims of the cup should be of equal depth relative to the cranial and caudal poles of the acetabulum. This is more difficult to evaluate in more severely deformed acetabula. In general, the number of rows of cup perforations that are visible dorsally, with an appropriate ALO, correspond to the cup size: 21.5-mm cup—one row; 23.5-mm cup—one to two rows; 26.5-mm cup—two to three rows; 29.5- or 32.5-mm cup—three to four rows. However, this is less reliable when substantial dorsal rim loss is present. The surgeon should confirm the stability of the press-fit with manual pressure and should confirm that full circumferential implant/bone contact is present. A trial reduction using an unfixed stem with a short neck is performed to confirm that reduction is possible. Even if the trial stem is not rotationally stable and can subside, it offers a rough guide to reduction as well as cup position. For the evaluation of cup positioning, with the hip in a weight-bearing position, the plane of the equator of the femoral head should be roughly parallel with the plane of the face of the cup. An alternative method for evaluation of the ability to reduce the hip involves placing the spherical impactor into the acetabulum. If a short head/

neck will be reducible, the upper portion of the small drill guide should fit between the osteotomy and the impactor shaft.

Femoral stem fixation

Screw fixation of the femoral stem is performed with the aid of a self-retaining jig attached to the threads within the stem trunion. Secure, well-aligned fixation is critical and jig-stem alignment is confirmed using the large drill guide at the distal stem hole, ensuring that the guide hole and stem hole are congruent. The 4.5-mm drill bit, used for the lateral cortical guide hole, is adjusted to ensure that it does not contact the stem during drilling. The femur is lateralized manually or using the Hohmann as described in the "Femoral Preparation" section. The stem is inserted into the medullary canal in an orientation similar to the orientation created by femoral canal preparation. Prior to screw fixation, stem position must be evaluated for medial cortical contact, appropriate anteversion angle and adequate seating depth. A gap between the medial cortex and the proximal part of the stem suggests one of three problems. First, the gluteal musculature may impinge on the jig and force the stem laterally. This is more common in well-muscled dogs, particularly those with large-diameter femoral canals. Second, the femoral osteotomy may be too proximal and the curvature of the femoral neck at the calcar is not aligned with the medial cortex. Third, there may have been inadequate removal of cancellous bone from the medial cortex during femoral canal preparation. With the limb held parallel to the table, stem anteversion is evaluated based on the angle of the jig relative to a vertical plane perpendicular to the femur (Figure 7.32). The angle should be approximately 20 degrees.

The order of screw placement is 3, 1, 2, 4, 5. Until the first screw is tightened, the assistant must not shift limb position and the surgeon must avoid shifting the position of the jig. The guide hole in the lateral cortex is made using a 4.5-mm drill bit through the large drill guide. While drilling (Figure 7.33), lavage is provided at the level of the hole located at the base of the drill guide. Next, the small drill guide is inserted into the guide hole and debris is flushed with pulsatile lavage through the drill guide. The drill guide is then placed into the stem hole and kept centered on the jig. A 3.0-mm bit is used to drill the medial cortex, taking care not to exert excessive force (Figure 7.33). The

hole is flushed again after removal of the drill. The 3.4-mm conical screw is then inserted and firmly tightened (Figure 7.33). Stem position is rechecked before proceeding. A bicortical screw is generally placed in the most proximal hole. A depth gauge on the drill guide is used to determine bicortical screw length and screws are available in 5-mm increments. The remaining holes are drilled as described above. The screws are retightened in the

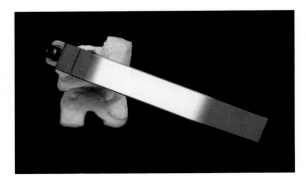

Figure 7.32 Axial proximal-distal image of the right femur with the attached jig. Anteversion of the femoral stem is established as the angle of the jig relative to a medial-to-lateral line perpendicular to the long axis of the femur. (Image courtesy of Kyon, Zurich, Switzerland)

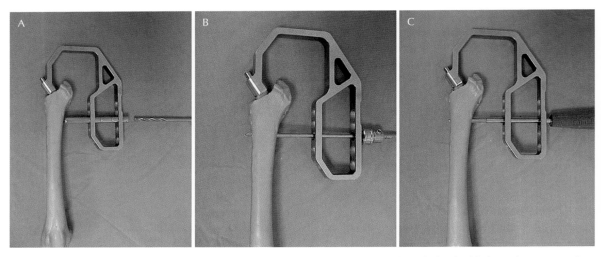

Figure 7.33 The first screw placed is screw number 3. The drill guide is inserted through the third hole in the jig. A guide hole is drilled in the lateral cortex using a 4.5-mm drill bit (A). The drill sleeve is inserted through the 4.5-mm guide hole and inserted into the hole in the femoral stem. A 3.0-mm drill bit is used to drill the hole in the medial cortex (B). The conical screw is then inserted and tightened (C).

order in which they were placed and the jig is removed.

Trial reduction

The length of the head/neck component is estimated by observing the distance between the trunion and the cup with moderate tension applied to the distal portion of the femur and with the femur perpendicular to the body. A trial set of head/neck components should be used to avoid damage to the implanted head/neck. The femur is externally rotated and the head/neck component is gently tapped using the head impactor. The hip can be reduced using the reduction hook. The head is positioned cranial to the acetabulum before pulling distally then caudally for reduction. Having an assistant pull on the limb seemingly makes reduction more difficult. An alternative method of reduction utilizes a small Hohmann retractor, with the tip placed as described for femoral retraction during acetabular preparation. The shaft of the Hohmann levers between the greater trochanter and the base of the femoral neck. Easy reduction does not imply an unstable hip. Likewise, a very tight reduction does not imply a stable hip. If appropriate steps are followed during the procedure, hip reduction should be possible. However, in the event that the hip cannot be reduced, several strategies are available. From simplest to most challenging, these include using a shorter femoral head/neck, performing a pectineal tenotomy, performing a tenotomy of internal obturator, removing the cup and reaming deeper, repositioning the cup to a more open or more anteverted position, and repositioning the stem in a more distal position. Following reduction of the hip, the construct must be evaluated for resistance to luxation. The hip is externally rotated in both weight-bearing and extended positions to evaluate for craniodorsal luxation. Osteophytes causing impingement should be removed. Next, the hip is placed in full flexion and internally rotated, as well as abducted, to evaluate for caudal/caudoventral luxation. The craniodorsal aspect of the acetabulum is evaluated for impingement while testing for caudal/caudoventral luxation. If impingement or luxation occurs during testing, the easiest option is to try a longer head/neck component, if possible. If that is not possible,

or is ineffective in controlling luxation, the cup will need to be repositioned.

Cup repositioning

Cup repositioning can be attempted without removing the cup. The head/neck component is removed by using the pointed impactor placed in the "dimple" on the reduction hook. The impactor is tapped and the head/neck component removed. If luxation is in a craniodorsal direction the cup should be further closed and/or retroverted. If the luxation is caudal/caudoventral, the cup should be opened and/or anteverted. The cup positioner is placed in the cup and moderate pressure is applied in the desired direction of correction while moderately tapping the impactor with the mallet. The pointed impactor can be applied to the titanium rim of the acetabular cup for repositioning as well. However, this risks damage or deformation of the cup, necessitating replacement with a new cup.

If the cup must be removed to achieve repositioning, or if additional reaming is necessary, several techniques may be used for cup removal. A small Hohmann can be hooked under the ventromedial aspect of the cup and leverage applied as described for reduction. Alternatively, the surgeon can attempt to wedge a Freer elevator between the acetabular bed and the shell to pry the cup loose. Finally, the pointed impactor can be applied to the dorsomedial aspect of the shell and tapped with moderate force. This final method risks damage to the cup, necessitating replacement with a new cup. If the press-fit is lost in the process of repositioning, options include increasing cup size (if possible), use of the Zurich Cementless revision cup, cementing a Zurich cup, or use of a custom femoral head with a CFX or BFX cup. After repositioning, the process of reduction and testing is repeated. Once the appropriate neck length has been determined, the head is assembled to the femoral stem. Wound closure is as described in the Universal Hip section. Postoperative radiographs are made using the same technique as described for the preoperative assessment and templating; however, the ventrodorsal projection of the pelvis is not used for evaluation of implant positioning because a complete assessment may be made using the lateral, craniocaudal

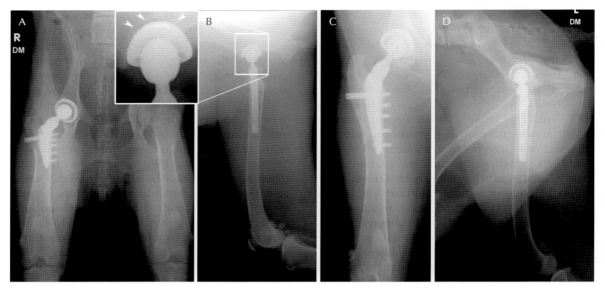

Figure 7.34 Postoperative radiographs of a Zurich Cementless hip replacement. The ventrodorsal, hip-extended view (A) is not utilized for evaluation of implant position. The open-leg medial-lateral view (B) is primarily used for evaluation of full seating of the acetabular component. The arrowheads on the inset indicate the lucent zone at the pole of the implant. The lucency is present because the prepared bed is a hemisphere, but the acetabular component is flattened at the pole. Also note the slight caudal tipping of the femoral component, which suggests that the initial opening of the femoral canal was more proximal than is ideal (B). Cross-table cranial-caudal view of the femur (C). This view is used to evaluate medial cortical contact of the prosthesis and to ensure that all screws are fully inserted. The tips of all screws should be aligned. The medial-lateral view of the pelvis (D) is the main view used to evaluate the angle of lateral opening of the acetabular component as well as its anteversion/retroversion angle.

horizontal beam, and open-leg lateral views (Figure 7.34).

Evaluation of acetabular component positioning for the universal hip system and zurich cementless hip

From the postoperative lateral pelvic radiograph, the anteversion/retroversion angle of the cup is determined based on a line connecting the center of the wing of the ilium to the center of the ischiatic tuberosity. The cup version angle is the angle created by the intersection of the above line with a line drawn through the long axis of the ellipse of the acetabular cup created by the lateral radiographic projection. The ALO is computed based on the $\sin^{-1}$ of the short axis (SA) of the ellipse divided by its long axis (LA) of the cup, forming the following equation:

$$\text{ALO} = \sin^{-1}\frac{\text{SA}}{\text{LA}}.$$

Several other methods for evaluation of acetabular component positioning have been described. They are described in Chapter 6.

Endnotes

1. Matis U, Holz I. Cemented total hip replacement in small dogs—The European experience. In: *Proceedings of the 2008 European Society of Veterinary Orthopaedics and Traumatology Meeting.* Munich, Germany, 2008, pp. 140–141.
2. Roe S, Marcellin-Little D, Lascelles D. Short-term outcome of uncemented THR. In: *Proceedings of the 2010 American College of Veterinary Surgeons Veterinary Symposium.* Seattle, WA, 2010.
3. Vezzoni A. Kyon cementless hip: My first 1000 cases. In: *Proceedings of the 2011 American College of Veterinary Surgeons Veterinary Symposium.* Chicago, IL, 2011.
4. Tepic S. Development and mechanical basis for Kyon THR. In: *Proceedings of the 2004 Annual American College of Veterinary Surgeons Forum.* Denver, CO, 2004, pp. 289–291.

5. Tepic S, Bresina S, Hintner M, et al. Reduced wear of UHMWPE THR liner with modified contact geometry (abstract). In: *Proceedings of the 2007 Orthopaedic Research Society Meeting*. San Diego, CA, 2007.

References

Andrews CM, Liska WD, Roberts DJ. Sciatic neurapraxia as a complication in 1000 consecutive canine total hip replacements. Vet Surg 2008;37:254–262.

Bergh MS, Gilley RS, Shofer FS, et al. Complications and radiographic findings following cemented total hip replacement: A retrospective evaluation of 97 dogs. Vet Comp Orthop Traumatol 2006;19:172–179.

Bishop NE, Waldow F, Morlock MM. Friction moments of large metal-on-metal hip joint bearings and other modern designs. Med Eng Phys 2008;30:1057–1064.

Bragdon CR, Jasty M, Greene M, et al. Biologic fixation of total hip implants. Insights gained from a series of canine studies. J Bone Joint Surg Am 2004;86(Suppl. 2):105–117.

Budsberg SC, Chambers JN, Lue SL, et al. Prospective evaluation of ground reaction forces in dogs undergoing unilateral total hip replacement. Am J Vet Res 1996;57:1781–1785.

Charnley J. Anchorage of the femoral head prosthesis to the shaft of the femur. J Bone Joint Surg Br 1960;42-B:28–30.

Charnley J. Total hip replacement by low-friction arthroplasty. Clin Orthop Relat Res 1970;72:7–21.

Chen PQ, Turner TM, Ronnigen H, et al. A canine cementless total hip prosthesis model. Clin Orthop Relat Res 1983;176:24–33.

Cross AR, Newell SM, Chambers JN, et al. Acetabular component orientation as an indicator of implant luxation in cemented total hip arthroplasty. Vet Surg 2000;29:517–523.

DeYoung DJ, Schiller RA. Radiographic criteria for evaluation of uncemented total hip replacement in dogs. Vet Surg 1992;21:88–98.

DeYoung DJ, DeYoung BA, Aberman HA, et al. Implantation of an uncemented total hip prosthesis. Technique and initial results of 100 arthroplasties. Vet Surg 1992;21:168–177.

DeYoung DJ, Schiller RA, DeYoung BA. Radiographic assessment of a canine uncemented porous-coated anatomic total hip prosthesis. Vet Surg 1993;22:473–481.

Dyce J, Wisner ER, Wang Q, et al. Evaluation of risk factors for luxation after total hip replacement in dogs. Vet Surg 2000;29:524–532.

Edwards MR, Egger EL, Schwarz PD. Aseptic loosening of the femoral implant after cemented total hip arthroplasty in dogs: 11 cases in 10 dogs (1991–1995). J Am Vet Med Assoc 1997;211:580–586.

Fitzpatrick N, Pratola L, Yeadon R et al. Total hip replacement after failed femoral head and neck excision in two dogs and two cats. Vet Surg 2012;41:136–142.

Gorman HA. A new prosthetic hip joint; experiences in its use in the dog, and its probable application to man. Mil Med 1957;121:91–93.

Guerrero TG, Montavon PM. Zurich cementless total hip replacement: Retrospective evaluation of 2nd generation implants in 60 dogs. Vet Surg 2009;38:70–80.

Hach V, Delfs G. Initial experience with a newly developed cementless hip endoprosthesis. Vet Comp Orthop Traumatol 2009;22:153–158.

Haney DR, Peck JN. Influence of canal preparation depth on the incidence of femoral medullary infarction with Zurich Cementless Canine Total Hip arthroplasty. Vet Surg 2009;38:673–676.

Hanson SP, Peck JN, Berry CR, et al. Radiographic evaluation of the Zurich cementless total hip acetabular component. Vet Surg 2006;35:550–558.

Hayes GM, Ramirez J, Langley Hobbs SJ. Does the degree of preoperative subluxation or soft tissue tension affect the incidence of postoperative luxation in dogs after total hip replacement? Vet Surg 2011a;40:6–13.

Hayes GM, Ramirez J, Langley Hobbs SJ. Use of the cumulative summation technique to quantitatively assess a surgical learning curve: Canine total hip replacement. Vet Surg 2011b;40:1–5.

Hummel DW, Lanz OI, Werre SR. Complications of cementless total hip replacement. A retrospective study of 163 cases. Vet Comp Orthop Traumatol 2010;23:424–432.

Ireifej S, Marino D, Laughin C. Nano total hip replacement in 12 dogs. Vet Surg 2012;41:130–135.

Jankovits DA, Liska WD, Kalis RH. Treatment of avascular necrosis of the femoral head in small dogs with micro total hip replacement. Vet Surg 2012;41:143–147.

Kalis RH, Liska WD, Jankovits DA. Total hip replacement as a treatment option for capital physeal fractures in dogs and cats. Vet Surg 2012;41:148–155.

Kim JY, Hayashi K, Garcia TC, et al. Biomechanical evaluation of screw-in femoral implant in cementless total hip system. Vet Surg 2012;41:94–102.

Lascelles BD, Freire M, Roe SC, et al. Evaluation of functional outcome after BFX total hip replacement using a pressure sensitive walkway. Vet Surg 2010;39:71–77.

Lauer SK, Nieves MA, Peck J, et al. Descriptive histomorphometric ingrowth analysis of the Zurich cementless canine total hip acetabular component. Vet Surg 2009;38:59–69.

Liska WD. Femur fractures associated with canine total hip replacement. Vet Surg 2004;33:164–172.

Liska WD. Micro total hip replacement for dogs and cats: Surgical technique and outcomes. Vet Surg 2010;39:797–810.

Liska WD, Poteet BA. Pulmonary embolism associated with canine total hip replacement. Vet Surg 2003;32:178–186.

Liska WD, Doyle N, Marcellin-Little DJ, et al. Total hip replacement in three cats: Surgical technique, short-term outcome and comparison to femoral head ostectomy. Vet Comp Orthop Traumatol 2009;22:505–510.

Liska WD, Doyle ND, Schwartz Z. Successful revision of a femoral head ostectomy (complicated by postoperative sciatic neurapraxia) to a total hip replacement in a cat. Vet Comp Orthop Traumatol 2010;23:119–123.

Magnuson PB. Technique of debridement of the knee joint for arthritis. Surg Clin North Am 1946;26:249–266.

Marcellin-Little DJ. Medical treatment of coxofemoral joint disease. In: Kirk's Current Veterinary Therapy XIV, Bonagura JD, Twedt DC (eds.). Philadelphia: Elsevier, 2008, pp. 1120–1125.

Marcellin-Little DJ, DeYoung BA, Doyens DH, et al. Canine uncemented porous-coated anatomic total hip arthroplasty: Results of a long-term prospective evaluation of 50 consecutive cases. Vet Surg 1999a;28:10–20.

Marcellin-Little DJ, DeYoung DJ, Thrall DE, et al. Osteosarcoma at the site of bone infarction associated with total hip arthroplasty in a dog. Vet Surg 1999b;28:54–60.

Marsolais GS, Peck JN, Berry CR et al. Femoral medullary infarction prevalence with the Zurich Cementless total hip arthroplasty. Vet Surg 2009;38:677–680.

Massat BJ, Vasseur PB. Clinical and radiographic results of total hip arthroplasty in dogs: 96 cases (1986–1992). J Am Vet Med Assoc 1994;205:448–454.

Massat BJ, Miller RT, DeYoung BA, et al. Single-stage revision using an uncemented, porous-coated, anatomic endoprosthesis in two dogs: Case report. Vet Surg 1998;27:268–277.

Mawby DI, Bartges JW, d'Avignon A, et al. Comparison of various methods for estimating body fat in dogs. J Am Anim Hosp Assoc 2004;40:109–114.

McCulloch RS, Roe SC, Marcellin-Little DJ, et al. Resistance to subsidence of an uncemented femoral stem after cerclage wiring of a fissure. Vet Surg 2012;41:163–167.

Montgomery RD, Milton JL, Pernell R, et al. Total hip arthroplasty for treatment of canine hip dysplasia. Vet Clin North Am Small Anim Pract 1992;22:703–719.

Nelson LL, Dyce J, Shott S. Risk factors for ventral luxation in canine total hip replacement. Vet Surg 2007;36:644–653.

Off W, Matis U. Excision arthroplasty of the hip joint in dogs and cats. Clinical, radiographic, and gait analysis findings from the Department of Surgery, Veterinary Faculty of the Ludwig-Maximilians-University of Munich, Germany. Vet Comp Orthop Traumatol 2010;23:297–305.

Olmstead ML. Total hip replacement in the dog. Semin Vet Med Surg (Small Anim) 1987;2:131–140.

Olmstead ML. Canine cemented total hip replacements: State of the art. J Small Anim Pract 1995a;36:395–399.

Olmstead ML. The canine cemented modular total hip prosthesis. J Am Anim Hosp Assoc 1995b;31:109–124.

Olmstead ML, Hohn RB, Turner TM. A five-year study of 221 total hip replacements in the dog. J Am Vet Med Assoc 1983;183:191–194.

Ota J, Cook JL, Lewis DD, et al. Short-term aseptic loosening of the femoral component in canine total hip replacement: Effects of cementing technique on cement mantle grade. Vet Surg 2005;34:345–352.

Otto K, Matis U. Changes in cardiopulmonary variables and platelet count during anesthesia for total hip replacement in dogs. Vet Surg 1994;23:266–273.

Paul HA, Bargar WL. Histologic changes in the dog femur following total hip replacement with current cementing techniques. J Arthroplasty 1986;1:5–9.

Paul HA, Bargar WL. Histologic changes in the dog acetabulum following total hip replacement with current cementing techniques. J Arthroplasty 1987;2:71–76.

Paul HA, Bargar WL, Mittlestadt B, et al. Development of a surgical robot for cementless total hip arthroplasty. Clin Orthop Relat Res 1992;285:57–66.

Piermattei DJ, Johnson KA. Approach to the craniodorsal aspect of the hip joint through a craniolateral incision. In: An Atlas of Surgical Approaches to the Bones and Joints of the Dog and Cat, Piermattei DJ, Johnson KA (eds.), 4th ed. Philadelphia: WB Saunders, 2004, pp. 290–295.

Pozzi A, Kowaleski MP, Dyce J, et al. Treatment of traumatic coxofemoral luxation by cemented total hip arthroplasty. Vet Comp Orthop Traumatol 2004;17:198–203.

Schiller TD, DeYoung DJ, Schiller RA, et al. Quantitative ingrowth analysis of a porous-coated acetabular component in a canine model. Vet Surg 1993;22:276–280.

Sebestyen P, Marcellin-Little DJ, DeYoung BA. Femoral medullary infarction secondary to canine total hip arthroplasty. Vet Surg 2000;29:227–236.

Shahar R, Banks-Sills L, Eliasy R. Mechanics of the canine femur with two types of hip replacement stems. Vet Comp Orthop Traumatol 2003;16:145–152.

Skurla CP, James SP. Postmortem retrieved canine THR: Femoral and acetabular component interaction. Biomed Sci Instrum 2004;40:255–260.

Skurla CP, James SP. Assessing the dog as a model for human total hip replacement: Analysis of 38 postmortem-retrieved canine cemented acetabular components. J Biomed Mater Res B Appl Biomater 2005;73:260–270.

Skurla CP, Pluhar GE, Frankel DJ, et al. Assessing the dog as a model for human total hip replacement. Analysis of 38 canine cemented femoral components retrieved at post-mortem. J Bone Joint Surg Br 2005;87:120–127.

Smith GK, Langenbach A, Green PA, et al. Evaluation of the association between medial patellar luxation and hip dysplasia in cats. J Am Vet Med Assoc 1999;215:40–45.

Stone MH, Wilkinson R, Stother IG. Some factors affecting the strength of the cement-metal interface. J Bone Joint Surg Br 1989;71:217–221.

Sumner DR, Turner TM, Pierson RH, et al. Effects of radiation on fixation of non-cemented porous-coated implants in a canine model. J Bone Joint Surg Am 1990;72:1527–1533.

Tidwell SA, Graham JP, Peck JN, et al. Incidence of pulmonary embolism after non-cemented total hip arthroplasty in eleven dogs: Computed tomographic pulmonary angiography and pulmonary perfusion scintigraphy. Vet Surg 2007;36:37–42.

Torres BT, Budsberg SC. Revision of cemented total hip arthroplasty with cementless components in three dogs. Vet Surg 2009;38:81–86.

Warnock JJ, Dyce J, Pooya H, et al. Retrospective analysis of canine miniature total hip prostheses. Vet Surg 2003;32:285–291.

8 Revision Strategies for Total Hip Replacement

Jeffrey N. Peck and Denis J. Marcellin-Little

Despite careful patient selection, preoperative planning, and skillful surgical execution, complications occur. An awareness of the risks of such complications and the means to correct the correctible complications is as important as the knowledge and ability to perform the initial surgery. In general, complications can be divided into those that are the result of either mechanical failure or biological failure. Subtle or obvious errors in surgical technique are often the root cause of complications, regardless of the mode of failure. Therefore, whenever possible, the revision strategy should correct, or at least not repeat, the original error. This requires that the surgeon recognize the factors that led to failure.

Mechanical failure

Complications associated with mechanical failure include femoral or acetabular fracture, luxation, cup or stem avulsion, stem subsidence, and implant failure.

Femur fracture

The Vancouver classification for periprosthetic femur fractures associated with human total hip replacement (THR) was described in 1999 (Table 8.1; Brady et al. 1999; Masri et al. 2004). This classification scheme is based on the location of the fracture, the stability of the implant, and the quality of the bone stock.

The etiology of femoral fracture varies with the implant system used and typical Vancouver fracture classifications illustrate the variation. Femur fractures that occur with the BFX stem (BioMedtrix, Boonton, NJ) are typically associated with subsidence of the femoral stem and are most often Vancouver classification B2 fractures. However, it may be unclear whether fractures occur because of stem subsidence or vice versa. Subsidence can occur due to undersizing or because of incomplete impaction (see Chapter 7). Noncatastrophic fractures can be managed with the use of multiple cerclage wires. The use of multiple, double-loop cerclage wires was recently reported to result in

Advances in Small Animal Total Joint Replacement, First Edition. Edited by Jeffrey N. Peck and Denis J. Marcellin-Little.
© 2013 John Wiley & Sons, Inc. Published 2013 by John Wiley & Sons, Inc.

Table 8.1   Vancouver periprosthetic fracture classification

Category	Fracture level	Stem stability	Bone quality
A$_G$	Greater trochanter	Stable	Good
A$_L$	Lesser trochanter	Stable	Good
B$_1$	Involves prosthesis	Stable	Good
B$_2$	Involves prosthesis	Unstable	Good
B$_3$	Involves prosthesis	Unstable	Poor
C	Distal to prosthesis	Stable	Good

Source: Adapted from Masri et al. (2004).

greater resistance to failure than the intact femur (McCulloch et al. 2012). The current recommendations for BFX implantation are to place double-loop cerclages prophylactically in patients who appear to be predisposed to fissures, including giant-breed dogs with thin cortices, older dogs, and dogs with "stovepipe" femora (DeYoung and Schiller 1992; Figure 8.1). For most dogs, the wire size is 18 gauge (1 mm). A double-loop cerclage is placed around the femoral shaft proximal to the lesser trochanter, making sure that the wire does not interfere with femoral canal opening on the caudal aspect of the trochanteric fossa. A second double-loop cerclage wire is placed around the femoral shaft distal to the lesser trochanter. If a fissure develops during broaching, the broach is removed and the vastus lateralis is reflected distally to identify the distal extent of the fissure. Double-loop cerclage wires are placed along the femoral shaft every 15 mm so that the most distal double-loop cerclage is distal to the distal aspect of the fissure. The sides of the fissure should contact each other (i.e., no fissure gap) after the cerclage wires are placed. The fissure should not open during broaching or during stem placement. The arms of the double-loop cerclage wires can lift off the bone during broaching or during stem placement. If this occurs, the arms should be fully bent back after stem placement. If a long fissure

occurs early in the broaching process, conversion to a cemented stem should be considered.

Femur fractures associated with the use of the CFX system (BioMedtrix) most often occur at the level of the tip of the stem and are associated with a stress riser at that location. These are most often Vancouver classification type C fractures that are generally oblique fractures and frequently have concurrent loss of the cement mantle at the tip of the stem. Alternatively, fractures after cemented THR can be associated with the lack of a cement mantle at the stem tip due to varus stem placement and direct stem contact with the endosteum.

Femoral fractures associated with the Zurich system (Kyon, Zurich, Switzerland) appear to be associated with torsional failure through either the lateral guide holes or through the medial screw holes (Figure 8.2). Most often, these fractures are Vancouver classification type B1 fractures. They are generally long-oblique or spiral fractures that most frequently originate at the level of the one or two most distal holes. Occasionally, the fracture will traverse the entire length of the implant and involve both the medial and lateral drill holes. Most often, anatomical reconstruction of the fracture can be achieved using cerclage wiring. With anatomical reconstruction and appropriate wire tension, stem screws in a fracture-involved screw hole can often be salvaged. Additionally, mono-cortical stem screws can be replaced with bicortical screws. However, inadequate medial screw purchase cannot be compensated for with the use of bicortical screws. Following anatomical reconstruction, the fracture is protected using a neutralization plate. It may not be feasible to apply even monocortical screws along the length of the femoral stem and the plate must extend from the most proximal aspect of the greater trochanter. Given the limited availability of proximal bone stock, use of a locking plate may be advisable (Fitzpatrick et al. 2012). However, the superiority of locking implants in this situation is not proven (Figure 8.3). If more than two stem screws are involved in the fracture, or if anatomical reconstruction is not feasible, explantation may be necessary.

Repositioning of the implant can be considered; however, the surgeon must balance the desire to maintain the femoral stem with the knowledge

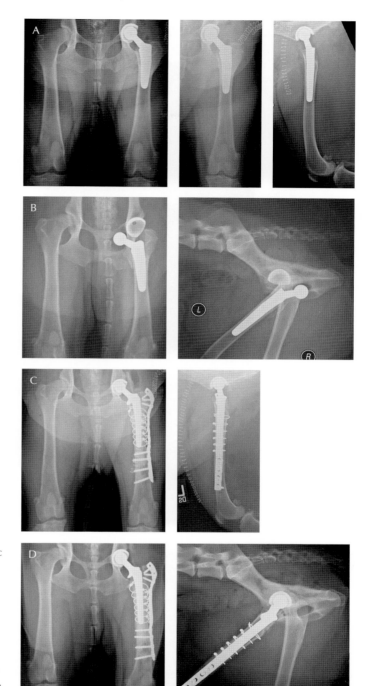

Figure 8.1 Immediate postoperative radiographic views (A) following BFX THR in a 5-year-old golden retriever; implant sizes were #9 stem, 28-mm cup, and 17 mm +3 head. Acute onset lameness occurred 2 weeks postoperatively and radiographs (B) revealed that stem subsidence, retroversion, and femoral fracture have occurred. The fracture was stabilized with single-loop cerclage wire; the stem was revised to a CFX #8 and a limited-contact dynamic compression plate (LC-DCP) was placed as a neutralization plate (C). Twelve weeks postoperatively, the fracture is healed, and the implants are stable (D).

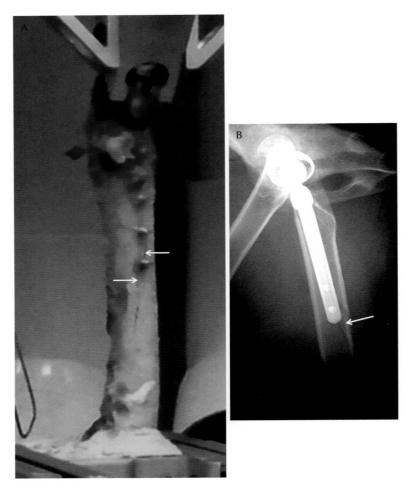

Figure 8.2 Photograph (A) made during torsional load-to-failure testing of Zurich Cementless femoral stem-femur construct with a Universal Testing machine (Instron, Norwood, MA). A fracture line is visible on the medial aspect of the femoral shaft (arrows). This fracture line is typically associated with the distal stem screw. On a radiograph of a clinical patient (B), a fissure is visible at the typical site of initiation of fracture.

that further weakening of the femur will occur with additional drill holes. Consideration should also be given to the feasibility of revision with either a BFX or CFX stem. Explantation with fracture repair and future reimplantation can be considered; however, the proximal femoral migration that occurs with femoral head and neck excision (FHNE) may complicate later reduction. Additionally, sclerosis may develop at the neck ostectomy site and great care will need to be taken with repreparation of the femoral canal.

For Vancouver classification type B3 fractures (i.e., unstable stem and poor bone quality), cortical strut allografts have been used in human patients to provide bone stock for fixation (Learmonth 2004). With this technique, two halves of an appropriately sized cortical allograft are applied to the host femur in a "clam shell" fashion and stabilized using cerclage wires. Plate fixation can then be applied to the graft, incorporating the host bone. Alternatively, a customized prosthesis can be fashioned for the patient, as described in Chapter 14.

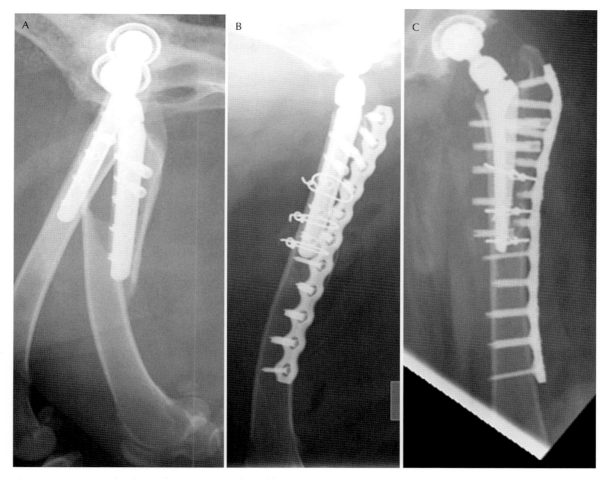

Figure 8.3   (A) Lateral radiographic projection of an oblique femur fracture following THR with a Zurich Cementless hip. (B and C) The femur was stabilized using a locking plate (ALPS, Kyon, Zurich, Switzerland) and single-loop cerclage wires. (Images courtesy of Dr. Aldo Vezzoni)

Acetabular fracture

Acetabular fracture after THR is far less common than femoral fracture, but is much more difficult to manage without reverting to FHNE. Reimpacting a press-fit acetabular component following fracture repair, in a single-stage procedure, is unlikely to achieve a stable prosthesis and is quite likely to result in failure of fixation. Cementing of the acetabular component is the most common method used in cases of single-stage revision of a press-fit component with acetabular fracture.

Custom femoral head/neck components are available from Kyon to allow the use of a CFX cup. Acetabular fractures occurring during implantation of a BFX press-fit cup have been anecdotally reported. In one instance, a fracture with minor displacement was successfully managed conservatively.[1] A single case report describes the use of a corticocancellous autograft from the wing of the ilium in the repair of a comminuted, periprosthetic acetabular fracture in a dog (Torres et al. 2009). A 2.7/3.5-mm reconstruction plate was anchored to the donor and recipient bone, and reaming and cup impaction were performed as usual. The dog reportedly had normal limb function at 19-month follow-up.

Luxation

Dorsal or ventral luxation of the replaced hip most often occurs in the first few weeks after hip replacement surgery. However, late luxations can occur months, or even years, later. Early luxations are most often associated with errors in implant positioning with secondary impingement, or in choice of neck length (i.e., too much laxity), while late luxations are most often, but not always, associated with trauma. Dorsal luxations can result from excessively large angles of lateral opening (ALOs) and ventral luxations can result from excessively small ALOs (see Chapter 7). Impingement of the prosthetic neck on the rim of the acetabular component, periarticular soft tissues, or periarticular osteophytes results in a levering of the femoral head from the acetabular cup. A further description of impingement is found in Chapter 6. Luxations secondary to laxity may occur in dogs with chronic dorsal displacement of the femur before surgery. At the time of surgery, tissue tightness may lead to the selection of a relatively short femoral neck. A few weeks later, with relaxation of the periarticular tissues, the prosthetic hip may be lax and may luxate. An additional risk factor for luxation is a contralateral hind limb amputation (Preston et al. 1999) because, in amputees, the pelvis is tilted down on the amputated side, resulting in decreased dorsal coverage of the prosthetic head by the cup. In addition to careful radiographic evaluation of implant position, the direction of luxation must be confirmed in surgery.

Management of THR luxations

Some THR luxations can be successfully managed with closed reduction and activity supervision for several weeks, but most THR luxations cannot be closed reduced or are managed surgically to eliminate the factors predisposing to luxation.

The joint should be reduced during surgery and the luxation should be recreated in order to determine the chain of events leading to that luxation. Caudoventral luxations can migrate such that, on

a lateral radiographic view, the femoral head is dorsal to the acetabulum. Increasing neck length is the simplest surgical method of dealing with luxation. Even in cases where cup positioning is not ideal, increasing neck length may adequately lateralize the femur and prevent impingement. However, increased neck length can result in a higher risk of femur fracture, greater postoperative discomfort, and in gait abnormalities (externally rotated limb) because of tension in the external rotator muscles.

Repositioning of the acetabular component, femoral component, or both is often the most appropriate means for preventing reluxation. Acetabular repositioning is most common. While techniques such as placement of an iliofemoral internal rotation suture or pelvic osteotomy (Dyce et al. 2000) may successfully prevent reluxation in some cases, the surgeon must critically evaluate implant positioning to determine the best course of action.

In general, craniodorsal luxation is associated with an increased ALO, excessive anteversion of the cup or stem, or any combination of these. Conversely, caudal or caudoventral luxation may be associated with the opposite positioning errors. Peculiarities of individual patient conformation can also contribute to luxation risk.

For BFX cups, if luxation occurs before bone ingrowth occurs (i.e., during the first few days that follow cup placement), the cup may be removed by tapping its most dorsal aspect and by rotating the cup out of its bone bed. If the cup is not damaged, it may be reimplanted with proper orientation (Figure 8.4). If bone ingrowth into the cup has occurred, the cup may be removed by tapping a thin osteotome on its medial aspect. Ideally, the osteotome should be curved to minimize bone loss (Hip Preservation Surgery Set, Synthes, West Chester, PA). For a BFX cup, the bone bed is most often reamed with a starter reamer that is 1 mm larger than the cup that was removed, followed by a finishing reamer that is 2 mm larger than the cup that was removed. A new cup is placed.

For cemented cups, the cup and polymethylmethacrylate (PMMA) may be removed with a large rongeur used to hold the cup and to rotate it ventrally or by placing a thin osteotome medial to the cement mantle. All PMMA should be removed from the bone bed and the keyholes. A new cemented cup is placed.

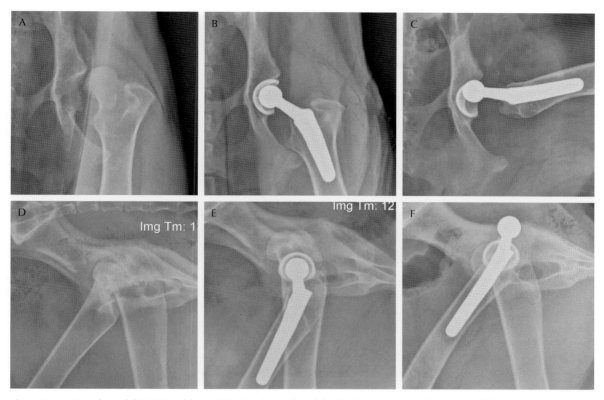

Figure 8.4   Cranial-caudal (A–C) and lateral (D–F) radiographs of the left hip joint of an 11-month-old Saint Bernard. Preoperatively (A and D), the hip joint is dorsally luxated. A cementless total hip replacement was performed (B and E). Postoperatively, the cup appears open (i.e., its angle of lateral opening [ALO] appears excessive). The prosthesis luxated dorsally after surgery (C and F). While the cause of luxation was not known, the large ALO and the preexisting luxation increased the likelihood of luxation. The luxation was successfully revised with an open reduction and the placement of monofilament nylon sutures connecting the greater trochanter to the iliopubic eminence.

Repositioning of the acetabular component with a well-seated Zurich prosthesis without damage to the previously placed cup can be challenging. The surgeon should be prepared to place a new acetabular component. If the cup is well seated, and if it has been in place for several weeks, cup repositioning will almost certainly require cup removal. However, the surgeon should first attempt to manipulate cup position as described in Chapter 7. If press-fit of the same size cup cannot be achieved, then a larger cup can be used, following appropriate reaming. Alternatively, a Zurich Cementless Revision Cup (discussed later) can be used. Prior to removal of a Zurich Cementless, anatomical landmarks should be identified, cup position should be assessed, and changes in cup position should be planned (Figure 8.5). For

example, if the ALO needs to be decreased, the surgeon should note the number of rows of visible shell holes at the dorsal rim (e.g., if only one row is visible, the cup should be repositioned such that two or three rows are visible). Cup removal can be accomplished in several ways. One method that is least likely to damage the component is the use of a small Hohmann retractor placed ventral to the ventral rim of the acetabular component and then applying distal force to the handle of the retractor. Alternatively, the pointed impactor or other tapered, blunt instrument can be placed at the exposed dorsal rim and blunt force used to dislodge the cup. Any deformation of the titanium shell or polyethylene liner necessitates placement of a new cup. A press-fit is imperative for long-term success. Kyon has

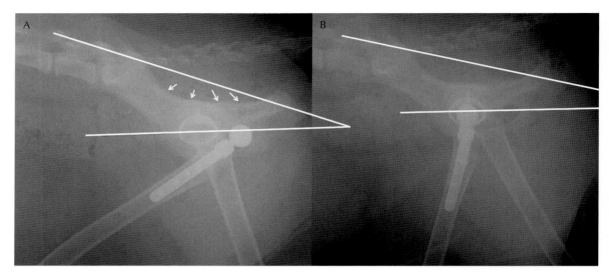

Figure 8.5　Caudoventral luxation (A), 1 week after total hip replacement in a 2-year-old Labrador retriever with a concave or "saddle-shaped" pelvis (arrows). The initial retroversion angle of the cup (21 degrees) does not appear excessive. However, this pelvic conformation may predispose to caudal or caudoventral luxation. The cup was repositioned to a greater ALO and was placed in less retroversion (B). After repositioning, the retroversion angle is 15 degrees.

recently developed a revision cup that has a titanium shell with multiple divergent screw holes that accommodate 2.4-mm screws (Figure 8.6). Once the shell is seated and screwed into place, the corresponding cup can be impacted into the shell. Long-term follow-up is not available for the revision cup.

In some cases, initial cup malpositioning (e.g., an excessively large ALO) may have been the result of recognition of inadequate dorsal rim or caudal rim bone support for the prosthesis. If repositioning is necessary in such cases, dorsal rim augmentation can be considered (Pooya et al. 2003; Torres et al. 2009). Caudal rim augmentation has not been described in the veterinary literature. If possible, reaming the acetabulum more deeply will improve coverage but it will increase laxity and will necessitate increased neck length. Reconstruction rings, as well as tantalum augments, are described in the aseptic loosening section of this chapter. Repositioning of the Zurich stem to a more anteverted or retroverted position should be undertaken with extreme caution because of the number of consequent open holes in the femur. If a femoral window was created for retrieval of the previous stem, the new stem should be placed prior to replacing the "coffin lid" in order to

minimize the number of drill holes. Protection of the femur using a bone plate in neutral fashion is advisable in cases of stem repositioning.

Stem avulsion

Avulsion of the femoral stem from the medial cortex has been described with the Zurich prosthesis (Figure 8.7). Manufacturer recommendations in the first several years after the release of this system included the use of monocortical screws in each screw hole. Stem avulsion occurs most often in giant-breed dogs, and this was the impetus for the use of the proximal bicortical screw. Surgeon error, particularly valgus stem placement where the proximal portion of the stem does not have intimate contact with the medial cortex, can also predispose to stem avulsion from the medial cortex. Avulsion will lead to a valgus shift, subsidence, or both. Since avulsion occurs in the first few weeks after surgery, the lateral guide holes remain open and screw removal is possible through these holes unless disarticulation at the stem–neck interface occurs, allowing extreme subsidence. Even in such cases, the stem can be gradually shifted

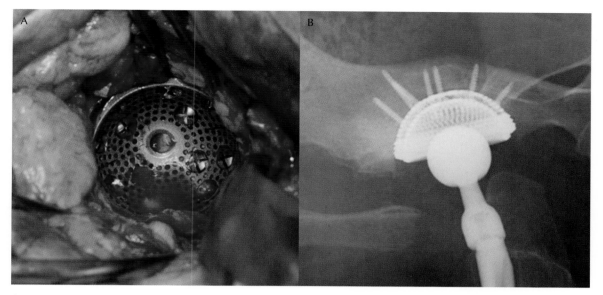

Figure 8.6   Intraoperative photograph of the shell of the Kyon revision cup. Note the use of multiple 2.4-mm screws (A). The corresponding Zurich Cementless cup is impacted into the revision cup shell as seen in the postoperative radiograph (B). (Images courtesy of Dr. Aldo Vezzoni)

proximally using a pin or other instrument introduced through the lateral guide holes.

Adequate medial screw purchase is unlikely to be achieved via the original screw holes. Although it may be tempting to replace the monocortical screws with bicortical screws, success with this technique has not been documented. A proximal or distal shift in implant position is likely necessary. This shift is challenging, as discussed above in the femoral fracture section. Alternatively, replacement of the Zurich stem with a BFX or CFX implant can be considered. If the surgeon chooses a CFX implant, cement that is extruded from the screw holes will need to be removed. The presence of the screw holes may create difficulty with pressurizing the cement during stem insertion. If a BFX stem is used, prophylactic application of double-loop cerclage wires prior to stem impaction is advisable (McCulloch et al. 2012). If a BFX or CFX stem is used, a modified head/neck component will be necessary because of differences in prosthetic head diameters. The femoral head of the Zurich hip is either 16 mm (for 21.5-, 23.5-, and 26.5-mm cups) or 19 mm (for 29.5- and 32.5-mm cups). The femoral head diameter for the Universal system (BioMedtrix) is 17 mm.

Cup avulsion

Avulsion of the acetabular component is most often due to inadequate initial press-fit, incomplete seating of the implant, inadequate reaming, or inadequate bony support for the implant. Treatment depends on the etiology. If inadequate initial press-fit was the result of a reaming error (e.g., excessive flare of the prepared bed), it may be necessary to implant the next larger cup size if adequate bone stock exists. If the initial reaming did not extend to the medial wall, deeper reaming may allow the surgeon to achieve a press-fit. Alternatively, switching from a cementless to a cemented cup may be considered. For the Zurich prosthesis, the revision shell, described above, can be considered.

Inadequate bone support poses a significant challenge. If recognized at the initial surgery, undersizing of the prosthesis may allow adequate support (Figure 8.8), but will sacrifice polyethylene thickness and possibly predispose to luxation.

Dorsal rim augmentation via screw fixation of autogenous cortical or corticocancellous graft from the iliac wing or the excised femoral head has

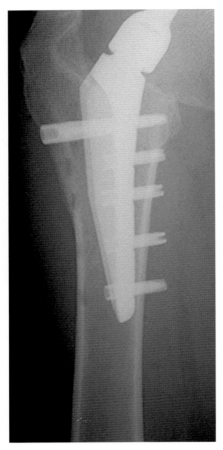

Figure 8.7 A 6-year-old Labrador retriever presented for routine 6-week follow-up radiographs following THR with a Zurich Cementless hip replacement. The stem is noted to have shifted into a valgus position and the femoral stem is no longer apposed to the medial cortex. The owner had noticed a gait change in the first week after surgery, but function continued to improve and no further change in implant position was noted at the 4-month and 1-year reevaluations. However, this radiographic finding implies instability and would most often suggest the need for revision.

been reported (Pooya et al. 2003; Torres et al. 2009). The sclerotic femoral head may have limited potential for osseointegration. After screw fixation of the graft, the graft and the acetabulum are prepared with appropriately sized reamers (Figure 8.9). It should be recognized, however, that much of the stability for press-fit is provided by the cranial and caudal poles of the acetabulum rather

than the dorsal rim or medial wall. In patients with very shallow acetabula, the controlled penetration of the medial wall may be considered in order to medialize the cup and to obtain adequate cranial and caudal support. This should be done with caution to avoid the complete protrusion of the cup through the medial wall.

Subsidence

Subsidence of cementless press-fit BFX stems may occur in the first weeks after implantation before bone ingrowth into the stem (Figure 8.10). Subsidence is often limited to a few millimeters (Marcellin-Little et al. 1999; Lascelles et al. 2010). This minor subsidence does not have clinical consequences. Major subsidence occurs in some instances. It may be associated with stem retroversion, femoral fissure or fracture, and luxation. Major subsidence is more likely to occur when the femur was prepared without much resistance to the progression of the broach (Rashmir-Raven et al. 1992). Most instances of major stem subsidence require stem revision. The stem is extracted. The femur is inspected for the presence of fissures or fracture. Any fissure or fracture is repaired and a new stem is implanted. The new stem may be a cementless stem if the original stem was undersized and the bone bed is normal. If the surgeon is concerned about further mechanical failure, a cemented stem is placed.

Subsidence of cemented stems may occur after failure of the implant–cement or the cement–bone interface. Fragmentation of the cement mantle and calcar bone resorption or calcar fracture is necessary before subsidence of a cemented stem occurs. Therefore, cemented stem subsidence is seen primarily in patients with chronic stem loosening. These chronic failures are most often managed with stem and cup extraction. Revision with another cemented hip could be considered, depending on the degree of bone change. This revision requires the removal of all cement and periprosthetic membranes and the reconstruction of the femur, followed by insertion of a new cemented stem. The incidence of aseptic loosening increases after the revision of a failed cemented stem, compared with primary cemented THR (Gramkow et al. 2001).

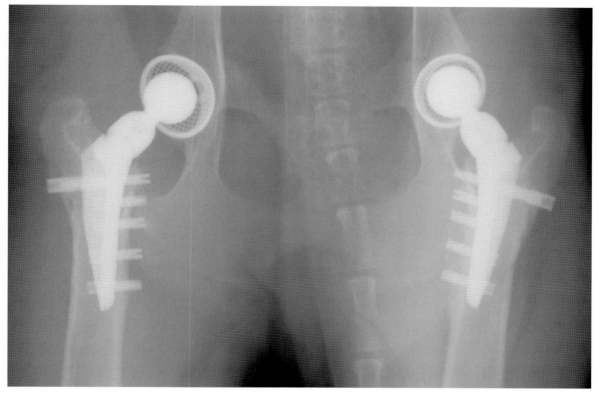

Figure 8.8   Radiograph from a mixed-breed dog with bilateral Zurich Cementless hip replacements. Extensive erosion of the left dorsal acetabular rim was noted on preoperative radiographs and confirmed intraoperatively. An undersized acetabular cup was used on the left side in order to ensure adequate bone support for the cup.

Stem failure

Failure of the femoral component as a result of accumulated fatigue stresses is uncommon. When stem failure occurs, replacement of the femoral component and removal of the prosthesis are the only options (Figure 8.11).

Failure of the BFX stem has not been reported or encountered to the authors' knowledge. Failure of cemented stems is rare and is the likely consequence of fatigue in stems with loose proximal portions, for example, when the distal aspect of the stem is rigidly fixed into the cement mantle but its proximal portion is not in contact with the calcar.

Failure of a Zurich Cementless stem is rare, but is most often associated with the use of an extra-small stem, particularly when a larger stem is more appropriate, based on patient size. Stem failure most often occurs at a screw hole; however, there were rare cases of failure at the trunion–stem interface prior to a design change in the early 2000s (Figure 8.12). Retrieval and replacement of a Zurich femoral stem can be accomplished via a lateral femoral window, also described as a "coffin lid," or by re-drilling the lateral femoral guide holes (presuming they have filled with bone) and unscrewing each of the stem screws. While the latter option is appealing, it can be quite challenging. Over time, a cold weld can form, particularly with titanium implants between the stem and the screw, making screw remove difficult (Fraitzl et al. 2011). The author has met with limited success with the use of various screw removal devices. The use of a new screwdriver, without rounding of the hexagonal head, is critical. If the screw head is damaged or stripped, it may be necessary to drill out the stem screw. This generates

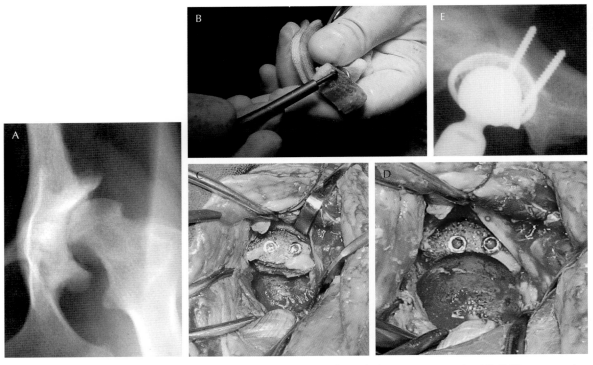

Figure 8.9 Radiograph from a 2-year-old Labrador retriever with dorsal acetabular rim (DAR) erosion (A). DAR augmentation was performed using a corticocancellous graft from excised femoral head that was shaped to fit the DAR using a high-speed bur (B). The graft is fixed to the DAR defect using two 2.7-mm screws in lag fashion (C). The graft and the acetabular bone bed are then reamed simultaneously using the appropriate-sized reamer (D). Radiograph made at 1-year follow-up is consistent with integration of the graft and a stable implant–bone interface (E). (Images courtesy of Dr. Aldo Vezzoni)

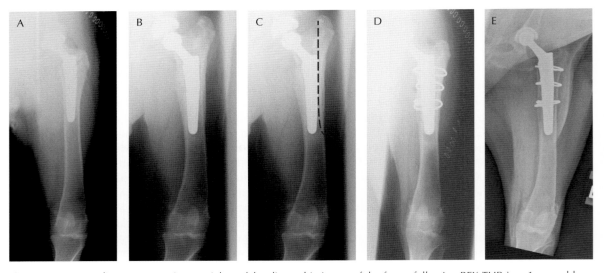

Figure 8.10 Immediate postoperative cranial-caudal radiographic image of the femur following BFX THR in a 1-year-old Labrador retriever (A). Three months postoperatively, significant subsidence of the stem is evident (B). An extended lateral femoral cortical window including the greater trochanter (dashed line) was planned for stem removal (C). The original #8 stem was removed, the femoral window was replaced and stabilized with three cable cerclage bands secured with crimps, the femur was broached, and a #10 stem was impacted (D). One year postoperatively the implants are stable (E). (Images courtesy of Dr. Michael Kowaleski)

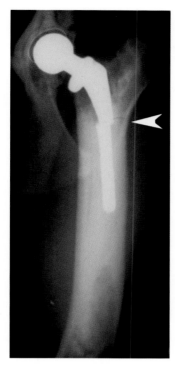

Figure 8.11 A cemented stem broke in its midshaft (arrowhead), most likely as a result of the lack of cement fill in the proximal portion of the femur that resulted in fatigue fracture of the stem. Also, the stem was undersized. This situation requires a revision of the stem with an extended trochanteric window or "coffin lid" femoral window, extraction of the well-fixed distal portion, and revision with another, larger cemented stem.

a substantial volume of debris and can increase the risk of loosening of the new stem.

Additionally, the screw hole will likely be compromised and the new stem screw will not achieve purchase in the medial cortex. It should also be noted that fatigue failure of the femoral component is more likely in cases where there is loosening associated with one or more stem screws, thus increasing stress adjacent to the loose screws. The surgeon must carefully evaluate the radiographs for evidence of bone resorption associated with the stem screws. Even with bone resorption, a "cold weld" can still make screw removal difficult.

A femoral window technique was described by Dyce and Olmstead (2002). Important aspects of creation of the window include adequate dimensions for access to the implant and rounding of the window "corners" to avoid creation of stress risers (Figure 8.13). In order to round the edges of the window, a narrow oscillating saw blade should be used. Alternatively, a 1.5-mm drill bit can be used to make holes at each corner. Ideally, the insertion of the adductor muscle is maintained along the caudal border of the bone flap. The saw blade is angled in order to bevel the edges of the flap for more secure replacement. Additionally, a thin blade is used in order to minimize the kerf. The flap is stabilized using three or more cerclage wires. The femoral window technique may be combined with an extended trochanteric osteotomy; with that technique, a cut is made on the cranial aspect of the femur extending distally from the greater trochanter. The length of the cut is adapted to the surgeon's needs (e.g., for removal of a loose cement mantle). The cut is rounded distally and extends proximally to the greater trochanter on the caudal aspect of the femur. The extended greater trochanteric flap represents approximately one-third of the circumference of the femur.

Cup failure (poly or metal backing)

Failure of the polyethylene liner as a result of wear-through is possible with any cup (Figure 8.14) but is unlikely, based on the low rate of cup wear in dogs (Skurla and James 2001). It is more likely to occur in cups with thin polyethylene liners measuring 2 mm or less. Oxidation may greatly accelerate polyethylene wear in cups that are exposed to oxygen for long periods of time (i.e., years) before implantation (Besong et al. 1997). To the author's knowledge, BFX cup wear-through or failure has not been encountered. If wear-through is encountered, it is possible to replace the polyethylene liner of a BFX cup without extracting the cup. The old liner is pulled using a rongeur. A new liner is aligned with the cup and impacted into place with a cup impactor. The failure of cemented polyethylene cup is most often the consequence of the failure of the cement mantle, described in the text below.

Wear-through of the ultrahigh-molecular-weight polyethylene (UHMWPE) liner of the

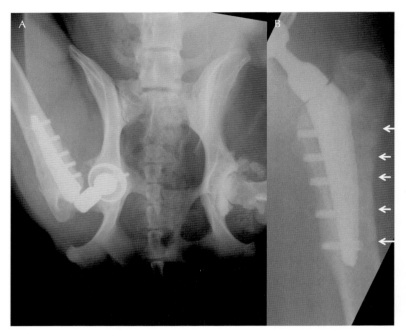

Figure 8.12   A mixed-breed dog presented for acute onset of lameness 4 years after THR. Failure of a Zurich Cementless stem at the trunion–stem interface occurred (A). The stem was revised by redrilling the lateral guide holes (arrows) to allow for removal, and then replacement, of the femoral stem (B). Extensive soft tissue debridement was required at the osteotomy site in order to allow retrieval of the implant. Note that there was no lucency associated with the original screws and all screw holes were reused.

acetabular component of the Zurich prosthesis is rare and is primarily limited to the 21.5-mm (i.e., the smallest) cup size (Figure 8.15). The UHMWPE liner in the 21.5-mm cup is 1.5mm thick in the load transfer zone. The risk of this complication is higher when a 21.5-mm cup is implanted in a very young patient. If wear-through occurs, excessive wear debris and osteolysis will make revision particularly challenging, unless the problem is noticed early. Revision strategies are similar to those for cup avulsion. Careful debridement of wear debris containing soft tissues is imperative.

Failure of the titanium shell of the Zurich acetabular prosthesis is rare as well. Shell failure with the current generation of double-shell acetabular components has not been reported; however, long-term follow-up of the current design is lacking.

Cement failure

Causes of cement failure in canine hip replacement were reported independently by Skurla

(Skurla et al. 2005) and Bergh (Bergh et al. 2004). They are described in detail in Chapter 6. In this section, we consider the mechanical causes of cement failure, including fracture of the cement mantle and debonding at the cement–implant interface (Figure 8.16). The implantation of a stem exposed to body fluids prior to implantation, the use of titanium stems, and varus stem orientation within the femoral canal have been shown to increase the risk of debonding. Exposing the stem to body fluid before insertion, for example, decreases the strength of the cement–implant interface by approximately 80% (Stone et al. 1989). Titanium stems have a higher debonding rate than cobalt-chromium stems with similar morphology (Tompkins et al. 1994). In dogs, debonding of titanium stems was described in 10 patients (Edwards et al. 1997). Debonding requires stem revision, and more specifically, cement-in-cement revision (Edwards et al. 1997; Duncan et al. 2009). Cement-in-cement revision is performed by doing a craniolateral approach to the hip joint, removing the loose stem, cleaning the cement mantle with a

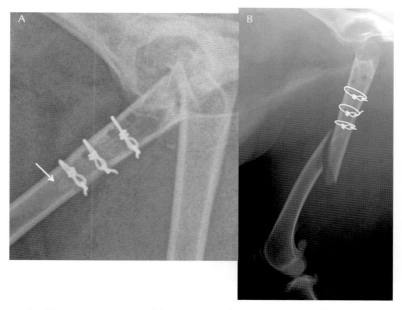

Figure 8.13   A 7-year-old golden retriever presented for progressive lameness 4 years following THR with a Zurich Cementless hip. Aseptic loosening of the acetabular component was found and owners elected to have the prosthesis explanted rather than pursue revision. A lateral femoral window ("coffin lid") was created for access to the femoral component. A sharp angle was inadvertently created at the cranial-distal corner of the window (arrow) (A). One week after the explant procedure, the owners reported an acute onset of pain and nonweight-bearing lameness. A femur fracture occurred at the distal aspect of the femoral window (B). Locking plate and cerclage wire fixation was performed (not pictured) and the fracture healed uneventfully.

high-speed bur without perforating it, drying it, and reimplanting a new stem with a clean and dry surface.

Biological failure

Biological failure includes failure of bone ingrowth or ongrowth for cementless prostheses, as well as loss of bone support (e.g., bone resorption, osteolysis, and osteonecrosis) with either cemented or cementless prostheses. Causes of biological failure include excessive micromotion, aseptic loosening, septic loosening, and stress protection. Excessive micromotion will result in a failure of osseointegration of cementless implants. It will also result in the generation of wear debris and is therefore intimately associated with aseptic loosening. Failure of osseointegration is typically a consequence of inadequate initial press-fit or other forms of initial fixation and is therefore

addressed in the "Mechanical Failure" section of this chapter. Management of the consequence of failure of integration (i.e., aseptic loosening) is discussed here.

Aseptic loosening

Wear debris-mediated osteolysis is described in detail in Chapter 6. Techniques for revision will be similar to those discussed above, with the addition of removal of the periprosthetic fibrous membrane. The periprosthetic fibrous membrane surrounding a loose prosthesis contains activated macrophages, as well as several mediators of osteolysis, including tumor necrosis factor-α (TNF-α) and oxygen-derived free radicals (Shanbhaq et al. 1995; Merkel et al. 1999; Kinov et al. 2006a). Therefore, revision of a loose implant should include removal of all grossly evident periprosthetic fibrous membrane. The removal of

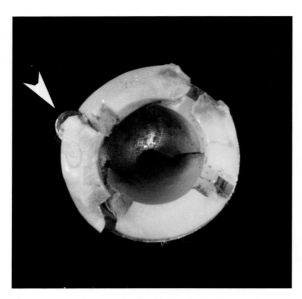

Figure 8.14 Photograph of a Canine PCA (Howmedica, Mahwah, NJ) that has been extracted from a dog during a cup revision. The cup had been in place for more than 4 years. The fixation peg (arrowhead) is on the cranial aspect of the cup. Wear-through of the polyethylene is visible in the craniodorsal aspect of the cup and the liner fragmented into several large pieces that were reconstructed before the cup was photographed. After extraction, the cup was replaced by another cup that was one size larger.

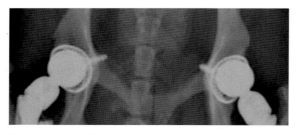

Figure 8.15 Radiograph of a pelvis from a dog with bilateral Zurich Cementless hips implanted 4 years earlier. The prosthetic heads are located eccentrically in the 21.5-mm acetabular components, indicating polyethylene wear (see Chapter 6—Figures 6.7D and 6.10 for images of the explanted implants). The left cup was removed and a BFX cup was implanted in the right hip. (Image courtesy of Dr. Michael Kowaleski)

the membrane is done using a periosteal elevator or a curette.

Early recognition is the key to successful revision in patients with aseptic loosening. This requires critical analysis of any report of diminished clinical function, as well as careful review of follow-up radiographs. In particular, follow-up radiographs should be compared with immediate postoperative radiographs. In addition to evaluation of lucency surrounding the implant, new bone deposition medial to the acetabulum is frequently noted in hips with aseptic loosening. This new bone formation may be useful if deeper reaming is necessary (Figure 8.17). Any nonartifactual radiolucency (e.g., Uberschwinger artifact in computed radiographs; Hanson et al. 2006) must be closely monitored. Owners should be made aware that any hip-associated lameness after full recovery from THR surgery is not normal. Nuclear scintigraphy can be utilized in evaluation for possible aseptic loosening; however, aseptic loosening cannot be distinguished from septic loosening with standard bone scan isotopes (Tc^{99} pertechnetate). Furthermore, increased radiopharmaceutical uptake is present for several months after THR surgery. Radiolabeled white blood cells have been used to distinguish aseptic loosening from septic loosening in humans and in one dog (Peremans et al. 2002; Love et al. 2009). Nuclear arthrography has also been used to evaluate potentially loose THR in humans (Oyen et al. 1996), but a meta-analysis found no advantage of nuclear arthrography, bone scintigraphy, or subtraction arthrography over plain radiography to diagnose aseptic loosening in humans (Temmerman et al. 2005).

Bisphosphonates decrease osteoclastic bone resorption, as well as regulate the proliferation of osteoblasts (Wise et al. 2005). Bisphosphonates include zolendronate, risedronate, etidronate, and alendronate. Multiple studies in the human literature support the use of bisphosphonates in the prevention and for the treatment of periprosthetic bone loss in the presence of wear debris or stress shielding (Sabokbar et al. 1998; Wise et al. 2005; Kinov et al. 2006b). Some studies suggest that bisphosphonates may actually encourage bone apposition (Wise et al. 2005). Sabokbar et al. added etidronate to PMMA at the time of the original THR surgery and concluded that bone resorption was inhibited in these cases. Wise et al. administered zolendronate for 26 weeks in a canine aseptic loosening model. In the Wise study,

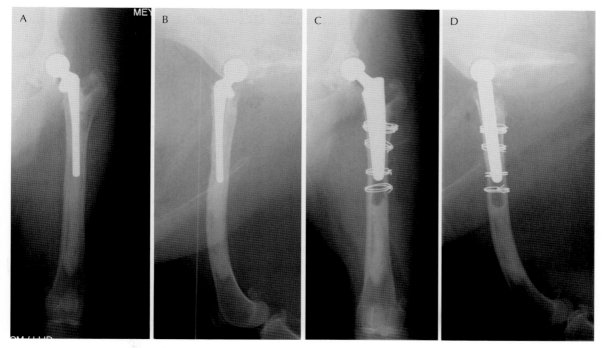

Figure 8.16 Cranial-caudal (A) and lateral (B) radiographs of the femur of a 3-year-old Labrador retriever who received a cemented total hip prosthesis at 9 months of age. A radiolucent line is visible on the caudal aspect of the stem–cement interface and the stem is retroverted, indicating that debonding has occurred (i.e., the stem is loose within its cement mantle). An extended trochanteric osteotomy was performed (C and D) and stabilized with four double-loop cerclage wires, the stem and proximal portion of the cement mantle were extracted, and a cementless stem was implanted. Bone ingrowth and long-term stem stability were confirmed in subsequent radiographs.

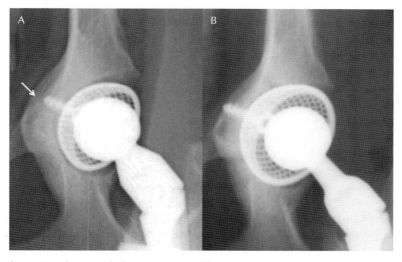

Figure 8.17 Aseptic loosening of an acetabular component with circumferential lucency surrounding the cup (A). New bone is visible medial to the acetabulum (arrow). The cup was revised using an acetabular component one size larger (B). All fibrous membrane tissue was debrided and removed at the time of revision surgery.

polyethylene particles were packed into the femoral component of a cementless femoral stem. Low-dose (2 µg/kg–10 dogs), high-dose (10 µg/kg–10 dogs), and control (10 dogs) groups were evaluated. In the 10 µg/kg group, bone resorption was prevented and bone quality, based on cortical porosity, mineralization, and failure strength, was maximized. In a randomized, prospective study, Kinov et al. found that administration of risedronate from day 20 to 6 months after surgery was associated with a significantly lower level of deoxypyridinoline, a resorption marker, in treated patients, versus control patients. The findings of the above studies suggest that bisphosphonates may be an underutilized tool in the prevention or early management of aseptic loosening and stress protection. However, long-term use of bisphosphonates may prevent adaptive bone remodeling. Many of the studies in the human literature utilize an approximately 6-month administration period.

Pentoxifylline, a TNF-α inhibitor, as well as recombinant human bone morphogenetic protein-2 (rh-BMP2) have each demonstrated capacity for prevention of aseptic loosening (Pollice et al. 2001; Thorey et al. 2010). rh-BMP2 has also demonstrated the ability to stimulate osseointegration.

Impaction allografting has been used in human THR revision in cases of periprosthetic bone loss (Board et al. 2006). This technique utilizes morselized cancellous bone chips that are progressively compacted into a bony defect. Board et al. concluded that the optimal size of the bone chips used for impaction allografting is 8–10 mm. After impaction of the bone chips, the prosthesis is cemented into the prepared bone bed.

Reconstruction rings/cages are well described in the human literature (Gross and Goodman 2004). These implants are used in cases with large bone defects and provide a scaffold for bone grafting. After ring placement, the acetabular component is cemented in place.

Tantalum acetabular augments have been described in the human literature (Siegmeth et al. 2009). Tantalum components are created to mimic the properties of trabecular bone and are useful for filling bone defects. The beneficial properties of

tantalum materials are discussed in detail in Chapter 3.

Septic loosening

Infection as a cause of implant loosening has been a major cause of patient morbidity since the development of joint prostheses. While many surgeons procure bacterial cultures at the time of THR surgery, positive cultures do not necessarily correlate with postsurgical infection (Lee and Kapatkin 2002; Ireifej et al. 2012). Attempting to salvage a joint replacement in the face of infection is a daunting challenge. In the presence of active infection, salvaging the implanted prosthesis with the use of systemic or locally implanted (e.g., antibiotic-impregnated PMMA beads) antibiotics is unlikely to succeed. The successful revision of an infected cemented prosthesis with a press-fit cementless stem was reported (Torres and Budsberg 2009). A successful single-stage revision of a loose, infected carbon composite stem was also reported (Massat et al. 1998).

Stress protection

THR involves the rigid fixation of a femoral component that has a higher elastic modulus than the proximal femoral metaphyseal/trabecular bone, as well as the diaphyseal cortical bone. This modulus mismatch and its role in bone resorption and implant loosening are discussed in detail in Chapter 6. Revision in the face of extensive bone loss resulting from stress shielding is a tremendous challenge. Early detection and close monitoring for progression are each critical if revision is to be successful.

General recommendations

Algorithms for general recommendations for a loose acetabular component and for a loose femoral component are presented in Figures 8.18 and 8.19, respectively.

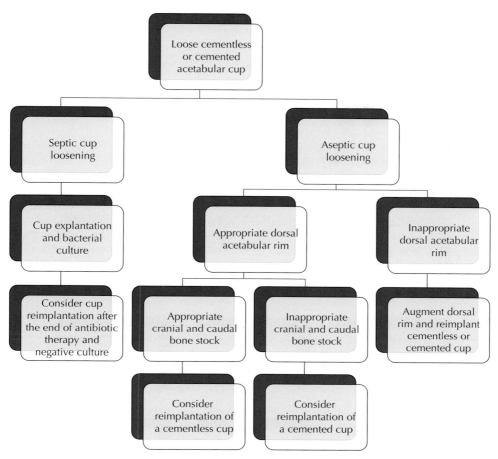

Figure 8.18 Algorithm of management recommendations for a loose acetabular component.

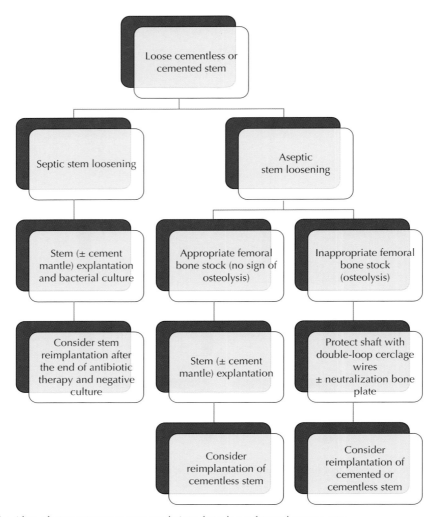

Figure 8.19 Algorithm of management recommendations for a loose femoral component.

Endnotes

1. Roe S, Marcellin-Little D, Lascelles D. Short-term outcome of uncemented THR. In: *Proceedings of the 2010 American College of Veterinary Surgeons Veterinary Symposium*. Seattle, WA, 2010.

References

Bergh MS, Muir P, Markel MD et al. Femoral bone adaptation to unstable long-term cemented total hip arthroplasty in dogs. Vet Surg 2004;33:238–245.

Besong AA, Hailey JL, Ingham E et al. A study of the combined effects of shelf ageing following irradiation in air and counterface roughness on the wear of UHMWPE. Biomed Mater Eng 1997;7:59–65.

Board TN, Rooney P, Kearney JN et al. Impaction allografting in revision total hip replacement. JBJS-Br 2006;88:852–857.

Brady OH, Kerry R, Masri BA, et al. The Vancouver classification of periprosthetic fractures of the hip: A rational approach to treatment. Tech Orthop 1999;14:107–114.

DeYoung DJ, Schiller RA. Radiographic criteria for evaluation of uncemented total hip replacement in dogs. Vet Surg 1992;21:88–98.

Duncan WW, Hubble MJ, Howell JR et al. Revision of the cemented femoral stem using a cement-in-cement technique: A five- to 15-year review. J Bone Joint Surg Br 2009;91:577–582.

Dyce J, Olmstead ML. Removal of infected canine cemented total hip prostheses using a femoral window technique. Vet Surg 2002;31:552–560.

Dyce J, Wisner ER, Wang Q, Olmstead ML. Evaluation of risk factors for luxation after total hip replacement in dogs. Vet Surg 2000;29:524–532.

Edwards MR, Egger EL, Schwarz PD. Aseptic loosening of the femoral implant after cemented total hip arthroplasty in dogs: 11 cases in 10 dogs (1991–1995). J Am Vet Med Assoc 1997;211:580–586.

Fitzpatrick N, Nikolaou C, Yeadon MA, et al. String-of-pearls locking plate and cerclage wire stabilization of periprosthetic femoral fractures after total hip replacement in six dogs. Vet Surg 2012;41(1):180–188.

Fraitzl CR, Moya LE, Castanelli L et al. Corrosion at the stem-sleeve interface of a modular titanium alloy femoral component as a reason for impaired disengagement. J Arthroplasty 2011;26:113–119.

Gramkow J, Jensen TH, Varmarken JE et al. Long-term results after cemented revision of the femoral component in total hip arthroplasty. J Arthroplasty 2001;16:777–783.

Gross AE, Goodman S. The current role of structural grafts and cages in revision arthroplasty of the hip. Clin Orthop Relat Res 2004;429:193–200.

Hanson SP, Peck JN, Berry CR. Radiographic evaluation of the Zurich Cementless total hip acetabular component. Vet Surg 2006;35:550–558.

Ireifej S, Marino D, Loughin CA et al. Risk factors and clinical relevance of positive intraoperative bacterial cultures in dogs with total hip replacement. Vet Surg 2012;41(1):63–68.

Kinov P, Leithner A, Radl R et al. Role of free radicals in aseptic loosening of hip arthroplasty. J Orthop Res 2006a;24:55–62.

Kinov P, Tircher P, Doukova P et al. Effect of risedronate on bone metabolism after total hip arthroplasty: A prospective randomized study. Acta Orthop Belg 2006b;72:44–50.

Lascelles BD, Freire M, Roe SC, et al. Evaluation of functional outcome after BFX total hip replacement using a pressure sensitive walkway. Vet Surg 2010;39: 71–77.

Learmonth ID. The management of periprosthetic fractures around the femoral stem. J Bone Joint Surg Br 2004;86:13–19.

Lee KC, Kapatkin AS. Positive intraoperative cultures and canine total hip replacement: Risk factors, periprosthetic infection, and surgical success. J Am Anim Hosp Assoc 2002;38:271–278.

Love C, Marwin SE, Palestro CJ. Nuclear medicine and the infected joint replacement. Semin Nucl Med 2009;39:66–78.

Marcellin-Little DJ, DeYoung BA, Doyens DH, et al. Canine uncemented porous-coated anatomic total hip arthroplasty: Results of a long-term prospective evaluation of 50 consecutive cases. Vet Surg 1999; 28:10–20.

Masri BA, Meek RMB, Duncan CP. Periprosthetic fractures evaluation and treatment. Clin Orthop Rel Res 2004;420:80–95.

Massat BJ, Miller RT, DeYoung BA, et al. Single-stage revision using an uncemented, porous-coated, anatomic endoprosthesis in two dogs: Case report. Vet Surg 1998;27:268–277.

McCulloch RS, Roe SC, Marcellin-Little DJ, Mente PL. Resistance to subsidence of an uncemented femoral stem after cerclage wiring of a fissure. Vet Surg 2012;41(1):163–167.

Merkel KD, Erdmann JM, McHugh KP et al. Tumor necrosis factor-α mediates orthopedic implant osteolysis. Am J Pathol 1999;154:203–210.

Oyen WJ, Lemmens JA, Claessens RA, et al. Nuclear arthrography: Combined scintigraphic and radiographic procedure for diagnosis of total hip prosthesis loosening. J Nucl Med 1996;37:62–70.

Peremans K, De Winter F, Janssens L et al. An infected hip prosthesis in a dog diagnosed with a 99mTc-ciprofloxacin (Infecton) scan. Vet Radiol Ultrasound 2002;43:178–182.

Pollice PF, Rosier RN, Looney JL et al. Oral pentoxifylline inhibits release of tumor necrosis factor-alpha from human peripheral blood monocytes: A potential treatment for aseptic loosening of total joint components. J Bone Joint Surg Am 2001;83:107–1061.

Pooya HA, Schulz KS, Wisner ER, et al. Short-term evaluation of dorsal acetabular rim augmentation in 10 canine total hip replacements. Vet Surg 2003;32: 142–152.

Preston CA, Schulz KS, Vasseur PB. Total hip replacement in 9 canine hind limb amputees: A retrospective study. Vet Surg 1999;28:341–347.

Rashmir-Raven AM, DeYoung DJ, Abrams CF Jr., et al. Subsidence of an uncemented canine femoral stem. Vet Surg 1992;21:327–331.

Sabokbar A, Fujikawa Y, Murray DW et al. Bisphosphonates in bone cement inhibit PMMA particle induced bone resorption. Ann Rheum Dis 1998;57:614–618.

Shanbhaq AS, Jacobs JJ, Black J et al. Cellular mediators secreted by interfacial membranes obtained at revision total hip arthroplasty. J Arthroplasty 1995;10:498–506.

Siegmeth A, Duncan CP, Bassam AM, et al. Modular tantalum augments for acetabular defect in revision hip arthroplasty. Clin Orthop Relat Res 2009;467: 199–205.

Skurla CT, James SP. A comparison of canine and human UHMWPE acetabular component wear. Biomed Sci Instrum 2001;37:245–250.

Skurla CP, Pluhar GE, Frankel DJ et al. Assessing the dog as a model for human total hip replacement. Analysis of 38 canine cemented femoral components retrieved at post-mortem. J Bone Joint Surg Br 2005;87: 120–127.

Stone MH, Wilkinson R, Stother IG. Some factors affecting the strength of the cement-metal interface. J Bone Joint Surg Br 1989;71:217–221.

Temmerman OPP, Raijmakers PGHM, Berkhof J et al. Accuracy of diagnostic imaging techniques in the diagnosis of aseptic loosening of the femoral component of a hip prosthesis. A meta-analysis. J Bone Joint Surg Br 2005;87:781–785.

Thorey F, Menzel H, Lorenz C et al. Enhancement of endoprosthesis anchoring using BMP-2. Technol Health Care 2010;18:217–229.

Tompkins GS, Lachiewicz PF, DeMasi R. A prospective study of a titanium femoral component for cemented total hip arthroplasty. J Arthroplasty 1994;9:623–630.

Torres BT, Budsberg SC. Revision of cemented total hip arthroplasty with cementless components in three dogs. Vet Surg 2009;38:81–86.

Torres BT, Chambers JN, Busdsberg SC. Successful cementless cup reimplantation using cortical bone graft augmentation after an acetabular fracture and cup displacement. Vet Surg 2009;38:87–91.

Wise LM, Waldman SD, Kasra M et al. Effect of zoledronate on bone quality in the treatment of aseptic loosening of hip arthroplasty in the dog. Calcif Tissue Int 2005;77:367–375.

9 Biomechanical Considerations in Total Knee Replacement

Matthew Allen and Kenneth Mann

Gait analysis and kinematics of the stifle joint

Gait analysis is used extensively in human and veterinary applications to quantify locomotion patterns for a wide range of activities. Gait analysis makes use of engineering kinematics to describe the motion of bodies (the skeleton in this case), without reference to the forces that cause the motion. Kinematic data are often collected using optical camera systems that track the two- and three-dimensional position of reflective markers placed on anatomical joints. For example, to study the kinematics of the stifle joint, reflective markers are placed on the skin at the hip, stifle, and hock joints. The kinematics of the femur are tracked by the hip and stifle markers, while the tibial motion is tracked by the stifle and hock joint markers (Figure 9.1).

The angular position of the stifle joint, in terms of flexion and extension, can be determined by calculating the relative angular position between the femur and the tibia. As shown in Figure 9.1, with the angular position measured on the flexion side of the joint, the value of the angle decreases during flexion and increases during extension. For a series of clinically normal Labrador retrievers (Ragetly et al. 2010) at a trotting pace (~2 m/s), the stifle joint flexion angle (with angle defined in Figure 9.1) was approximately 155 degrees at paw strike, decreasing to 130 degrees at 30% of the gait cycle, and then increased to 135 degrees at the end of stance phase. During the swing phase, the stifle joint flexion decreased to ~90-degree flexion at 70% of the gait cycle, before increasing to 155-degree flexion at the next paw strike. The angular excursion experienced by the stifle joint in the sagittal plane would then be about 65 degrees for this dog breed performing a trot activity. Other activities, such as sitting, would increase the magnitude of flexion (~46-degree flexion; Feeney et al. 2007). In any total knee design, an excursion that accommodates the full range of motion of the stifle joint is required to restore normal function. However, the periarticular changes in an end-stage stifle will likely preclude normal stifle excursion.

Extending two-dimensional descriptions of joint kinematics to three-dimensional cases adds substantially to the complexity of the kinematic analysis. Grood and Suntay (1983) defined a joint coordinate system for the knee joint described by a set of three clinically relevant rotations and three

Advances in Small Animal Total Joint Replacement, First Edition. Edited by Jeffrey N. Peck and Denis J. Marcellin-Little.
© 2013 John Wiley & Sons, Inc. Published 2013 by John Wiley & Sons, Inc.

translations. This coordinate system has been extrapolated for use in the stifle joint in dogs (Korvick et al. 1994). Flexion/extension rotations are defined with respect to a coordinate system fixed to the femur, while internal/external rotations are defined with respect to the long axis of the tibia. Adduction/abduction is defined on a "floating axis" that is perpendicular to the

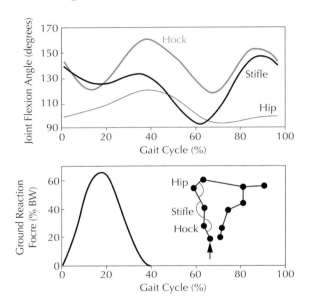

Figure 9.1 Figure illustrating joint angles at hip, stifle, and hock joints and ground reaction forces from a gait lab analysis for a trotting 32.5-kg dog. (Graphs courtesy of the J.D. Wheat Veterinary Orthopaedic Laboratory, University of California—Davis)

two fixed-bone axes. Translations are measured between the femur and tibia along these three rotation axes and include medial/lateral, cranial/caudal, and compression/distraction. These three rotations and three translations of the tibia relative to the femur describe the six degrees of freedom (6 dof) of motion. Examples for the rotations and translations for trotting dogs (Table 9.1) show that flexion motion is largest during the swing phase. Abduction/adduction and external/internal rotations are smaller, but are not negligible. Translations are also larger during the swing phase, with the largest motions in the cranial/caudal direction. During the first half of the stance phase, the angular position of the stifle increases from 40 to 55 degrees and there is a subtle cranial translation of the tibia (~2 mm, according to Korvick et al. [1994]). During the swing phase, there is a caudal displacement of −5 mm, followed by a 3-mm cranial displacement in the second half.

In addition to the traditional clinical gait laboratory evaluations, there have been developments to more accurately measure motion at the stifle joint using radiostereometric analysis (RSA). With the RSA approach, small tantalum beads (~1-mm diameter) are implanted in the distal femur and proximal tibia. The beads are set into the bone and a pair of radiographic images, fitted to a calibration cage, is captured to determine the three-dimensional position of the beads. Because one set of beads tracks the kinematics of the femur and another set of beads tracks the kinematics of the tibia, the 6-dof relative motion between the two

Table 9.1   Ranges of rotation and translations during swing and stance phases for the stifle joint of the dog

| | | Intact | | CrCL deficient | |
	Motion	Swing	Stance	Swing	Stance
Rotation (degrees)	Flexion (+)/extension (−)	+38 to +101	+40 to +55	+45 to +103	+46 to +55
	Abduct (+)/adduct (−)	0 to +6	0 to +2	+2 to +8	+1 to +4
	External (+)/internal (−)	−8 to +5	−2 to +2	−6 to +4	−4 to +1
Translation (mm)	Cranial (+)/caudal (−)	−5 to +3	0 to +3	−2 to +4	+4 to +14
	Lateral (+)/medial (−)	−2 to 0	0	−5 to −2	−6 to −2
	Distraction (+)/compression (−)	−4 to +2.5	−2 to 0	−4 to 0	−10 to 0

Source: Adapted from Korvick et al. (1994), with permission from Pergamon Press.
Joint kinematics were measured using a six-degrees-of-freedom linkage system attached between the tibia and femur. Results for intact and cranial cruciate ligament (CrCL)-deficient cases are shown. A plus sign (+) indicates motion in a positive direction.

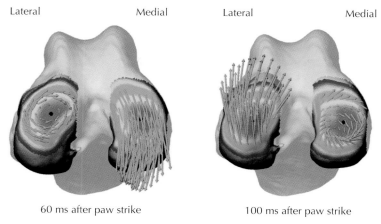

Lateral   Medial   Lateral   Medial

60 ms after paw strike   100 ms after paw strike

Figure 9.2   Relative velocity vectors indicate initial rotation about the lateral condyle early in the stance phase (60 ms after paw strike). This is followed by a rotation about the medial condyle at 100 ms after paw strike. (Adapted from Anderst and Tashman [2010], with permission from Elsevier)

bones can be determined. Using foxhounds on a treadmill at 1.5 m/s, Anderst and Tashman (2010) found that there was 5 degrees of tibial external rotation during the peak loading phase. Early in the loading phase (60 ms after paw strike), the rotation was about the lateral condyle (Figure 9.2). Later (at 100 ms), this center of rotation shifted to the medial condyle. This illustrates how internal/external rotation is an important component of natural joint kinematics and how articulating surfaces will experience sliding and nonsliding load transfers during the gait cycle.

Stifle joint loading

The forces that act on the stifle joint could be considered in terms of external and internal forces (Andriacchi et al. 1986). External forces would include the weight of the dog, inertial forces from acceleration and deceleration of the limb segments, and the ground reaction forces acting on the paw. Internal forces will balance the external forces and include muscle forces that act across the joint during contraction, ligament forces, and joint contact forces. External forces can be measured or estimated using force plates and gait analysis. Internal forces are much more challenging to measure and are most often estimated using mathematical modeling or directly measured using *in vitro* cadaver studies to simulate *in vivo* conditions

(Shahar and Banks-Sills 2004; Shahar and Milgram 2006; Kim et al. 2009).

Forces that act across joints of the musculoskeletal system can be quite large. In humans, it is common for these forces to reach several times body weight (BW) for activities of daily living such as walking (gait), rising from a chair, and stair climbing. Even single-legged stance can cause hip joint forces of two times BW. A very simple static force analysis is instructive to illustrate some key features of the stifle joint in terms of magnitude of the force across the joint. If we consider the hind limb of a dog near the end of the stance phase (Figure 9.3), there is a ground reaction force (GRF) acting on the paw from the ground. In this example, we are illustrating only the vertical reaction force. There are also cranial/caudal and medial/lateral directed forces during the gait cycle. At the stifle joint, a tensile force acts on the patellar tendon (PT), and this force is aligned with the tendon structure from its point of insertion on the tibial tuberosity to its origin on the patella. The joint force (JF) is the compressive force acting on the proximal tibial surface from the distal femoral condyles.

In this example, the ground reaction force creates a counterclockwise moment (or torque) about the stifle joint because the line of action is caudal to the stifle joint. The perpendicular distance from this line of action (shown as "*a*") is the moment "arm" of the ground reaction force. The

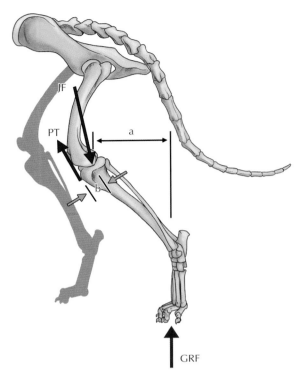

Figure 9.3 Free body diagram of the dog stifle joint illustrating ground reaction force (GRF), patellar tendon force (PT), and joint reaction force (JF). The GRF acts through a moment arm (a) and PT acts through a moment arm (b) relative to the joint center. (Image courtesy Karen Howard, MS [SUNY Upstate Medical University, Syracuse, NY])

patellar tendon also creates a moment about the joint (shown as "b"), but in this case the moment is clockwise with respect to the stifle joint. To maintain static equilibrium, these moments will balance each other such that

$$PT \times b = GRF \times a$$

$$\text{with } \frac{a}{b} = 3, \quad \text{then } PT = 3\,GRF.$$

If, for example, the ground reaction force were 1/2 BW for the dog, the patellar tendon force would be 1.5 BW. Continuing with the example, we will assume that the patellar tendon force acts at a 30-degree angle relative to the vertical axis. Again, invoking static equilibrium with forces in the x and y directions, we can calculate the

components of the joint force (JF_x and JF_y) as well as the overall joint force magnitude (JF):

$$JF_x = \frac{a}{b} \times GRF \times \sin(30°) = 0.75\,BW$$

$$JF_y = GRF + \frac{a}{b} \times GRF \times \cos(30°) = 1.8\,BW$$

$$JF = \sqrt{JF_x^2 + JF_y^2} = 1.95\,BW.$$

This simple example shows that the force on the proximal tibial surface could approach two times BW, even though the ground reaction force was only 1/2 BW.

More complicated three-dimensional mathematical models of the canine stifle joint during slow gait including the femur, tibia, and patella have been constructed (Shahar and Banks-Sills 2004). These models include a full complement of muscles and tendon forces along with time-varying ground reaction forces. Results show that the medial and lateral femoral condyles each exert 1 BW force on the tibia near the end of the stance phase of slow gait, for a total tibial force of 2 BW. Femoral trochlea forces are approximately 0.3 BW from the articulation with the patella. The cranial cruciate ligament (CrCL) is loaded through the first 80% of the stance phase and reaches a tensile force of 0.12 BW during mid-stance. The caudal cruciate ligament (CaCL) is loaded to a much lesser extent (0.02 BW) and only near the end of the stance phase. It should be noted that trotting and running gait, along with jumping, would create larger ground reaction forces and larger muscle forces. These, combined with greater acceleration and deceleration of the hind limb segments, would result in larger joint reaction forces.

Mechanical versus anatomical axes

Several different schemes have been developed to quantify the frontal alignment of the stifle joint in the dog (Dismukes et al. 2007, 2008; Tomlinson et al. 2007). An anatomical axis system (Figure 9.4A) at the stifle joint is determined by drawing axes along the medullary canal of the tibia and femur through the condylar notch in the femur. A mechanical axis system uses the joint centers to

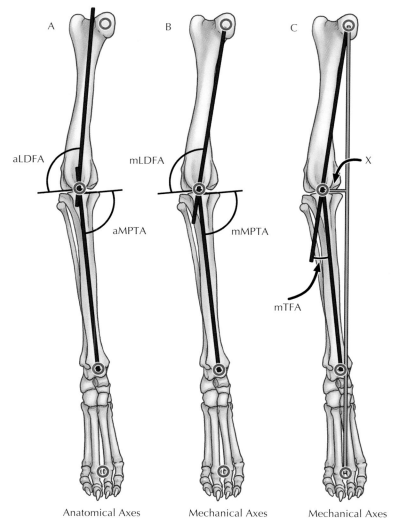

Figure 9.4 Frontal view of hind limb illustrating anatomical axes (A), mechanical axes (B), and mechanical axes showing pelvic limb line (C). Anatomical and mechanical axes as described by Dismukes et al. (2008). (Image courtesy Karen Howard, MS [SUNY Upstate Medical University, Syracuse, NY])

define the femoral and tibial axes (Figure 9.4B). Recreation of the mechanical axis system is important in total knee replacement (TKR) preoperative planning, component insertion, and ligamentous balancing to recreate the natural kinematics of the joint and to minimize excessive stresses on the implant and soft tissue components. For example, making component cuts that place the joint in an increased varus position would increase external moments on the joint resulting in higher joint

medial condyle contact forces that could contribute to loosening of the implant components.

A number of parameters have been developed to describe the angular and mechanical axes at the stifle joint (Figure 9.4). Anatomical lateral distal femoral angles (aLDFA) for four dog breeds (Labrador retrievers, golden retrievers, German shepherd dogs, and Rottweilers) averaged 97, 97, 94, and 98 degrees, respectively (Tomlinson et al. 2007). Use of mechanical axes (mechanical lateral distal femoral angle [mLDFA]) resulted in a slight increase in mean angles to 100, 100, 97, and 100 degrees. For normal tibiae, the mechanical and anatomical axes would not differ. The mechanical medial proximal tibia angle (mMPTA) has been reported to be 93 degrees (average) for Labrador retrievers (Dismukes et al. 2007). The mechanical tibiofemoral angle (mTFA) is 9.1 degrees (95% confidence interval [CI] of mean: 8.5–9.7 degrees) for mid- to large-size dogs (Dismukes et al. 2008) with a varus orientation (Figure 9.4C). In contrast, humans have normal mTFA of about 1 degree (Cooke et al. 2007). The ramifications of this become apparent by constructing the pelvic limb line that passes from the femoral head center to the location of the ground reaction force, which is located between the distal third and fourth metatarsal (Dismukes et al. 2008). Loads applied to the paw will tend to cause a varus moment about the stifle joint. This has been quantified as the mechanical axis deviation (MAD), calculated as the deviation distance (marked "X" in Figure 9.4C) divided by the length of the constructed pelvis limb line. For mid- to large-size dogs, the MAD is 3.6% at the stifle joint (Dismukes et al. 2008).

Role of ligaments

The stifle joint has 15 ligaments (Carpenter and Cooper 2000) and four of these are most important in terms of joint stability. These four are the medial and lateral collateral ligaments and the cranial and caudal cruciate ligaments. The ligaments act as passive constraints to provide joint stability. The collateral ligaments stabilize the joint against abduction and adduction torques when the joint is in extension. During limb abduction (valgus angulation of the stifle), a moment couple at the joint is created to resist the externally applied torque consisting of a tensile force in the medial collateral ligament combined with a compressive load across the lateral condyle. Tensile loading of the patellar tendon from active muscle contraction can also contribute to the moment couple and decrease the tensile forces in the medial collateral ligament. This active muscle contraction can protect the collateral ligaments from excessive loading. During limb adduction (varus angulation of the stifle), the opposite occurs. Tensile force

increases in the lateral collateral ligament and compression increases across the medial condyle of the joint. Again, tension forces acting through the patellar tendon can decrease tensile forces on the lateral collateral ligament. In extension, both collateral ligaments are taut (Carpenter and Cooper 2000) and they can resist internal rotation. During flexion, the lateral collateral ligament becomes lax, allowing for internal rotation of the tibia relative to the femur.

The cranial and caudal cruciate ligaments are the primary structures that control cranial and caudal translation of the tibia with respect to the femur. The CrCL functions to prevent cranial translation of the tibia relative to the femur and carries substantial tensile loads during the stance phase as described above. With an internal rotation torque, the CrCL can twist about the CaCL to minimize internal rotation of the tibia. The CaCL acts against caudal translation of the tibia with respect to the femur. However, the estimated loads on the CaCL are substantially lower than the CrCL. There has been a large body of research focused on disruption of the CrCL as this is a common clinical issue in dogs. From a research perspective, disruption of the CrCL has also been used as a model for degenerative arthritis (Pond and Nuki 1973). As shown in Table 9.1 rupture of the CrCL causes cranial translation of the tibia on the order of 10 mm (in a 35-kg dog). In addition, loss of CrCL function increases internal rotation in the stance phase of gait.

TKR surgery that removes the effective function of the cruciate ligaments requires additional passive constraints to prevent excessive cranial/caudal translation. One approach to achieve this is to add additional conformity between the tibial and femoral components. Increasing conformity can be effectively designed to improve joint stability, but will also increase stresses at the fixation interfaces due to lack of the anatomical passive constraints provided by the ligaments. In contrast, knee replacement designs that retain the cruciate ligaments require articular surfaces that are similar to the natural surfaces being replaced. Excessive forces in the cruciate ligaments could occur if the conformity of the articular surface is increased for a cruciate sparing TKR because the articular surface could force the joint into a supraphysiological kinematic state.

Stifle joint contact pressures

Contact between the articular surfaces of the tibial and femoral components is the primary mechanism of load transfer across the joint and these forces are compressive in nature. In the well-functioning joint, there is negligible friction between the articulating surfaces so that forces act perpendicular to the articulating surface. Depending on the conformity between the two contacting surfaces, the contact area and contact pressures can change. It is generally not possible to measure contact areas or pressures directly *in vivo*. Computer simulations using sophisticated finite element modeling methods and *in vitro* experiments using cadaver material are often used to determine contact mechanics. Using a mechanical loading device with pelvic limbs from dog

cadavers, Kim et al. (2009) placed thin digital pressure sensors subjacent to the menisci to measure the distribution of contact pressure. With a load of 30% BW and a stifle angle of 135 degrees, they found average contact areas of 316 mm^2 with greater contact on the medial condyle (179 mm^2) than the lateral condyle (137 mm^2). Peak pressures were 2.7 MPa and 2.4 MPa in the medial and lateral compartments, respectively. Peak pressure locations were located at a fractional distance of 48% from the caudal edge for the medial tibial plateau and 64% for the lateral tibial plateau (Figure 9.5). Following CrCL sectioning, there was a substantial caudal shift in position of the contact zone, a large increase in contact pressure (peak of 4.9 MPa, an increase of 81%) and a large reduction in contact area (total of 178 mm^2, a decrease of 44%). In human knees, the tibiofemoral contact moves

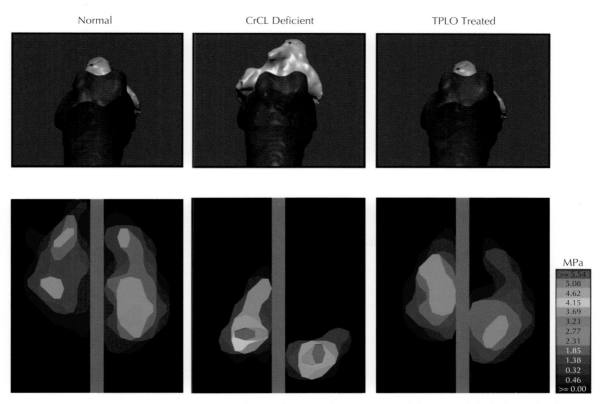

Figure 9.5 Axial view of the stifle joint for normal, cranial cruciate ligament (CrCL) deficient, and tibial plateau leveling osteotomy (TPLO) treatments. Top panel row shows distal femur in dark gray and proximal tibia in silver. The bottom panel row illustrates contact pressure distributions for the three cases in terms of pressure magnitude and distribution. (Reproduced from Kim et al. [2009], with permission from John Wiley & Sons)

posteriorly with increasing knee flexion (Andriacchi et al. 1986).

The menisci are C-shaped fibrocartilaginous discs located between the femoral condyles and tibia (Carpenter and Cooper 2000), and they increase the stability of the stifle joint by functionally increasing the conformity between the femoral and tibial contact surfaces. This increased conformity increases the contact area and reduces contact stresses. Thieman et al. (2010) showed that a partial meniscectomy of the medial meniscus in the canine stifle joint reduced contact area by 38% and increased peak contact stress by 86%.

Design considerations for TKR implants

The design of contemporary TKR implants is based on the goal of restoring normal motions of the knee, especially flexion-extension and internal-external rotation, while resisting varus-valgus angulation and cranial-caudal translation.

Restoring joint motion

Flexion-extension is controlled by the sagittal plane geometries of the femoral component and the ultra-high molecular weight polyethylene (UHMWPE) tibial component. In the BioMedtrix (Boonton, NJ) system, the femoral component incorporates two distinct radii of curvature (Figure 9.6A); a larger radius that recapitulates the curvature of the patellofemoral joint, and a smaller radius that is based on the center of rotation of the femoral condyle. By incorporating both radii into one smooth curvature, it is possible to achieve smooth motion and stable femorotibial contact during the flexion-extension arc. The medial and lateral condyles have the same radii of curvature in the sagittal plane, and their radii of curvature in the frontal plane are also matched (Figure 9.6B). When combined with a symmetrical femoral trochlea, this allows for the manufacture of a single implant design to accommodate both left and right stifle joints in the dog. Ultimately, this

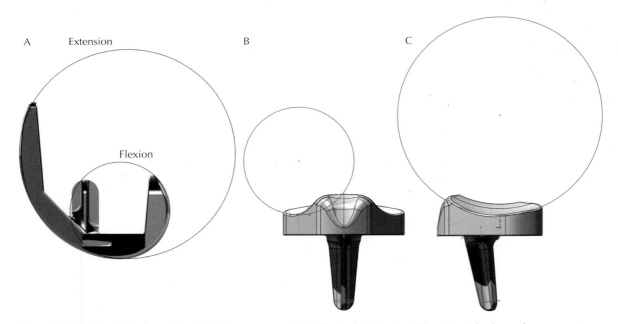

Figure 9.6   Design of the femoral and tibial components of the BioMedtrix Canine TKR system. The femoral component incorporates two radii of curvature, one for extension and the other for flexion (A). Medial-lateral and cranial-caudal translations of the femoral component are limited by the geometry of the tibial component in the frontal (B) and sagittal (C) planes respectively. (Images courtesy of Greg van der Meulen, MS [BioMedtrix LLC])

eliminates the need for separate left and right instrumentation, as well as reducing the implant inventory required to undertake these surgeries.

Rotational constraint within a condylar TKR is also determined by the geometry of the implants. For a conforming articulation, rotational constraint is proportional to the relative radii of the femoral and tibial components. If the radii are closely matched, less rotation will be allowed than for a less conforming design (Wright 2003). It should be noted that the degree of rotational stability also changes with knee position. For semi-constrained canine TKR components (as described in the following section), rotational stability is lower at high flexion angles when there is less conformity between the femoral and tibial surfaces. The BioMedtrix canine TKR implant is designed to allow −15 to +15 degrees of rotation. Rotation in the intact stifle is reported to be −8 to +5 degrees (Korvick et al. 1994; see Table 9.1).

Patellofemoral tracking is a significant issue in human TKR and a concern in canine TKR, especially in light of the significant variations in distal femoral geometry that are evident in dogs. The normal canine femoral trochlea is asymmetric in the transverse plane but the trochlea on the femoral component is usually symmetric. Although the prosthetic trochlea is relatively deep as compared with the natural trochlea, errors in the rotational alignment of the femoral component have the potential to increase the risk of patellar luxation. Varus-valgus misalignment of the femoral component can also result in patellar maltracking. It is critically important to assess patellar tracking at the time of surgery so that any problems can be identified and resolved. If there is mild patellar instability, it may be sufficient to imbricate the joint capsule, but more significant instability may necessitate revision of the femoral ostectomy in order to restore optimal alignment of the trochlea and extensor mechanism.

Restoring joint stability: Constrained, semiconstrained, and minimally constrained TKR implants

The majority of dogs presenting for TKR surgery have experienced rupture of the CrCL. The mechanical consequences of CrCL rupture have been studied and described extensively (Pozzi and Kim 2010) and will not be restated here. However, it is important to note that loss of the CrCL alone results in a clinically unstable stifle joint. During non-cruciate ligament-sparing TKR surgery, both the cranial and caudal cruciate ligaments are excised, along with the menisci. Consequently, the stability of the stifle joint is significantly compromised when TKR is performed. Following TKR, stability of the stifle joint is determined by the inherent stability of the "new" joint, consisting of the articulating TKR implant and the surrounding ligaments (medial and lateral collateral ligaments) and soft tissues (patellar tendon, popliteal tendon, and joint capsule). The relative contributions of the implant and the periarticular soft tissue to knee stability vary according to knee design, and are best described in terms of *degrees of constraint*.

The earliest TKR designs focused on recreating the hinge (ginglymus) function of the joint. The clinical performance of these early *constrained linked* implants was poor, with survival rates of only ~65% at 5–6 years as a result of complications such as loosening, infection, and fracture (Knutson et al. 1986). The use of a fixed hinge allowed flexion-extension but effectively prevented varus-valgus tilt, internal-external rotation, and axial joint distraction. Loads applied to the implant therefore resulted in high stresses through the hinge joint and increased load transfer across the interfaces between the implant, cement, and bone, resulting in loss of implant fixation. Newer versions of these linked devices, including rotating-hinge designs, have been developed to overcome the limitations of the earlier fixed-hinge designs (Callaghan et al. 2000). In humans, these implants are used in patients with significant bone or soft tissue deficits secondary to aseptic or septic loosening, trauma, or neoplasia. In the veterinary arena, there have now been a limited number of reports on the use of custom fixed and rotating-hinge designs in the management of dogs with stifle joint derangement and primary bone neoplasms (Figure 9.7).[1]

Constrained, unlinked condylar TKR implants have been used in humans but have yet to find an application in canine TKR. In these implants, a central spine made of UHMWPE projects up from the tibial component and engages a recess in the

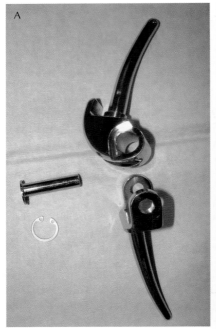
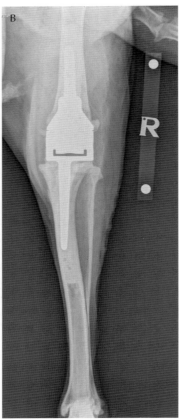

Figure 9.7   Use of a constrained, fixed-hinge TKR implant in a dog. The femoral and tibial components are linked with a bushing that is inserted at the time of implantation (A). The long stems on the femoral and tibial components are intended for cemented fixation (B). (Images courtesy of Noel Fitzpatrick, MVB, MRCVS [Fitzpatrick Referrals])

intercondylar region of the femoral component. Varus-valgus and anterior-posterior movements are constrained by contact between the plastic eminence and its enclosure. Although popular for a while, these implants have generally fallen out of favor as a consequence of retrieval studies that showed consistent patterns of UHMWPE wear and deformation on the central spine (Haman et al. 2005).

Recognition that it was not feasible to use materials alone to constrain the movements of the knee led to the development of *semiconstrained* condylar knee designs in which stability is imparted both through the geometry of the articulation and through the contributions of the local soft tissues, especially the collateral ligaments, patellar tendon, and the joint capsule.

The commercial canine TKR implants that are currently available incorporate a semiconstrained design (Figure 9.8). The radius of curvature of the concavity in the UHMWPE tibial components is slightly larger than that of the femoral counterface in both the sagittal plane and the frontal plane, resulting in an articulation that allows for some degree of stifle joint rotation, especially in flexion. The sloped contours of the cranial and caudal surfaces of the tibial concavities serve to reduce the ability of the femoral component to translate out of the articulation. Medial-lateral translation is resisted primarily by the presence of a raised ridge of UHMWPE between the medial and lateral tibial concavities (Figure 9.8B).

Minimally constrained TKR implants are used in humans but are not available in dogs. The most

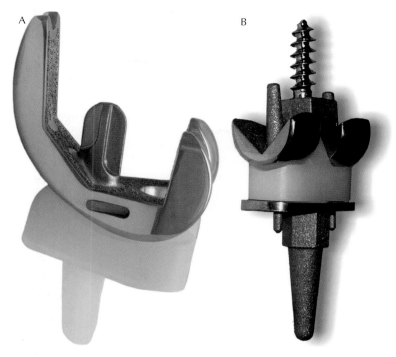

Figure 9.8   Commercial canine TKR designs: (A) BioMedtrix Canine TKR and (B) GenuSys Knee System. Both implants incorporate a semiconstrained femorotibial articulation. (Image of the GenuSys knee courtesy of Manssur Arbabian [INNOPLANT Medizintechnik, Hannover, Germany])

common of these is the cruciate-retaining (CR) implant that spares the posterior cruciate ligament (PCL). Proposed benefits of CR implants include better preservation of bone stock and improved kinematics following surgery. However, maintenance of the PCL reduces the surgeon's ability to balance soft tissues and to manage deformity (Morgan et al. 2005), so many surgeons prefer to use either an unlinked constrained implant that restores PCL function or a semiconstrained, cruciate-sacrificing implant of the type used in dogs.

Patellar resurfacing

The issue of whether or not to resurface the patella during TKR surgery remains contentious. Proponents of patellar resurfacing believe that replacement of the patellar cartilage with a UHMWPE button provides for an optimal articulation against the metal trochlea. They also argue that

replacement at the time of surgery prevents the need for a second surgery in the event of subsequent cartilage degeneration as a result of either natural disease that was not diagnosed at the time of surgery, or of damage caused by abrasion against the metal femoral counterface. However, recent data from a prospective study of over 1700 patients failed to demonstrate any significant difference in knee function following TKR with or without patellar resurfacing (Breeman et al. 2011).

In dogs, patellar resurfacing has not been included in TKR for a number of reasons. First, the size and geometry of the canine patella would make resection and replacement with a cemented UHMWPE button quite challenging. Second, introduction of another implant and another interface increases the risk of implant-related complications such as loosening or wear. Unless long-term clinical data indicate that patellofemoral complications limit the survival of canine TKR implants, it is unlikely that patellar resurfacing will be widely adopted as a standard procedure for dogs undergoing TKR.

Less invasive TKR solutions

In humans, isolated degeneration and/or collapse of the medial or lateral femorotibial compartment results in a varus or valgus knee deformity. In these patients, unicondylar knee arthroplasty (UKA) is a logical and economic alternative to TKR. The procedure is less invasive than TKR and does not preclude subsequent revision to a TKR. Since only one joint compartment is replaced and the associated soft tissues are maintained, it is possible to use minimally constrained articulations to ensure optimal range of motion. Clinical data indicate that UKA produces reliable 8–10-year results in appropriately selected patients (Deshmukh and Scott 2001).

UKA has not been explored in dogs and, given the nature of the pathology that is normally seen in dogs evaluated for TKR, it is unlikely that this will be adopted in the veterinary field. However, there is great potential for the development of minimally invasive condylar implants that can be implanted through smaller incisions and simpler instrumentation.

Mechanical factors at the femorotibial articulation

The knee joint is the largest joint in the body and, as described earlier in this chapter, load transfer across the canine stifle joint may approach two times BW, depending on the activity and the angle at which the joint is loaded.

From a practical perspective, any consideration of load transfer through an implant must consider three factors. First, what is the relative distribution of the load across the surface of the implant? Second, what is the mechanical response of the implant to the loads that are experienced? Third, what proportion of the load does the implant transmit across the implant–bone or cement–bone interface?

Although there have been a number of studies on load distribution in the normal stifle joint, information on the relative distribution of loads

following TKR is lacking. Nevertheless, some important lessons can be learned from human TKR and these can be used to inform the design of canine TKR implants and the surgical techniques used to implant these devices.

Contact pressures and UHMWPE stresses

Contact pressures play an important role in determining the long-term survival of the UHMWPE bearing surface. Bartel et al. (1986) used finite element analysis to explore the impact of knee component constraint and UHMWPE thickness on the contact stresses in the UHMWPE. An unconstrained knee implant, with limited conformity between the femoral and tibial components, transfers load across a small contact area, resulting in contact stresses that can exceed the yield stress of the UHMWPE, which is reported to range from 13 to 32 MPa (D'Lima et al. 2001; Figure 9.9). Conversely, load transfer in a semiconstrained implant with increased conformity occurs over a much larger surface area and results in lower contact stresses when the knee is appropriately aligned. Interestingly, peak contact stresses do not occur at the surface of the UHMWPE but in the subsurface; this observation likely explains the observation of subsurface material failure and delamination that has been reported in certain designs of TKR implant (Sathasivam and Walker 1998).

Data from the human literature indicate that contact stresses decrease as the thickness of the UHMWPE increases. For contemporary condylar knee designs, a minimum thickness of 6 mm of UHMWPE is recommended (Bartel et al. 1986). This means that the tibial insert is usually at least 8–10 mm in thickness. In dogs, removal of a centimeter of bone from the proximal tibia is not practical as it would risk injury to the insertion sites of the collateral ligaments. In addition, implantation of a cemented or cementless implant into the relatively spongiform bone of the proximal tibia would likely increase the risk of device subsidence or liftoff, especially when subjected to off-axis loading. Additional work is needed to determine contact stresses in the UHMWPE implants that are currently used in dogs, but reductions in contact stress are more likely to come from changes in implant conformity and modifications to the

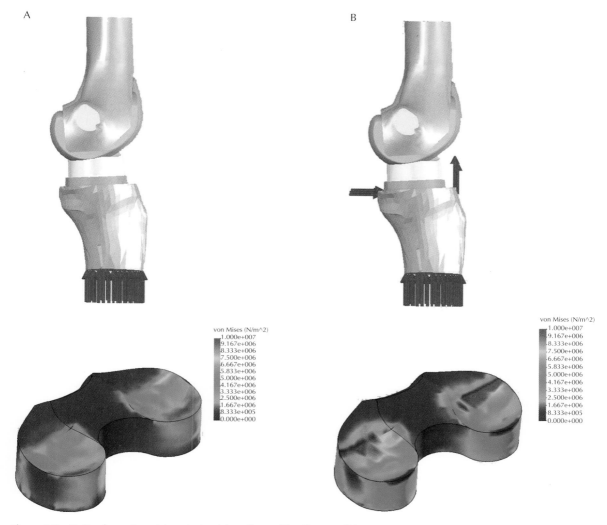

Figure 9.9   Finite element model analysis of the effects of loading conditions on contact stresses in a UHMWPE tibial insert. Under static loading (A), contact stresses are relatively low and evenly distributed. With application of quadriceps load and a shear force (B), the contact pressures increase substantially. Similar increases are seen when the joint is flexed and the contact area decreases. (Images courtesy of Evangelos Magnissalis, PhD [Biohexagon Ltd., Athens, Greece])

material properties of the bearing surfaces than from increases in the thickness of the UHMWPE components.

Deformation of the implant

The mechanical response to loading is dictated both by the geometry of the implant and the material from which it is fabricated. In human TKR, all-polyethylene tibial components were largely abandoned back in the 1980s in favor of metal-backed components with an enclosed UHMWPE articular insert. The primary concern at that time was that the all-polyethylene implants experienced increased deformation when subjected to varus-valgus or anterior-posterior loading (Reilly et al. 1982) and that this deformation would result in an increased incidence of implant loosening and revision surgery. Metal-backed trays were shown to more effectively distribute and reduce the maximum compressive loads seen in the cancellous bone bed adjacent to the implant and it was postulated that they would result in reduced early implant migration and subsequent loosening (Taylor et al. 1998). Additional benefits of metal-backed tibial components include modularity (including the use of long stems), cementless fixation with porous or beaded coatings, and the potential for revision of a worn UHMWPE insert without need for removal of the entire implant. However, these advantages are offset by the increased cost of a metal-backed component, the requirement for a deeper tibial bone cut for a given UHMWPE thickness with a metal backing, and by the potential for backside wear of the UHMWPE insert.

The use of all-polyethylene tibial implants is now being revisited in human TKR. Despite the predictions from the laboratory, a number of all-polyethylene designs have demonstrated performance that is equivalent or superior to that of metal-backed components of the same design (Browne et al. 2011).

Both cemented, all-polyethylene and cementless, metal-backed tibial implants are now available for canine TKR. In the long-term, it will be interesting to see whether the perceived advantages of the metal-backed components are reflected in differences in clinical performance and implant survival.

Importance of cut geometry and soft tissue balance

The functional stability of a TKR implant is determined by the inherent geometry of the implant and the surgeon's ability to restore correct joint alignment and soft tissue balance. Although ligament balancing procedures, including ligament releases and/or lengthening, are commonly used in human TKR, these procedures have not been evaluated in dogs. Unless a dog presents with significant joint deformity, it is usually possible to maintain alignment and soft tissue balance by paying careful attention to the bone cuts that are used to prepare the femur and tibia.

The tibial osteotomy, which traditionally precedes the femoral osteotomy in a TKR procedure,

should result in a bone surface that is perpendicular to the mechanical axis of the tibia. The femoral osteotomies are then made, using the tibial osteotomy as a reference. The goal is to produce a joint space that is rectangular in geometry in both extension and flexion (the so-called flexion and extension gaps; Figure 9.10A). Failure to create flexion and/or extension gaps with a parallel relationship between femur and tibia will lead to varus or valgus angulation of the implants (Figure 9.10B). In a laboratory setting, malalignment of the femoral and/or tibial components results in increased load transfer and contact pressures on the tibial UHMWPE (Werner et al. 2005). These effects are even more pronounced when a highly conforming implant design is used, especially one with closely matched radii in the mediolateral plane. One potential solution to this issue is the use of condylar geometries that prevent edge loading if they are subjected to off-axis loading. In a clinical setting, malalignment results in increased wear and an increased risk of implant failure (Ritter et al. 1994).

Materials selection and the problem of implant wear

The materials used in TKR are similar to those available in THR. The most common bearing surfaces are cobalt-chromium (CoCr), titanium alloy (Ti6Al4V), and UHMWPE. In humans, ceramics such as alumina and zirconia have been shown to result in less wear of the UHMWPE counterface, and are starting to see increased clinical application (Oonishi et al. 2005).

The femoral component of the BioMedtrix Canine TKR system has an ingrowth surface composed of two to three layers of CoCr beads with a mean diameter of 250–300 μm. The femoral component of the GenuSys implant (INNOPLANT, Hannover, Germany) is fabricated from titanium-coated CoCr and stabilized using a single screw into the femoral metaphysis.

The tibial component of the BioMedtrix implant is fabricated as a monobloc of UHMWPE that is designed for cemented fixation. A cementless fixation option, consisting of a CoCr tibial tray with a snap-fit UHMWPE insert, has undergone preclinical evaluation (Allen et al. 2010) and is now

A B

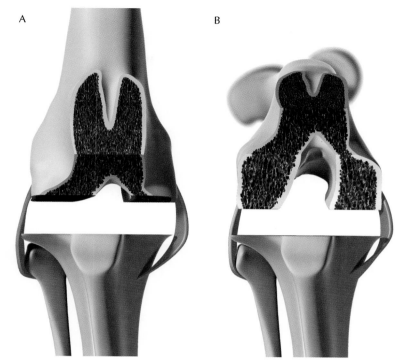

Figure 9.10   Flexion and extension gaps in total knee replacement. In extension (A), the tibial ostectomy and the distal femoral ostectomy are parallel. In flexion (B), the tibial ostectomy and the caudal femoral ostectomy are parallel. (Image courtesy of Tim Vojt.)

available for clinical use. A metal-backed tibial tray (titanium-coated CoCr) is also used in the GenuSys knee.

Wear of the UHMWPE component is inevitable given the loads to which the implants are subjected *in vivo*. Wear is an important cause of implant failure in TKR. Particulate debris (metal, UHMWPE, or polymethylmethacrylate [PMMA]) from the articular or nonarticular surfaces of the implant are liberated into the joint tissues, where they incite inflammatory reactions that result in periprosthetic inflammation and bone resorption (Harris 2001). In both cemented and cementless components, bone loss compromises the fixation of the implant and initiates mechanical loosening. Micromotion at the implant–bone, cement–bone, or stem–cement interface serves to exacerbate the release of particulate debris, which are forced along the interface by the pumping of synovial fluid (Konttinen et al. 2005).

The mechanisms responsible for the generation of wear debris appear to be different in TKR as compared with THR. In THR, wear occurs predominantly as a result of surface phenomena such as abrasive or adhesive wear. In TKR, wear is more commonly the result of fatigue phenomena that manifest as pitting or delamination. Wear particles generated from TKR have been shown to be larger than those from THR, and it has been suggested that this is one reason why the periprosthetic tissue response is often more aggressive in failed THR than in failed TKR (Schmalzried et al. 1994).

We recently reported the results of a study of implant wear following TKR in the dog (Rudinsky et al. 2010). Although the results from this study should be considered preliminary, they indicated that the common wear mechanisms seen in human TKR specimens (Hood et al. 1983) are also evident in canine TKR retrievals. Pitting was evident in six of six implants and delamination was seen in three of six implants. Additional, longer-term studies will be needed to more completely quantify the incidence and significance of both articular surface and backside wear mechanisms in canine TKR, as well as to determine the relationship between wear and implant survival.

Mechanical factors at the implant–bone or cement–bone interface

Cemented versus cementless fixation

Data from the Swedish Knee Arthroplasty Registry indicate that the relative risk of implant revision is 1.6 times higher for implants with a cementless tibial component as compared with a cemented tibial component (Robertsson et al. 2001). The primary cause of implant failure in these cases is aseptic loosening of the tibial component. Femoral component survival does not appear to be different in cemented, versus cementless, components (Robertsson et al. 2001). It should be noted, however, that these data come exclusively from the human literature. There have not been any prospective clinical trials of cemented versus cementless fixation in canine TKR, but a recent preclinical study indicated that fixation with a cementless, hydroxyapatite-coated tibial component was as effective as that achieved with bone cement at time points out to 6 months (Allen et al. 2007). More recently, we used a novel *in vitro* loading regimen and direct analysis of implant micromotion to characterize the mechanical performance of the cement–bone interface in UHMWPE tibial components from a series of canine TKR retrievals (Mann et al. 2011). The results from this study confirmed the stability of these cemented implants, with interface motions that were similar to those seen from a series of clinically successful human retrieval specimens. However, histological analysis of specimens from these animals highlighted the potential for cement cracking and the development of cavitary defects at the cement–bone interface. Even with appropriate cement technique, it may be difficult to ensure optimal interdigitation of bone cement into the dense cancellous bone that typically predominates in the subchondral bone of the proximal portion of the tibia (Figure 9.11).

Cementless tibial fixation has been used successfully in preclinical models of canine TKR (Turner et al. 1989; Sumner et al. 1994), as well as

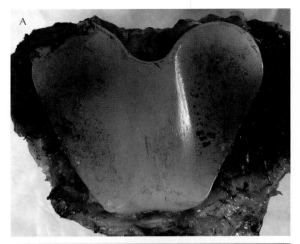

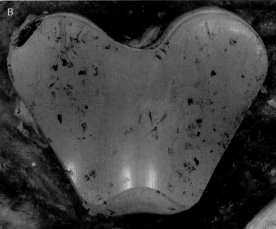

Figure 9.11   UHMWPE components retrieved from a dog that had undergone bilateral TKR. Wear scores were higher for the implant retrieved from the right stifle (A). This implant had been in service for 14 months (A) as compared with only 3 months for the left stifle (B). Pits and scratches are evident on both implants. Damage at the caudal edge of the implant (A) represents delamination. (Images courtesy of Mark Miller, MS [SUNY Upstate Medical University]; retrieval specimens kindly provided by Melvyn Pond, BVMS, MRCVS)

in select clinical cases.[2] The GenuSys TKR system incorporates a cementless CoCr tibial component that is secured to the tibia with screws, and a cementless, metal-backed tibial component is now available for the BioMedtrix TKR implant system (Allen et al. 2010).

Fixation in primary versus revision TKR

In a revision setting, particularly when implant failure is associated with significant bone loss or when revision surgery requires the removal of an extensive cement mantle from the proximal tibia, bone loss can be a major challenge. Long stems that extend beyond the region of bone loss can be used to ensure fixation with solid bone (Liska et al. 2007); these stems support effective load transfer to cortical bone, and they can be used with or without cement. In humans, fixation may also be achieved through the use of conical metallic augments that are press-fit into the proximal tibia and into which a standard tibial implant can be cemented (Meneghini et al. 2008).

Mechanical factors in periprosthetic tissues

Stress shielding

The alloys used most commonly in joint replacement implants (CoCr and Ti6Al4V) have material properties that far exceed those of the native bone into which they are implanted (see Chapter 2). As a consequence, loads are preferentially transferred through the implant, resulting in a significant reduction in the loads "seen" by periprosthetic bone. In accordance with the postulates embodied in Wolff's law, the skeletal response to reduced loading involves net bone resorption. In canine TKR, stress shielding has been identified in the distal femur, adjacent to the craniodistal chamfer cut (Allen et al. 2009). Bone densitometry studies have demonstrated stress shielding in similar locations in human TKR patients (Abu-Rajab et al. 2006).

Kinematics after TKR

Although a number of studies have documented joint function and functional loading of the operated limb after TKR in the dog (Allen et al. 2009; Liska and Doyle 2009), there is currently a near-complete lack of detailed information regarding the effectiveness of TKR surgery in restoring joint kinematics in dogs. A number of research groups are actively working to develop methods for assessing TKR kinematics through the use of standard three-dimensional motion capture (Hatfield et al. 2011), biplanar fluoroscopy (Dennis et al. 2003), or uniplanar fluoroscopy combined with image matching (Okamoto et al. 2011).

The available data from human TKR indicate that although gait patterns change following TKR, they do not return to normal (Noble et al. 2005). In particular, the functional gait adaptations that are seen in patients with advanced osteoarthrosis (OA) are retained. Data addressing this issue are clearly needed in dogs since it will be important to be able to determine whether residual gait abnormalities are the result of ongoing postoperative pain or of chronic adaptations in the patient's gait.

Summary and conclusions

Much remains to be learned about the mechanical performance of canine TKR implants. Particular areas of interest include the kinematics of TKR implants and the significance of wear mechanisms in the development of implant-related complications. These questions are best answered through a combination of controlled clinical trials and laboratory investigations, including systematic analysis of retrieval specimens.

Endnote

1. Fitzpatrick N, Asher K. Constrained total knee replacement: A novel prosthesis for salvage arthroplasty in the dog and cat. Vet Surg 2010;39:E36.
2. Turner T. Personal communication.

References

Abu-Rajab RB, Watson WS, Walker B, et al. Periprosthetic bone mineral density after total knee arthroplasty. Cemented versus, cementless fixation. J Bone Joint Surg Br 2006;88:606–613.

Allen M, Leone K, Zhang R, et al. Histomorphometric and mechanical evaluation of a peri-apatite coated tibial baseplate in a canine total knee arthroplasty model. Trans Orthop Res Soc 2007;32:1864.

Allen MJ, Leone KA, Lamonte K, et al. Cemented total knee replacement in 24 dogs: Surgical technique, clinical results, and complications. Vet Surg 2009;38: 555–567.

Allen MJ, Rudinsky A, Shah S, et al. Preclinical assessment of cementless total knee replacement in the dog. Vet Comp Orthop Traumatol 2010;23:A1.

Anderst WJ, Tashman S. Using relative velocity vectors to reveal axial rotation about the medial and lateral compartment of the knee. J Biomech 2010;43: 994–997.

Andriacchi TP, Stanwyck TS, Galante JO. Knee biomechanics and total knee replacement. J Arthroplasty 1986;1:211–219.

Bartel DL, Bicknell VL, Wright TM. The effect of conformity, thickness, and material on stresses in ultra-high molecular weight components for total joint replacement. J Bone Joint Surg Am 1986;68:1041–1051.

Breeman S, Campbell M, Dakin H, et al. Patellar resurfacing in total knee replacement: Five-year clinical and economic results of a large randomized controlled trial. J Bone Joint Surg Am 2011;93:1473–1481.

Browne JA, Gall-Sims SE, Giuseffi SA, et al. All-polyethylene tibial components in modern total knee arthroplasty. J Am Acad Orthop Surg 2011;19: 527–535.

Callaghan JJ, Squire MW, Goetz DD, et al. Cemented rotating-platform total knee replacement. A nine to twelve-year follow-up study. J Bone Joint Surg Am 2000;82:705–711.

Carpenter DH, Jr, Cooper RC. Mini review of canine stifle joint anatomy. Anat Histol Embryol 2000;29: 321–329.

Cooke TD, Sled EA, Scudamore RA. Frontal plane knee alignment: A call for standardized measurement. J Rheumatol 2007;34:1796–1801.

D'Lima DD, Chen PC, Colwell CW Jr. Polyethylene contact stresses, articular congruity, and knee alignment. Clin Orthop Relat Res 2001;392:232–238.

Dennis DA, Komistek RD, Mahfouz MR, et al. Multicenter determination of in vivo kinematics after total knee arthroplasty. Clin Orthop Relat Res 2003;416: 37–57.

Deshmukh RV, Scott RD. Unicompartmental knee arthroplasty: Long-term results. Clin Orthop Relat Res 2001;392:272–278.

Dismukes DI, Tomlinson JL, Fox DB, et al. Radiographic measurement of the proximal and distal mechanical joint angles in the canine tibia. Vet Surg 2007;36: 699–704.

Dismukes DI, Fox DB, Tomlinson JL, et al. Determination of pelvic limb alignment in the large-breed dog: A cadaveric radiographic study in the frontal plane. Vet Surg 2008;37:674–682.

Feeney LC, Lin CF, Marcellin-Little DJ, et al. Validation of two-dimensional kinematic analysis of walk and sit-to-stand motions in dogs. Am J Vet Res 2007;68:277–282.

Grood ES, Suntay WJ. A joint coordinate system for the clinical description of three-dimensional motions: Application to the knee. J Biomech Eng 1983;105: 136–144.

Haman JD, Wimmer MA, Galante JO. Surface damage and wear in fixed, modular tibial inserts: The effects of conformity and constraint. In: Total Knee Arthroplasty: A Guide to Get Better Performance, Bellemans J, Ries MD, Victor J (eds.). Heidelberg: Springer, 2005, pp. 85–89.

Harris WH. Wear and periprosthetic osteolysis: The problem. Clin Orthop Relat Res 2001;293:66–70.

Hatfield GL, Hubley-Kozey CL, Astephen Wilson JL, et al. The effect of total knee arthroplasty on knee joint kinematics and kinetics during gait. J Arthroplasty 2011;26:309–318.

Hood RW, Wright TM, Burstein AH. Retrieval analysis of total knee prostheses: A method and its application to 48 total condylar prostheses. J Biomed Mater Res 1983;17:829–842.

Kim SE, Pozzi A, Banks SA, et al. Effect of tibial plateau leveling osteotomy on femorotibial contact mechanics and stifle kinematics. Vet Surg 2009;38:23–32.

Knutson K, Lindstrand A, Lidgren L. Survival of knee arthroplasties. A nation-wide multicentre investigation of 8000 cases. J Bone Joint Surg Br 1986;68: 795–803.

Konttinen YT, Zhao D, Beklen A, et al. The microenvironment around total hip replacement prostheses. Clin Orthop Relat Res 2005;430:28–38.

Korvick DL, Pijanowski GJ, Schaeffer DJ. Three-dimensional kinematics of the intact and cranial cruciate ligament-deficient stifle of dogs. J Biomech 1994;27:77–87.

Liska WD, Doyle ND. Canine total knee replacement: Surgical technique and one-year outcome. Vet Surg 2009;38:568–582.

Liska WD, Marcellin-Little DJ, Eskelinen EV, et al. Custom total knee replacement in a dog with femoral condylar bone loss. Vet Surg 2007;36:293–301.

Mann KA, Miller MA, Townsend KL, et al. The dog as a preclinical model to evaluate interface morphology and micro-motion in cemented total knee replacement. Vet Comp Orthop Traumatol 2011;25:1–10.

Meneghini RM, Lewallen DG, Hanssen AD. Use of porous tantalum metaphyseal cones for severe tibial bone loss during revision total knee replacement. J Bone Joint Surg Am 2008;90:78–84.

Morgan H, Battista V, Leopold SS. Constraint in primary total knee arthroplasty. J Am Acad Orthop Surg 2005;13:515–524.

Noble PC, Gordon MJ, Weiss JM, et al. Does total knee replacement restore normal knee function? Clin Orthop Relat Res 2005;431:157–165.

Okamoto N, Breslauer L, Hedley AK, et al. In vivo knee kinematics in patients with bilateral total knee arthroplasty of 2 designs. J Arthroplasty 2011;26: 914–918.

Oonishi H, Kim SC, Kyomoto M, et al. Change in UHMWPE properties of retrieved ceramic total knee prosthesis in clinical use for 23 years. J Biomed Mater Res B Appl Biomater 2005;74:754–759.

Pond MJ, Nuki G. Experimentally-induced osteoarthritis in the dog. Ann Rheum Dis 1973;32:387–388.

Pozzi A, Kim SE. Biomechanics of the normal and cranial cruciate-deficient stifle treated by tibial osteotomies. In: *Advances in the Canine Cranial Cruciate Ligament*, Muir P (ed.). Ames, IA: Wiley-Blackwell, 2010, pp. 195–199.

Ragetly CA, Griffon DJ, Mostafa AA, et al. Inverse dynamics analysis of the pelvic limbs in Labrador retrievers with and without cranial cruciate ligament disease. Vet Surg 2010;39:513–522.

Reilly D, Walker PS, Ben-Dov M, et al. Effects of tibial components on load transfer in the upper tibia. Clin Orthop Relat Res 1982;165:273–282.

Ritter MA, Faris PM, Keating EM, et al. Postoperative alignment of total knee replacement. Its effect on survival. Clin Orthop Relat Res 1994;299:153–156.

Robertsson O, Knutson K, Lewold S, et al. The Swedish Knee Arthroplasty Register 1975–1997: An update with special emphasis on 41,223 knees operated on in 1988–1997. Acta Orthop Scand 2001;72:503–513.

Rudinsky A, Townsend KL, Thurston S, et al. Wear analysis is retrieved canine total knee replacement implants. Vet Comp Orthop Traumatol 2010;23: A21.

Sathasivam S, Walker PS. Computer model to predict subsurface damage in tibial inserts of total knees. J Orthop Res 1998;16:564–571.

Schmalzried TP, Jasty M, Rosenberg A, et al. Polyethylene wear debris and tissue reactions in knee as compared to hip replacement prostheses. J Appl Biomater 1994;5:185–190.

Shahar R, Banks-Sills L. A quasi-static three-dimensional, mathematical, three-body segment model of the canine knee. J Biomech 2004;37:1849–1859.

Shahar R, Milgram J. Biomechanics of tibial plateau leveling of the canine cruciate-deficient stifle joint: A theoretical model. Vet Surg 2006;35:144–149.

Sumner DR, Turner TM, Dawson D, et al. Effect of pegs and screws on bone ingrowth in cementless total knee arthroplasty. Clin Orthop Relat Res 1994;309: 150–155.

Taylor M, Tanner KE, Freeman MA. Finite element analysis of the implanted proximal tibia: A relationship between the initial cancellous bone stresses and implant migration. J Biomech 1998;31:303–310.

Thieman KM, Pozzi A, Ling HY, et al. Comparison of contact mechanics of three meniscal repair techniques and partial meniscectomy in cadaveric dog stifles. Vet Surg 2010;39:355–362.

Tomlinson J, Fox D, Cook JL, et al. Measurement of femoral angles in four dog breeds. Vet Surg 2007;36:593–598.

Turner TM, Urban RM, Sumner DR, et al. Bone ingrowth into the tibial component of a canine total condylar knee replacement prosthesis. J Orthop Res 1989;7: 893–901.

Werner FW, Ayers DC, Maletsky LP, et al. The effect of valgus/varus malalignment on load distribution in total knee replacements. J Biomech 2005;38:349–355.

Wright TM. Knee biomechanics and implant design. In: *The Adult Knee*, Callaghan JJ, Rosenberg AG, Rubash HE, Simonian PT, Wickiewicz TL (eds.). Philadelphia: Lippincott, Williams & Wilkins, 2003, pp. 145–161.

10 Clinical Application of Total Knee Replacement

Melvyn Pond

Introduction

Since the 1950s, the canine stifle joint has been the subject of a considerable number of publications in the veterinary literature. Issues addressed include medial patellar luxation, osteochondroses, fractures, and ligament deficiency. The topic of the majority of these publications is cranial cruciate ligament (CrCL) disease. Despite many improvements in the management of stifle joint problems, the end result is very often osteoarthritis. Canine patients with osteoarthritis of the stifle joint show a wide range of clinical signs, but many develop disease that can limit the ability to lead a life of acceptable quality, despite medications, physical therapy, acupuncture, and other conservative means. Surgical techniques for management of osteoarthritis of the stifle have traditionally been limited to arthrodesis and amputation, but in recent years, the development of implants and instrumentation for replacing the canine stifle joint has given veterinarians another option for helping patients with this debilitating problem.

Historical perspectives

The human orthopedic literature abounds with descriptions of arthroplasty to treat intractable pain and loss of function due to pathology of the knee.

During the 1890s, Themistocles Gluck replaced knees affected by tuberculosis with a hinged prosthesis made of ivory. He performed the procedure on 14 patients, all of which failed (Eynon-Lewis et al. 1992). It was almost 100 years before further attempts were made to replace the human knee, but during that time much work was published on resurfacing and interposing a wide variety of materials between the joint surfaces. Verneuil, in 1860, considered interposing soft tissues to restore the articular surfaces of the knee joint and this stimulated the use of fat, fascia lata, prepatellar bursa, and pig bladder (Verneuil 1860). Even as late as 1958, Brown and colleagues used skin as interpositional tissue (Brown et al. 1958). Many synthetic materials were also used, including nylon and cellophane, but, as with the soft tissues,

Advances in Small Animal Total Joint Replacement, First Edition. Edited by Jeffrey N. Peck and Denis J. Marcellin-Little.
© 2013 John Wiley & Sons, Inc. Published 2013 by John Wiley & Sons, Inc.

all had poor results. Arthrodesis was the surgical treatment of choice for severe knee pain until joint replacements began to be developed in the 1950s. Metal-on-metal implants were initially in vogue, until metal-on-plastic prostheses evolved as experience was obtained in the use of such materials in total hip arthroplasty.

During the 1960s, Gunston developed a system of metal runners cemented to the femoral condyles and polyethylene implants cemented to the tibial plateau (Gunston 1971).

Stability of the replaced knee joint is of major concern and a variety of hinged prostheses were developed with modifications to allow some degree of rotation. Following patients over the long term showed the hinged prostheses to have a high rate of infection, loosening, and implant failure (Deburge et al. 1979).

During the 1960s and early 1970s three basic designs were developed that have had great influence on modern total knee replacements (TKRs). First, unicompartmental prostheses resurfaced either the lateral or medial articulation. Next, duocompartmental designs were essentially joined unicompartmental femoral components with separate tibial components. The femoral component was curved in two planes, but the tibial component was flat in the sagittal plane. Thus, there was no constraint built into the designs and cruciate ligament retention was essential for joint stability. The third concept was the Geomedic prosthesis (Mayo Clinic, Minneapolis, MN), which had a constant radius femoral component and separate dished tibial components. The constraint in this design was so great that the cemented implants rapidly loosened soon after weight bearing commenced.

At the time of the development of the Geomedic prosthesis, Freeman and colleagues in London developed a design with components that reduced shear forces at the bone–cement interface, minimized friction, and reduced wear by allowing contact over a wide area. In addition, this design allowed for minimal bone resection to allow salvage by arthrodesis (Freeman et al. 1973).

Ranawat and Shine, as well as Walker et al., were the first to introduce instrumentation to aid the insertion of the femoral and tibial components and laid the groundwork for precision in implant positioning and articulation (Ranawat and Shine

1973; Walker et al. 1983). Further precision in component insertion has been made necessary by the development of porous-coated (PCA), press-fit implants, which require accurate preparation of the bone surfaces to receive implants and, as a result, more consistent and reproducible implant positioning.

Knee arthroplasty developed into true TKR with the introduction of patellar resurfacing in 1955. At the time, the femoral component designs were condylar and the articulation of the initial metal resurfaced patella with the articular cartilage of the trochlear groove resulted in severe wear and very poor results.

With cemented polyethylene resurfacing of the patella and femoral component designs incorporating a trochlear groove, the modern concept of the TKR evolved. Patellar resurfacing is not performed routinely by all surgeons and precise indications as to when it may be beneficial have not been developed.

In human medicine two basic designs are in use: cruciate sparing and cruciate sacrificing. There is considerable debate as to the merits of each system, especially with regard to soft tissue balancing and implant contact over the full range of motion (ROM) of the joint. Increasing conformation between the implants results in less contact stress and less wear of the tibial component. This degree of conformation is simpler to achieve in cruciate sacrificing designs. Increasing sophistication in design of the tibial component has reduced rotational and craniocaudal instability in cruciate deficient joints. This type of highly conformed prosthesis is used in the canine TKR system described below.

The number of knees replaced in human medicine now far exceed the number of hips replaced and in data published by the Centers for Disease Control and Prevention, it is seen that during 2007, 534,000 TKRs were performed in the United States, compared with 235,000 total hip replacements (THRs).[1] Patient expectations after a TKR are expanding beyond simple relief of pain and many people expect to return to some degree of athletic activity beyond basic activities of daily living that, by itself, can subject the replaced joint to substantial forces. For example, the repetitive climbing flights of stairs can place considerable loads on a resurfaced patella and high-flexion designs have become necessary for patients in cultures who require more than 130 degrees of flexion in the knees for sitting cross-legged or kneeling to pray.

The current design of the canine TKR is based on the lessons learned from the history of human total knee arthroplasty as it evolved from Gluck's first attempt in 1890 to the advanced materials and nonhinged designs of today.

The first reported veterinary application of TKR involved implantation of a cementless TKR in cats. The prosthesis was used as a model for human finger joint prostheses. The prosthesis was implanted in 42 cats (Walker et al. 1983).

In 1989, Turner reported on a condylar total joint arthroplasty (TJA) of the canine stifle in experiments to investigate bone apposition and bone ingrowth in cementless tibial components (Turner et al. 1989).

These implants were subsequently used with subjectively assessed success in a few clinical cases.[2] These results, however, were not reported in the peer-reviewed literature.

In 2007, Liska et al. used a custom-designed TJA to reconstruct a canine stifle joint that had loss of the medial femoral condyle, medial patellar luxation, angular limb deformity, and severe muscle contracture following a gunshot injury. Standard femoral and tibial components were augmented by a titanium implant stabilized by a stem cemented into the medullary cavity of the femur. The procedure resulted in a greatly improved ROM in the stifle joint and the patient returned to full activity following intensive rehabilitation (Liska et al. 2007).

Allen et al. described the use of a cemented TKR system in 24 purpose-bred dogs followed up to 52 weeks after surgery. Despite encouraging results, the articulation was not thought to be optimal for long-term implantation because it was noted that 6 out of 24 stifle joints were unstable when internally and externally rotated with the joints in greater than 60 degrees of flexion (Allen et al. 2009).

In 2009, Liska and Doyle published the surgical technique and results of the use of a modular TKR (Canine Total Knee System, BioMedtrix LLC, Boonton, NJ). Six clinical patients were followed for 12 months after TKR implantation. These patients had TKR surgery to relieve the symptoms of end-stage osteoarthritis (Liska and Doyle 2009).

The dogs ranged in weight between 22 and 58 kg, and three had had previous surgery on the joint to be replaced. The dogs underwent supervised and home-based rehabilitation, and regular objective assessment of postoperative progress included force plate gait analysis. The most significant complication was in a seventh patient that could not be followed in the same manner because the owner allowed inappropriate activity that resulted in collateral ligament damage, further surgery, sepsis, and eventually amputation. The overall results of this detailed study were extremely encouraging and the current use of this system in many veterinary centers throughout the world will allow the collection of data to fully evaluate the system with special reference to technique modifications, implant fixation, complications, and expectations over the long term.

The implants include a cobalt-chromium (CoCr) femoral component that replaces the femoral condyles and trochlear groove. The femoral component articulates with a tibial surface manufactured from a block of ultrahigh-molecular-weight polyethylene (UHMWPE).

The implant design prevents rotation and translation of the surfaces but the construct is not fully constrained, so as to reduce stress at the bone–implant interface.

The surface of the femoral component in contact with the bone is covered with three layers of CoCr beads and bone ingrowth is expected to occur to achieve permanent fixation of the implant. The UHMWPE tibial component is secured with polymethylmethacrylate (PMMA) bone cement (Figure 10.1).

Indications for TKR

Osteoarthritis of the canine stifle is a common reason for patient visits to primary care veterinarians and veterinary referral centers. It can result in severe joint disease and loss of quality of life, particularly in instances of bilateral disease.

The most common cause of degenerative joint disease of the canine stifle is CrCL disease. The inflammation and joint instability associated with partial or complete tear of the CrCL results in osteoarthritis with varying degrees of pathology in the synovium, articular surfaces, and menisci.

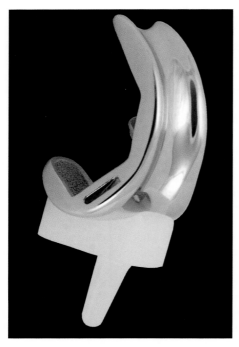

Figure 10.1 The CoCr femoral component and the monoblock UHMWPE tibial component. (Courtesy of BioMedtrix LLC, Boonton, NJ)

Left untreated, and sometimes despite conservative and or surgical management, the end result can be a degree of joint disease that limits the patient's use of the limb and interferes with the ability to work or to enjoy day-to-day activities. Other conditions that can result in osteoarthritis in the stifle include injuries to the collateral ligaments or menisci, the osteochondroses (e.g., osteochondritis dissecans), avulsion of the tendon of origin of the long digital extensor (LDE) muscle from the lateral femoral condyle, fractures, luxation of the patella, and femoral and or tibial deformities.

If the osteoarthritis is too advanced for management of the primary etiology to be successful, or if treatment fails and the osteoarthritis becomes the most significant problem, then the goals of treatment are relief of pain and restoration of weight bearing ability, ROM, and muscle mass. Conservative management with analgesics, nonsteroidal anti-inflammatory drugs, chondroprotectants, acupuncture, shockwave therapy, or physical therapy is often helpful. Intra-articular

injection of long-acting methylprednisolone and hyaluronate can also be useful in alleviating symptoms.

Patients presented with a history of unsuccessful conservative treatment may be candidates for a TKR. The radiographs of a stifle joint of such a patient are shown before surgery in Figure 10.2 and then after a TKR in Figure 10.3.

Preoperative considerations

Arriving at the decision to recommend a TKR should be based on a detailed history. Concurrent medical, neurological, or musculoskeletal issues may impact the success of TKR surgery. In particular, a complete review of prior treatment of the stifle joint in question is essential. This component of the history is generally more significant with TKR compared with THR. Patients evaluated for THR have rarely had surgical procedures performed on the hip prior to presentation, whereas many patients presented with severe stifle osteoarthritis frequently had surgical intervention on the stifle. Prior surgical intervention increases the risk of infection after TKR (Peersman et al. 2001).

Because CrCL disease is the most common cause of stifle osteoarthritis, a large number of patients being considered for a TKR will have had previous surgical procedures performed that have not resulted in the desired long-term results. These procedures could include arthroscopy and/or the insertion of implants such as the crimps and nonabsorbable materials used in a variety of extracapsular stabilization techniques or the metallic implants inserted during a tibial plateau leveling osteotomy (TPLO) or a tibial tuberosity advancement (TTA) or similar procedure.

If there have been repeated surgical attempts to stabilize a CrCL-deficient joint, then there is an increased likelihood of infection being present, in addition to the presence of severely inflamed bone and periarticular tissues. The radiographs shown in Figure 10.4 illustrate severe osteoarthritis despite a TPLO procedure in one patient and, in the other, after multiple attempts at extracapsular stabilization.

Surgery may also have been performed to repair fractures and collateral ligaments or to manage osteochondrosis. Luxation of the patella and

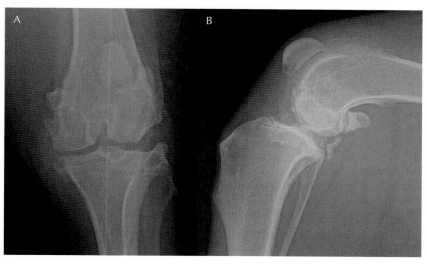

Figure 10.2   Preoperative radiographs of a canine stifle joint with severe degenerative joint disease.

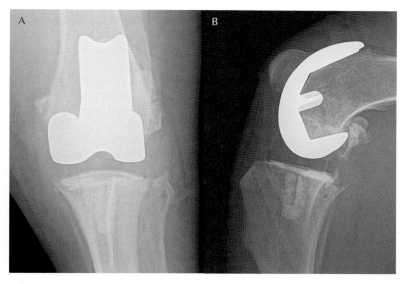

Figure 10.3   Radiographs of the joint shown in Figure 10.2, made immediately after replacement with a cementless femoral component and a cemented tibial component. (A) The CaCr view shows the condyles of the femoral component aligned with the cut surface of the tibia. (B) The lateral view demonstrates the slope of the cut surface of the tibia, bone cement around the keel of the tibial component, and the femoral component impacted onto the four ostectomy sites.

deformities of the femur or tibia often are present when patients are presented for evaluation for a TKR.

Many patients will have problems in other joints of the fore and hind limbs. These problems are rarely a contraindication to performing a TKR and, in fact, may be a reason for having the severely affected joint replaced. However, management during the immediate postoperative period may be more difficult and consideration should be given to this issue when planning short-term and long-term rehabilitation.

As well as the usual preanesthetic medical evaluation, it is accepted practice to obtain a urine

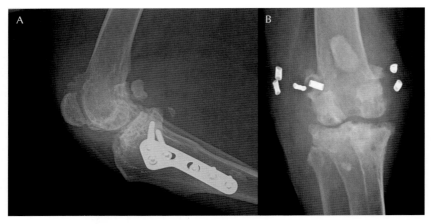

Figure 10.4   Mediolateral radiograph of the left stifle (A) and CaCr radiograph of the right stifle (B) of a dog that had a tibial plateau leveling osteotomy on one stifle (A) and extracapsular suture stabilization on the other stifle (B). Severe osteoarthritis is present, despite tibial plateau leveling (A) or extracapsular suture stabilization (B). The presence of implants necessitates staged procedures to reduce the risk of bacterial infection.

culture, and synovial fluid aspiration for cytology, culture, and antibiotic sensitivity.

Staging

If any implants, such as plates, screws, crimps, or nonabsorbable sutures are present, these should be removed during an initial procedure and cultures obtained from the tissues and the implants. If an infection is detected, the TKR should be delayed until repeated cultures obtained by fine-needle aspiration of tissues and fluid show that the infection is resolved.

Implant selection

Radiographs of the stifle joint are obtained as follows:

1. Mediolateral (M-L) view with the stifle joint flexed to 90 degrees and the hock rotated slightly to ensure that the femoral condyles are superimposed.
2. A true caudocranial (CaCr) view of the stifle with the patella centered in the trochlear groove.
3. Additional views may be necessary if there are bony deformities that will need correcting during the procedure.

All radiographs should include a magnification marker. Acetate templates are placed over the radiographs to assess the implant sizes to be used. As will be described later, final decisions regarding the sizes are made using trial implants, but accurate preoperative templating is especially important with regard to the femoral component because, once the femur is prepared, the only change possible is to remove more bone and use a smaller femoral implant (Figure 10.5).

The current canine total knee system has femoral components ranging in size from 30 to 42 mm, in 2-mm increments, and tibial components ranging in size from 30 to 38 mm, also in 2-mm increments. These sizes of implants are appropriate for dogs with a normal breed weight above 18 kg. The author's series of dogs undergoing TKR range in weight from 18 to 80 kg. It is important to note the femoral and tibial components do not have to be matching in size (e.g., a 36-mm femoral component will have a satisfactory articulation with a 30-mm tibial component).

Surgical procedure

The following is an outline of the procedure described in detail by other authors (Allen et al. 2009; Liska and Doyle 2009), with modifications that are based on the author's experience.

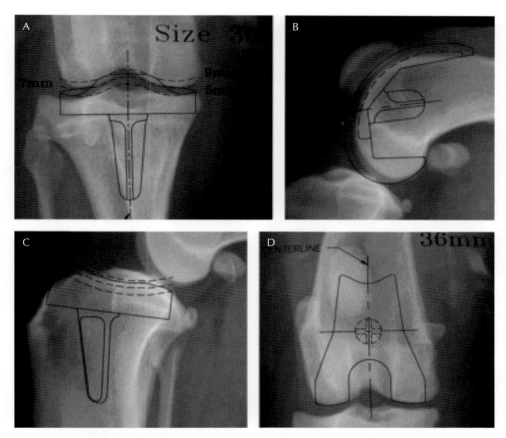

Figure 10.5   Templates are used to select the appropriately sized implants. (Courtesy of Dr. W. Liska)

The patient is placed in dorsal recumbency and positioned to allow free movement of the hip and stifle, such that when the stifle is fully flexed the hock is close to the end of the table. Iodine-impregnated adhesive film is used to cover all exposed skin and intravenous antibiotics are administered during the procedure. The joint can be approached either medially or laterally and the patella is luxated and flipped to lock it in position to fully expose the distal femur and tibial plateau. The bursa between the tibia and straight patellar tendon (SPT) is opened and the menisci and cruciate ligaments are excised, leaving a small tag of meniscus attached to the medial collateral ligament to facilitate identification and protection. The tibial plateau is further exposed by elevating the joint capsule and periarticular tissues from the edges of the tibial plateau (Figure 10.6).

An extramedullary tibial alignment guide (ETAG) is attached and positioned to obtain a final slope to the proximal tibial surface of approximately 6 degrees (Figure 10.7). Vasculature caudal to the stifle joint is protected by full flexion of the joint and the use of an instrument such as a Hohmann retractor to create cranial tibial translation. The collateral ligaments and SPT are protected with retractors and an oscillating saw is used to expose cancellous and cortical bone to the level of the caudal osteochondral junction (Figure 10.8). A keel-less tibial trial is used to ensure that the final implant will have maximum peripheral cortical bone support and will fit in a centralized position caudal to the SPT. There is often an overhang of the implant at the point where the LDE passes over the tibial plateau.

The author delays further preparation of the tibia until the femoral ostectomies have been completed and the femoral trial and tibial trial implants can be used in concert to assure that final alignment is satisfactory.

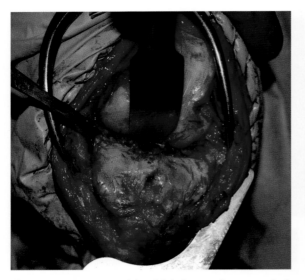

Figure 10.6 Exposure of the tibial plateau after removal of the cruciate ligaments and menisci. A large Hohmann retractor translates the tibia craniad and a small Hohmann retractor protects the medial collateral ligament. (Courtesy of Dr. Christopher Preston)

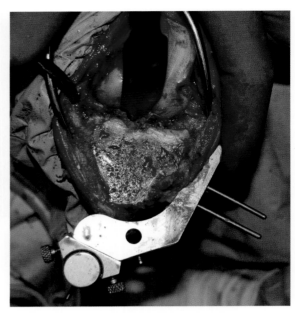

Figure 10.8 The tibial plateau has been removed and cancellous and cortical bone exposed. (Courtesy of Dr. Christopher Preston)

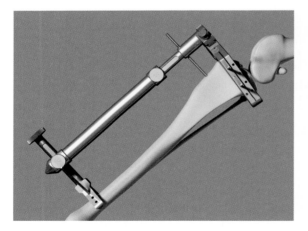

Figure 10.7 The extramedullary tibial alignment guide (ETAG) positioned to control the ostectomy of the tibial plateau. (Courtesy of BioMedtrix LLC, Boonton, NJ)

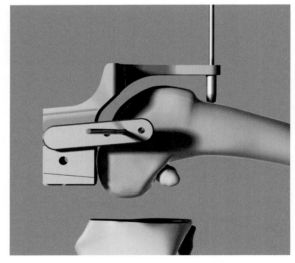

Figure 10.9 Femoral cutting block (FCB) positioned to guide the four femoral ostectomies. (Courtesy of BioMedtrix LLC, Boonton, NJ)

The femoral cutting block (FCB) is centered on the distal femur using two reference points: first, the middle of the trochlear groove adjacent to the origin of the LDE; and second, the middle of the most proximal extent of the trochlear groove (Figures 10.9 and 10.10). Minor adjustments in position may be necessary to ensure that the FCB is parallel to the cut surface of the tibia and then it is attached with fixation pins. The FCB has four slots through which an oscillating saw blade is inserted to make ostectomies in the sequence of cranial, caudal, distal, and cranioproximal. All cut

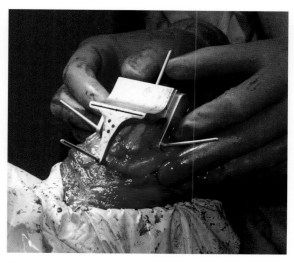

Figure 10.10 The FCB in place showing the fixation pins, the datum hole in the FCB, and the slot for directing the oscillating saw during the resection of the distal portion of the femoral condyles. (Courtesy of Dr. Christopher Preston)

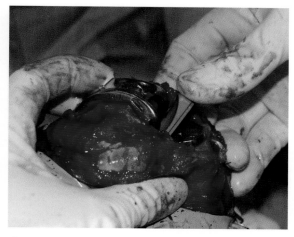

Figure 10.11 The trial femoral and tibial components are in place and a 5-mm-thick trial tibial component is being inserted. The articular surface of the patella can be seen medial to the ridge of the trochlea. The patella has been flipped to increase exposure of the joint surfaces. (Courtesy of Dr. Christopher Preston)

surfaces will be in contact with the beaded surface of the femoral component and precision is critical. Thus, there should be minimal "chattering" of the blade during cutting and the blade used must be 0.9 mm in thickness for a precise fit in the slots. Prior to removal of the FCB, a hole is drilled into the bone at the datum hole on the FCB. This will allow accurate positioning if the use of a smaller femoral component than the size selected during preoperative measurements becomes necessary.

Trial femoral and tibial components are used to make a final selection of the implants to be used and to evaluate positioning. The selected femoral trial implant is impacted into place and the bone–implant interface checked for satisfactory contact. The keel-less tibial trial is placed as before to obtain maximum cortical contact and the articulation between the femoral and tibial components assessed. If the femoral condyles are not accurately centered on the tibial component, the femoral component can be reapplied slightly medial or lateral to the previous position. Alternatively, the tibial component can be similarly repositioned, but it is important to maintain cortical bone support for the tibial component and there may not be much latitude for adjusting the position of this component.

When satisfactory alignment between the components has been attained, the trial femoral component is removed. The tibia is prepared by drilling and reaming to accept the keel and 2-mm-diameter holes are drilled in the tibial plateau as peg holes for the PMMA cement.

To assess the correct thickness of the tibial component, the metal form is placed on the tibial plateau with the peg inserted into the hole prepared for the final implant. With the trial femoral component in place, 5-, 7-, or 9-mm-thick tibial plateau trials are inserted into the metal form (Figure 10.11).

The correct choice of thickness of the tibial trial will allow a full ROM without medial or lateral instability. Instability is assessed by attempting to "open" the joint medially and laterally while the joint is held in extension and by attempting to translate the tibia relative to the femur in the M-L and a craniocaudal planes.

If full flexion is inhibited by collateral ligament tightness with the thinnest (5 mm) tibial trial in place, then a smaller femoral component will be necessary. A further 2 mm of bone is removed at the caudal femoral ostectomy. To achieve this, an FCB one size smaller than that previously used is positioned with the first fixation pin passing

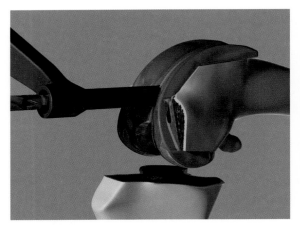

Figure 10.12 Use of the trial femoral prosthesis to drill the femur to accommodate the peg on the femoral component. (Courtesy of BioMedtrix LLC, Boonton, NJ)

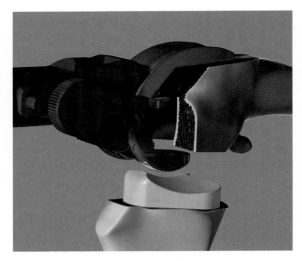

Figure 10.13 Implantation of the femoral component using the femoral impactor. Note the peg on the proximal aspect of the femoral component. (Courtesy of BioMedtrix LLC, Boonton, NJ)

through the datum hole drilled during fixation of the original FCB. This ensures that the smaller implant will fit precisely to all ostectomy sites.

When satisfied with the joint stability, ROM, and accuracy of fit of the femoral component, the final step in preparation is to drill a hole through a guide placed in the centrally located hole in the femoral trial. This hole will accept the peg of the final implant (Figure 10.12). The selected tibial implant is cemented into place using current-generation cementing techniques (see Chapter 5) and then the femoral component is impacted on to the distal femur (Figure 10.13). Care is taken to attain maximum contact between the bone and the implant. After copious lavage and removal of excess cement, the patella is repositioned and the soft tissues closed.

Postoperative radiographs

Lateral and CaCr views are obtained and the implants assessed for femoral bone contact, the caudal slope of the tibial plateau relative to the long axis of the tibia, and, in the CaCr view, overall alignment of the implants (Figure 10.3)

Cold packing and gentle physical therapy begins immediately and the patients are usually discharged 2 days after surgery with detailed instructions for home-based and clinic-based rehabilitation.

Results

As described in the "Historical Perspectives" section of this chapter, Liska and Doyle published a study describing six clinical patients followed for 12 months after surgery (Liska and Doyle 2009). This objective study confirmed the subjective assessment of significant improvement to almost normal use of the legs despite severe preoperative osteoarthritis.

Complications

The most significant complications in the author's experience and as reported in personal communications from Dr. William Liska and Dr. Christopher Preston are infection and damage to the collateral ligaments.[3,4]

Infection is catastrophic if it cannot be controlled with appropriate antibiotics. Implant removal may have to be considered if the infection cannot be resolved and temporary stability of the deconstructed joint with external skeletal fixation would then be necessary while attempting to manage the infection prior to reimplantation or arthrodesis.

This complicated and unpredictable staged treatment makes amputation the more likely scenario following unresolved infection of a TKR. It cannot be overemphasized that, if a patient selected for TKR has implants in place from previous surgical procedures, implants must be removed and bacterial cultures collected before undertaking the TKR.

Either of the collateral ligaments can be damaged during the TKR procedure, usually during the ostectomy of the proximal tibia. Every effort should be made to protect the collateral ligaments and it should be noted that the oscillating edges of the saw blade can be as damaging to the soft tissues as the cutting end. The amount of bone removed during the tibial and femoral ostectomies results in significant instability due to decreased ligament tension, even without damage to the collateral ligaments, and assessment of actual ligamentous integrity is made during the evaluation with the trial implants.

If the joint space can be opened medially or laterally with appropriately sized implants in place, then ligamentous damage has likely occurred and the joint should be supported by ligament repair or reconstruction using a suitable material attached to the femur and tibia with bone anchors or screws and spiked washers.

The author has used ligament reconstruction successfully in one patient that had obvious medial collateral ligament instability detected during the TKR procedure. A second patient developed medial joint instability 1 month following the TKR and was treated successfully in a similar manner.

Future directions

As experience is gained with the technique, and if clinical outcomes continue to be encouraging, then it is probable that TKR will come to be used earlier in the course of the development of osteoarthritis. TKR may also be used to correct skeletal abnormalities that may be the cause or result of severe joint disease. Illustrated in Figure 10.14 is a patient in which there has been collapse of the lateral aspect of the stifle joint and a subsequent malalignment of the long axis of the femur and tibia. This was corrected by ostectomy of 15 mm from the distal medial femoral condyle prior to placement of the FCB and the tibial ostectomy being made below the collapsed plateau. The result is alignment of the tibial axis and the femoral axis, and this patient recovered to full use of the leg in agility work.

Since the Canine Total Knee system (BioMedtrix LLC) has been in use in a number of veterinary centers throughout the world, reports from personal communications indicate that data is accumulating to support the continued use of TKR as a viable method of treating canine stifle joint disease, and it is anticipated that objective data will accumulate to guide the use and development of the technique.

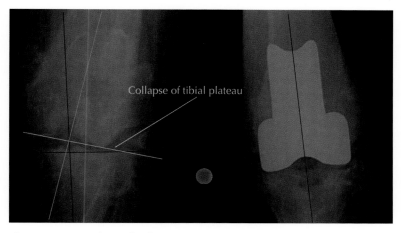

Collapse of tibial plateau

Figure 10.14   Pre- and postoperative radiographs illustrating correction of malalignment of the axis of the femur and the tibia following collapse of the lateral tibial plateau.

Endnotes

1. DeFrances CJ, Hall MJ. National Hospital Discharge Survey. U.S. Department of Health and Human Services, Centers for Disease Control and Prevention, National Center for Health and Human Statistics, 2009.
2. Turner T. Personal communication, 2011.
3. Liska B. Personal communication, 2011.
4. Preston C. Personal communication, 2011.

References

Allen MJ, Leone KA, Lamonte K, et al. Cemented total knee replacement in 24 dogs: Surgical technique, clinical results and complications. Vet Surg 2009;38: 555–567.

Brown JE, McCaw WH, Shaw DT. Use of cutis as an interposing membrane in arthroplasty of the knee. J Bone Joint Surg Am 1958;40:1003–1018.

Deburge A, Aubriot JH, Genet JP. Current status of a hinge prosthesis. Clin Orthop Relat Res 1979;145: 91–93.

Eynon-Lewis NJ, Pearse MF, Ferry D. Themistocles Gluck: An unrecognized genius. Br Med J 1992;305: 1534–1536.

Freeman MAR, Swanson SAV, Todd RC. Total replacement of the knee using the Freeman-Swanson knee prosthesis. Clin Orthop Relat Res 1973;94:153–170.

Gunston FH. Polycentric knee arthroplasty: Prosthetic simulation of normal knee movement. J Bone Joint Surg Br 1971;53:272–277.

Liska W, Doyle N. Canine total knee replacement: Surgical technique and 1 year outcome. Vet Surg 2009;38:568–582.

Liska W, Marcellin-Little D, Eskelinen E, et al. Custom total knee replacement in a dog with femoral condyle loss. Vet Surg 2007;36:293–301.

Peersman G, Laskin R, Davis J, et al. Infection in total knee replacement: A retrospective review of 6489 total knee replacements. Clin Orthop Relat Res 2001;392:15–23.

Ranawat CS, and Shine JJ. Duo-Condylar total knee arthroplasty. Clin Orthop Rel Res 1973;94:185–193.

Turner TM, Urban RM, Sumner DR, et al. Bone ingrowth into the tibial component of a canine total knee replacement prosthesis. J Orthop Res 1989;7:893–901.

Verneuil A. De la création d'une fausse articulation par section ou résection partielle de l'os maxillaire inferieur, comme moyen de remédier à l'ankylose vraie ou fausse de la mâchoire inférieure. Arch Gén Méd 1860;15(Sec 5):174, 284–288.

Walker PS, Nunamaker D, Huiskes R, et al. A new approach to the fixation of a metacarpophalangeal joint prosthesis. Eng Med 1983;12(3):135–140.

11 Biomechanical Considerations in Total Elbow Development

Greg Van Der Meulen

History of total elbow replacements

The elbow, a complex trochleoginglymoid joint encompassing three articulations, is an inherently difficult joint to replicate. The limited success of conservative management and arthroscopic surgeries to treat end-stage elbow osteoarthritis (OA) has stimulated a genuine interest in the development of a total elbow replacement (TER) over the last 20 years.

The first TER implants used in custom clinical cases tended to be fully constrained (i.e., hinged) cemented designs with little to no success. The early 1990s brought about the first attempts at developing a TER to treat end-stage OA. BioMedtrix (Boonton, NJ) began research and development into a cemented three-component resurfacing design that was then passed on to Vasseur (University of California—Davis; Figure 11.1). Ultimately, this implant design did not proceed into clinical trials due to an inability to biomechanically align all three components during preliminary testing.[1] In 1996, Lewis reported on the use of a cemented hinge design in 10 clinical cases, which had little success.[2] Lewis continued to revise his design throughout the late 1990s,

ultimately arriving at a three-component semiconstrained system, but was never able to achieve repeatable success (Figure 11.2). Conzemius began clinical testing on a cemented two-component semiconstrained design (Iowa State Elbow), which fused the radius and ulna, in an attempt to reduce the joint to a simple hinge. In 1998, Conzemius reported positive results on the use of this system in six normal dogs (Conzemius and Aper 1998), and then, 2 years later, on 20 dogs afflicted with naturally occurring OA (Conzemius et al. 2001).[3] In 2003, Cook also explored the potential of a two-component design using a transolecranon surgical approach that ultimately had little to no success in clinical cases.[4] In 2005, after further refinement, the Iowa State Elbow became the first commercially available TER, offered through BioMedtrix (Figure 11.3). In 2008, Acker and Van Der Meulen reported satisfactory results on a biologically fixed two-component system, known as the TATE Elbow™, on six clinical cases with end-stage elbow OA.[5] This system was also licensed to BioMedtrix and was released in 2009 to a select group of surgeons for further review. The TATE is commercially available and a second-generation implant has been introduced, focusing on improved

Advances in Small Animal Total Joint Replacement, First Edition. Edited by Jeffrey N. Peck and Denis J. Marcellin-Little.
© 2013 John Wiley & Sons, Inc. Published 2013 by John Wiley & Sons, Inc.

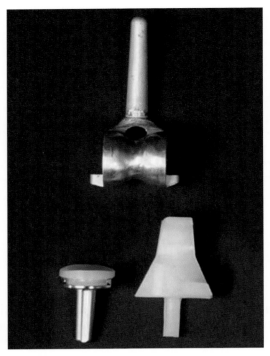

Figure 11.1 Chris Sidebotham (president of BioMedtrix LLC) gave this TER to Vasseur in the early 1990s. Unfortunately neither group was able to attain a satisfactory result due to an inability to biomechanically align all three components, and as a result the project was discontinued. (Courtesy of Chris Sidebotham)

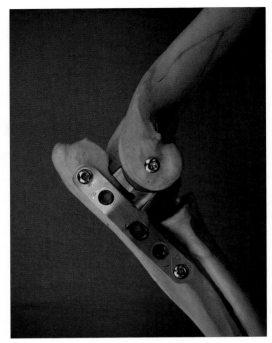

Figure 11.2 Lewis's third-generation semiconstrained three-component design with a cemented UHMWPE radial head in order to retain pronation and supination. The radioulnar component was attached much like a standard bone plate. (Courtesy of Dr. Loïc M. Déjardin)

osseointegration through an improved bone-ingrowth surface and a reduction in articular constraints (Figure 11.4). A two-component system developed by Innes, known as the Sirius Elbow, uses a hybrid fixation system. The Sirius Elbow uses both cement and biological fixation for the humeral component and screw fixation with biological apposition surfaces for the radioulnar component.[6]

As our understanding of OA in the elbow has advanced, attempts have been made to develop medial unicompartmental replacements in an attempt to deter the progression of OA. Cook and Schulz, working with Arthrex, developed the Canine Unicompartmental Elbow (CUE), which functions much like an Osteochondral Autograft Transfer System (OATS), but with metal and polyethylene implants substituted for osteochondral autograft. This system has completed a multicenter clinical study[7] and is now commercially available. Another medial unicompartmental system is currently under development by Wendelburg and Tepic and is also undergoing clinical testing.[8]

Chapter overview

The purpose of this chapter is to provide a foundation of the anatomy, biomechanics, and implant design principles to better understand TERs. The anatomy is briefly reviewed, including the osteology of the distal humerus, proximal radius, and ulna, the ligamentous structures, the surrounding musculature, and pertinent nerves and vasculature. The anatomical review is followed by an overview of our current understanding of the biomechanics of the elbow and the transarticular

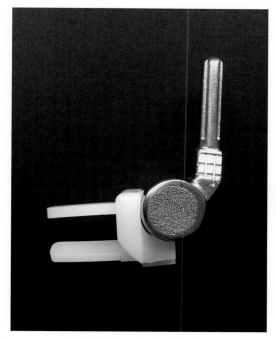

Figure 11.3   The fifth-generation of the Iowa State implant shows the addition of sintered beads to the medial and lateral surfaces of the humeral component in place of cement pockets.

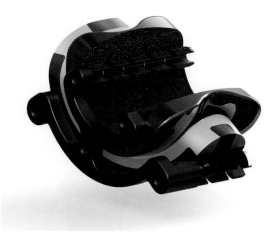

Figure 11.4   The second-generation TATE Elbow™ implant components: the humeral component, the radioulnar component, and the set plate insert as a single unit, or "cartridge," simultaneously. The set plate, in blue, is removed after insertion, allowing the joint to articulate.

forces. In addition, a review of the common surgical approaches used for elbow replacements are discussed as they pertain to the necessary exposure of the elbow joint for establishing a repeatable, accurate surgical technique. This knowledge base is the foundation for the discussion of establishing the basic design principles for successful elbow replacement.

The elbow: Anatomy

The elbow is a complex trochleoginglymoid synovial joint encompassing the articular surfaces of the distal portion of the humerus, the proximal portion of the radius, and the proximal portion of the ulna. It comprises the humeroulnar, humeroradial, and radioulnar articulations. Flexion and extension is the primary function of the humeroulnar joint, while pronation and supination occur primarily at the humeroradial and the radioulnar joints (Figure 11.5).

The distal humerus

The humeral condyle essentially consists of the diaphysis splitting into two bony columns that support the humeral articular surfaces. The sagittally circular humeral articular surface may be further described as two distinct surfaces. The capitulum, which includes the nearly spherical lateral articular surface, and the trochlea, a pulley-shaped surface located medially. The humeral capitulum articulates with the radial head, forming the humeroradial joint. The humeral trochlea articulates with the trochlear notch of the ulna, forming the primary articulation of the elbow, the humeroulnar joint, an inherently stable hinge joint. The lateral epicondyle, located caudolateral to the capitulum, is the origin of the extensor muscle group (functionally referred to as the extensor epicondyle) and the proximal end of the lateral collateral ligament (LCL). The medial epicondyle gives origin to the flexor muscle group in addition to the proximal end of the medial

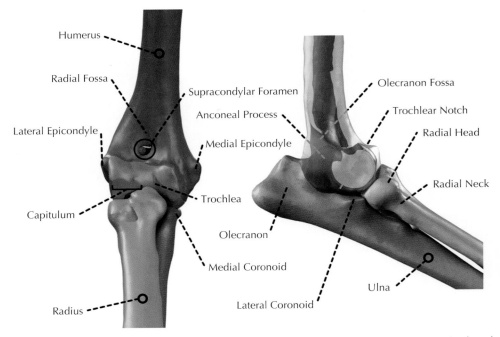

Figure 11.5　Cranial and lateral views of the elbow joint, showing anatomical structures pertinent to an implant designer.

collateral ligament. Although the medial and lateral epicondyles are not coincident with the central axis of rotation, an important reference with some implant designs, they are commonly used as anatomical references during surgery. Cranially and caudally, there are two fossae, the radial fossa, which accepts the radial head while in deep flexion, and the olecranon fossa, which accepts the anconeal process of the ulna when the joint is in extension. The radial and olecranon fossa partially overlap, creating the supratrochlear foramen and thus the separation of the humeral shaft into the aforementioned two bony columns.

The radius

The proximal portion of the radius consists of the radial head, which is an irregular semicircular shape in the transverse plane, and quickly tapers distally, forming the radial neck. The articular surface has a slightly concave surface that functionally mirrors that of the humeral capitulum and thus forms the aforementioned humeroradial joint. Extending distally, along the mediocaudal

aspect of the radial head, is the articular surface that articulates against the radial notch of the ulna forming the radioulnar joint. The radioulnar joint, which allows pronation and supination, previously has been thought to provide very little to the overall function of the elbow and has therefore led to the fusion of this joint in an effort to simplify implants and surgical techniques. The radial head has a bulbous protuberance that extends laterally and does not have any muscular or ligamentous attachments, but does function as a visual reference for some surgical techniques. The radial tuberosity, which is located along the medial aspect of the radius just distal to the radial neck, is a roughened area that functions as an insertion point for the biceps brachii and the brachialis muscles.

The ulna

The proximal portion of the ulna, unlike its human equivalent, has a large olecranon that extends proximally, away from the joint surface, and functions as a lever arm for amplifying the forces generated primarily by the triceps muscle. The articular surface of the ulna, a semilunar notch that faces cranially, encompasses three primary structures: the trochlear notch, the coronoid process, and the anconeal process. The trochlear notch mirrors the pulley-like shape of the humeral trochlea and thus creates a highly constrained articulation. The coronoid process, just distal to the trochlear notch, is divided into medial and lateral surfaces, with the medial surface significantly more prominent. The anconeal process, which extends cranially and makes up the proximal articular surface, inserts into the olecranon fossa and supratrochlear foramen of the humerus when the elbow is in extension.

Ligaments

The healthy elbow is a very stable joint not only because of the high congruency of its articular surfaces but also because of the surrounding ligamentous structures and joint capsule. The elbow has two collateral ligaments, one medial and one lateral, that each originate proximally to either epicondyle and divide into two crura just distal to the annular ligament where they insert on the radius and ulna. Within the cranial aspect of the elbow resides the annular ligament. It lies deep to the collateral ligaments, attaches to the medial and lateral extremities of the radial notch, and wraps around the radial head. Attaching proximally to the annular ligament, along the dorsal edge of the supratrochlear foramen of the humerus and crossing the flexor surface of the elbow, in a distomedial direction, is the oblique ligament. At the point that the oblique ligament crosses the annular ligament, the oblique ligament divides into two separate branches. The shorter of the two branches blends with the cranial branch of the medial collateral ligament and the longer branch attaches to the medial edge of the radius, after looping around the tendons of the biceps brachii and brachialis. The caudally located olecranon ligament attaches to the caudolateral ridge of the lateral epicondyle and into the olecranon fossa and distally to the distolateral margin of anconeal process. The function of the olecranon ligament is to prevent elbow hyperflexion.

Musculature

The musculature that inserts and originates around the elbow can be divided into two groups: musculature responsible for the primary function of the elbow (i.e., flexion and extension), located within the brachium; and musculature that controls the carpus, found in the antebrachium.

The muscles of the brachium encompass the entire humerus, except for a small exposed region located mediodistally. The primary cranial muscles, responsible for flexion of the elbow, are the biceps brachii and the brachialis. The biceps brachii tendon of insertion divides distally into two distinct branches attaching to the previously mentioned radial and ulnar tuberosities. The brachialis tendon of insertion travels between the branches of the biceps brachii tendons and inserts at the ulnar tuberosity. The primary extensor muscles of the brachium are the triceps brachii and the anconeus. The triceps muscle, located caudal to the humerus, has four separate heads: the lateral, long, medial, and accessory heads that share a common insertion along the most proximal edge of the olecranon process. The anconeus muscle originates primarily along the caudal edge of the lateral epicondyle; however, the origin continues proximally and medially over the perimeter of the supratrochlear foramen along the caudal edge of the medial epicondyle as well. The anconeus inserts along the cranial and lateral surfaces of the proximal ulna.

The muscles of the antebrachium, although numerous, have few attachment points that need to be considered when evaluating an elbow replacement. Medially, the primary flexor group attaches to the distal surface of the epicondyle. The pronator teres, responsible for flexion of the carpus and pronation of the elbow, originates at the tip of the medial epicondyle. The extensor muscle group and the supinator muscle arise from the lateral epicondyle of the humerus, with the origin of the extensor carpi radialis extending proximally along the lateral aspect of the humerus. The supinator extends distally, inserting on the craniolateral surface of the radius, distal to the radial head. The proximal portion of the ulna has two ancillary muscle origins that should be considered: the flexor carpi ulnaris, located along the medial concave surface and caudal aspect of the olecranon; and the ulnar origin of the deep digital flexor that extends distally down the ulnar diaphysis.

Nerves and vasculature

An understanding of the primary nerves and vasculature in the immediate vicinity of the elbow joint is critical when deciding upon and performing a surgical exposure. The medial aspect of the elbow has multiple critical structures: the ulnar nerve, the median nerve, and the median artery and vein. The ulnar nerve, which runs just cranial to the medial head of the triceps muscle, passes the elbow just caudal to the medial epicondyle. The median nerve runs parallel to the ulnar nerve through the brachium, but diverges cranially, along with the median artery, just proximal to the elbow and crosses the joint at the flexor surface. The deep branch of the radial nerve runs along the lateral aspect of the brachium. Like the median nerve, the deep branch transitions the elbow at the flexor surface, but on the lateral side.

Elbow biomechanics

Motion

The canine elbow has two degrees of freedom: flexion–extension and axial rotation. The range of motion (ROM) of the elbow, established through a

goniometric study, is 36 ± 2 degrees in flexion and up to 165 ± 2 degrees in extension (Jaegger et al. 2002). In addition, the elbow, measured with the forelimb and palmar surfaces in neutral extension, is able to supinate 50 degrees and pronate up to 90 degrees (Newton and Nunamaker 1985).

The use of gait analysis has led to an evolution in the understanding of the elbow and how the functional ROM is utilized. Two-dimensional analysis of a series of clinically normal mixed-breed dogs at a walk was collected via force platform and three-dimensional (3D) videography (Nielsen et al. 2003). The elbow joint was at an angle of 112 ± 12 degrees of flexion at the point of initial ground contact. After initial ground strike, the elbow extended slightly and then flexed to its starting angle as it was loaded. It then extended steadily throughout the stance phase to a maximum angle of 136 ± 10 degrees and flexed slightly prior to liftoff.

In order to achieve a more comprehensive understanding of the complexities of the canine elbow, Guillou et al. implanted radiopaque markers in the right humerus, radius, and ulna of six adult dogs.[9] The dogs were then walked and trotted on a gait analysis track equipped with a dynamic radiostereometric analysis (RSA) system. Using custom software to track the individual markers that had been merged with individual 3D reconstructions from computed tomography (CT) scans, they were able to establish kinematic curves of the elbow in 3D space (Figure 11.6). Through the individual examination of the humerus, ulna,

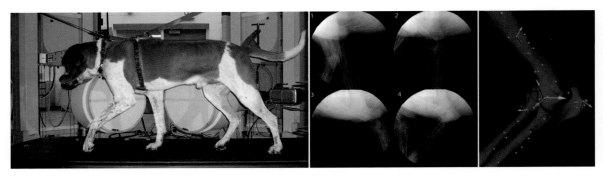

Figure 11.6   After having tantalum beads implanted in the humerus, radius, and ulna, the dogs were walked and trotted on a motion analysis track equipped with a biplanar radiographic system (*left* and *center*). This data was then merged with the three-dimensional reconstructions of each elbow (*right*) and, using proprietary software, the relative motion was tracked. (Courtesy of Dr. Reunan Guillou)

Table 11.1   Three-dimensional kinematics of the normal canine elbow at the walk and trot

	Max extension[a]	Max flexion[a]	Min varus during midstance[a]	Varus amplitude[a]	Pronation/ supination	Proximal/distal translation of radial head[a]
Walk	151.3 ± 3.9[a]	80.6 ± 4.2[a]	4.9 ± 3.4[a]	16.6 ± 3.4[a]	15.2 ± 4.1[a]	0.93 ± 0.16 mm
Trot	148.3 ± 4.5[a]	77.1 ± 7.5[a]	4.8 ± 4.0[a]	19.6 ± 3.4[a]	17.4 ± 4.4[a]	0.9 ± 0.16 mm

Data compiled from the work of Dr. Reunan Guillou et al., Michigan State University.
[a]No significant difference between the walk and trot.

and radius, the study identified significant aspects of how each bone contributes to the overall kinematics of the joint (Table 11.1). The varus angle fluctuated through an ROM. Specifically, the varus was minimal through the stance phase, at an angle of 4.9 ± 3.4 degrees, but continued to increase through the swing phase with a varus amplitude of 16.6 ± 3.4 degrees for the walk and 19.6 ± 3.4 degrees for the trot, which were not significantly different. In addition, at the point of ground contact, the elbow quickly pronated: 5 degrees during the walk and 8 degrees during the trot, and returned to neutral just prior to liftoff. Entering the swing phase, the elbow supinates approximately 7 degrees for both the walk and the trot, returning back to neutral just before ground strike.

The Guillou study illustrated the subtle complexities of the elbow joint. The study also demonstrated the challenges to be faced in the attempt to achieve the natural kinematics of the joint.

Axis of rotation

The axis of rotation of flexion–extension in the human elbow occurs around a tight locus of points only 2–3 mm wide at the broadest dimension (Morrey and Chao 1976). This axis can be identified at two points within the human and canine humerus: (1) the center of the humeral trochlea and (2) the center of the capitulum. If this axis were to extend outside of the humerus, it would emerge just distal and cranial to both the medial and lateral epicondyles (Figure 11.7). If the canine elbow functions in a manner similar to the human elbow, this axis is one of the most critical features of the biomechanics of the joint. Therefore, any implant design concerned with the balancing of the surrounding soft tissues, specifically unlinked

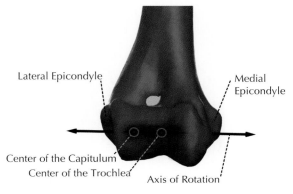

Figure 11.7   Axis of rotation. A cranial view of the distal humerus showing the two consistent reference points for establishing the axis of rotation of the elbow.

joint replacements, must accurately replicate this axis in order to achieve a ROM free of conflict with periarticular soft tissues. The ability to replicate the axis is most commonly dictated by the repeatability of the surgical technique and how consistently a surgeon can implant the prosthesis.

Varus angle/mechanical axis deviation

The canine elbow, much like the human knee, has a naturally occurring varus angulation.[10] Saviori et al. found that this angulation in the frontal plane can be evaluated by establishing the mechanical axes of the humerus[11] and radius–ulna[12] and measuring their angle of intersection at the elbow.[13] In a study performed on 100 adult canine forelimbs they found this angle, the mechanical humeral radial–ulnar angle, to be 9.0 ± 3.6 degrees (Figure 11.8). When compared with the mechanical axis of the overall limb, the mechanical axis deviation

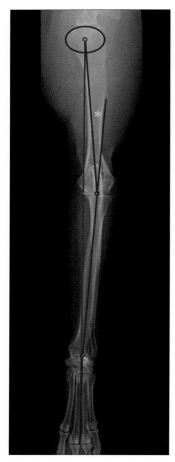

Figure 11.8 Varus angle and mechanical axis deviation (MAD). The blue lines represent the three mechanical axes of the forelimb, the red line shows the mechanical axis of the entire limb, the orange line represents the MAD, and the asterisk represents the location of the varus angle measurement. (Courtesy of Dr. Derek B. Fox)

(MAD) is described as the shortest distance from the mediolateral center of the articulating surface of the distal humerus to the limb mechanical axis. Expressed as a percentage of overall limb length, to normalize the effect of dog size, this value was 2.6% ± 0.02%. Therefore, a dog, for example, with a limb length of 45 cm would have a MAD measurement of 12 mm.

This varus angulation or MAD creates a medial to lateral shear force at the level of the elbow due to the eccentricity of the limb mechanical axis. The intrinsic and extrinsic stabilizers in a healthy joint counter this transarticular shear force and allow it to function as normal. However, if one or more of the stabilizers are compromised (the medial coronoid, LCL, etc.), then the eccentric loading of the joint results in an increase in transarticular forces in the medial compartment. Over time, this increased load could erode the articular cartilage of the medial compartment resulting in an increased varus angle and an off-loading of the lateral compartment.

Transarticular forces

The radial head, once thought to carry "practically all the weight transmitted from the arm to the forearm" (Evans 1993), actually carries approximately 52% (Mason et al. 2005) of the total transarticular forces, thus sharing a substantial amount with the humeroulnar articulation. This is contrary to initial assumptions based on the relative limited size of the articular surface of the distal ulnar styloid process when compared with the distal radial articular surface. A partial understanding of this near-equal load sharing came through an understanding of the human elbow. When a compressive force is transmitted through the hand, the majority of this load is transmitted through the radiocarpal joint and, thus, into the radius. As this force moves proximally—up the radial diaphysis—it stretches the interosseous membrane and transfers a portion of this compressive force to the ulna and, as a result, across the elbow at the humeroulnar joint (Figure 11.9; Pfaeffle et al. 2000). This results in a nearly equal loading of the humeroradial and humeroulnar joints in the human elbow when a compressive force is transmitted from the palm. Assuming the canine interosseous ligament has similar function, we conclude that the humeroulnar joint is loaded in a similar manner.

Stability

Complete joint stability can be broken down into two different facets: intrinsic stability, which is provided by the shape of the articular surfaces;

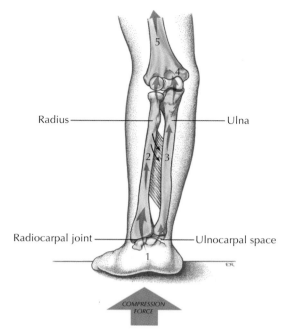

Radius

Ulna

Radiocarpal joint

Ulnocarpal space

Figure 11.9 A human arm in compression, much like a canine forelimb, transmits forces through the wrist (1) and into the distal radius, (2) proximally up the radial diaphysis and across the interosseous ligament, (3) into the ulna, and (4) across the humeroradial and humeroulnar joints as balanced loads. (Reproduced with permission from Pfaeffle et al. [2000], copyright Elsevier)

and extrinsic stability, which is provided by the periarticular soft tissues. The intrinsic stability of the elbow is substantial compared with other joints such as the knee or shoulder due to the trochlear features of the humerus and ulna. The primary extrinsic stabilizers in the elbow are the medial collateral ligament, the LCL, and the anconeal process. According to Talcott et al., when the elbow is at 135 degrees (i.e., angle of extension during peak vertical force of trotting dogs), the anconeal process, which inserts into the supratrochlear foramen, is the primary rotational stabilizer in pronation and the LCL is a primary stabilizer in supination (Talcott et al. 2002).

Incorporating the varus nature of the elbow, and thus the naturally occurring mediolateral shear force, it is possible to conclude that the anconeal process would be the primary stabilizer in extension opposing luxation. In addition, the LCL would, if intrinsic stabilizers were reduced, be

under increased tension. Therefore, any disruption to either of these two primary extrinsic structures could lead to instability capable of joint luxation.

The radioulnar articulation, responsible for pronation and supination, is not as intrinsically stable as the humeroulnar articulation. The radius relies heavily upon extrinsic structures such as the interosseous ligament and the annular ligament to refrain the radial head from luxating.

Surgical approaches

Over the years, the preferred surgical approach for an elbow replacement was through a lateral incision (i.e., Lewis, Iowa State Elbow, etc.); however, in recent years, with the introduction of the TATE Elbow, a medial approach has become a viable option. This is a result of a number of factors, but the primary reason is that most indications for an elbow replacement start in the medial compartment, with what is now referred to as medial compartment disease (MCD). Therefore, to accurately excise and replace the diseased tissue in the medial compartment, the medial approach becomes the clear option, as it is the most direct approach to the afflicted region.

The medial and lateral approaches, described below, are very similar but with subtle differences that are worth noting. The lateral approach is easily accessed and has few critical structures (nerves and arteries) that need to be identified and isolated; however, it has a number of muscular insertions in the vicinity that need to be negotiated. The use of a medial approach requires the identification and translocation of the ulnar nerve as it crosses directly over the medial aspect of the joint, but has no musculature covering the distocaudal surface of the humerus resulting in less muscle damage. Ultimately, due to the varus angulation of the elbow and its potential to increase as the medial compartment collapses, the medial collateral ligament carries less of a load than the LCL. As a result, whether a desmotomy or an osteotomy is used to release the elbow, the method for closing the joint and reconstructing the collateral ligament must not become the weak link.

Although other surgical approaches have been used for TER (i.e., transolecranon process osteotomy, etc.), they will not be discussed here due to the lack of postoperative success.

Design principles of TER

An ideal TER is fundamentally designed to provide the patient with a pain-free joint that kinematically and mechanically replicates the original articulation. As previously mentioned, over the last 20 years, multiple teams have worked on accomplishing these objectives. These designs have ranged from fully constrained, cemented, hinged prostheses to minimally invasive, biologically fixed, resurfacing implants. Every joint, in this case the elbow, has its own "window of acceptance." To fall within that window, the designer must consider the following: the articular surface as it relates to motion and stability, possible biomaterials, method of fixation, and how the implant will interact with periarticular tissues.

The articulation

The articulation of any joint replacement is a complicated balance between three intertwined factors: (1) joint kinematics, (2) intrinsic stability, and (3) implant wear potential. Although the primary articulation of the elbow (i.e., flexion and extension) appears to be a simple hinge, it is much more complex than that. Extensive research in the human field found that the elbow did not rotate about a fixed axis and that slight "out-of-plane" motion does occur throughout flexion and extension (Armstrong et al. 2005). Therefore, the articular surfaces of the implant must either reproduce or compensate for these motions. This is accomplished through a compromise between conformity—how geometrically similar the two surfaces are—and constraint— how restrictive the two surfaces are in relative motion (Figure 11.10). These features are balanced with the surrounding soft tissues to further stabilize the joint and minimize the stresses imposed on the bone–implant interfaces. Excessive articular constraint (i.e., hinge) or misalignment of the implant and anatomical axes (i.e., malpositioned

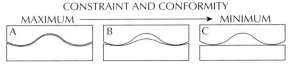

CONSTRAINT AND CONFORMITY

Figure 11.10   Like most ginglymoid joints, the elbow has a complex articulation that can be described through varying degrees of constraint and conformity. The image depicts three different potential articular surfaces decreasing, from left to right, in constraint and conformity. The first articulation, which is highly constrained (A), would result in a high kinematic control, high surface contact minimizing wear through load distribution, and minimal soft tissue involvement resulting in high implant fixation stresses. The second articulation (B) shows medium constraint and is closer to what one might expect in an implant. It has some kinematic restriction but allows for out-of-plane motion, has reduced articular surface contact, and relies upon soft tissue contributions for joint stability. The third articulation (C) provides no kinematic restrictions and has minimal articular surface contact. As a result, it would rely solely on the surrounding soft tissue for stability and the minimal articular surface contact would greatly increase the potential for wear decreasing the life span of the implant.

implant) results in excessive interfacial stresses at the bone–implant interfaces. Early hinged elbow designs, in both human and canine applications, failed to utilize the extrinsic stabilizers, which led to implant failure at the bone–implant interfaces (Dee 1972).

The manner in which the articular surface constrains the motion of the joint must be done gradually. As elbow motion moves through multiple planes, it is important that the articular surfaces guide this movement and, upon reaching the limits, engage the extrinsic stabilizers through a gradual tensioning in order to limit this motion. In contrast, abrupt limits imposed by articular surfaces will result in high stresses and, in the case of ultra-high molecular weight polyethylene (UHMWPE), could lead to cold flow and wear debris.

Implant fixation, either cemented or cementless, is also affected by the design of the articular surfaces. The articular surfaces of the two commercially available implants, the Iowa and the TATE, are quite similar; however, the Iowa is more constrained in torsion than the TATE.[14] As a result, this would theoretically lead to an increase in stress at the bone–implant interfaces. However, the Iowa, being a fully cemented implant, may be able to tolerate these higher stresses. In contrast, the TATE, which relies on biological fixation, works in concert with the surrounding soft tissues to assist in stabilizing the implant in the early post-op period. This is critical for bone ingrowth and long-term stability.

Pronation and supination

In an attempt to simplify the implant design, the articulation between the radius and ulna (i.e., pronation and supination) has been eliminated in several implant designs. The synostosis is typically created by removing the radioulnar articulation and attempting to eliminate relative motion through placing an interosseous screw or plating. In some surgical techniques, a distal ulnar ostectomy is performed. While there are benefits to synostosis—the reduction from a three- to a two-component design and the resulting simplification of the surgery—there are also drawbacks. The radioulnar articulation contributes to the overall motion and stability of the elbow; however, this has only recently been evaluated and defined. Based on the clinical follow-up of total elbow patients, an elbow with a radioulnar synostosis can still achieve a functional range of flexion and extension, and therefore, the implant can still provide functional motion for daily activities. However, from a biomechanical standpoint, the elbow motion has been compromised. The repercussions of this fusion are not fully understood and may potentially result in an unpredictable gait abnormality (i.e., lameness). Another potential complication arises when a synostosis fails and relative motion remains. Depending on implant design, persistent relative radioulnar motion could lead to complications. A failed synostosis would result in unpredictable motion between the radius and ulna, possibly jeopardizing osseointegration and producing a fibrous bone–implant interface.

The decision to fuse the radioulnar articulation is a critical decision in the implant design process and is done with the knowledge of compromising motion for the simplification of the implant and the surgical technique. This design approach takes into consideration both the patient and the surgical indications. If the primary goal is to provide a limb salvage technique for dogs suffering from end-stage elbow OA, then the use of a two-component elbow implant, requiring synostosis of the radius and ulna, can provide a successful clinical result.

Mechanical fixation

The methods for stabilizing any joint replacement design can be divided into two techniques: cemented fixation or biological fixation. The use of polymethylmethacrylate (PMMA) for "cementing" joint replacements has existed since the 1940s and still exists today as a proven and viable option for fixing implant components. Biological fixation, which is the use of biocompatible materials with rough or porous surfaces allowing for bone apposition or integration, came about in the 1950s. Both methods of fixation can result in a lasting stable implant, but both have potential complications.

Cemented fixation

Cemented fixation has been successfully used in canine total joint applications since the early 1970s. This fixation method is a very different model compared with biological fixation. While biological fixation may take over a year to develop its maximum interface strength, the cemented implant reaches its maximum within the first 24 hours. Cement fixation therefore affords the patient a quick return to activity. This early return to activity is even more beneficial in the veterinary field, where patient compliance to postoperative care protocol is commonly neglected.

Although the cemented implant is typically very stable immediately after surgery, the quality and consistency of the cement mantle will be tested over the longevity of the implant (see Chapter 5). The cemented implant introduces a unique element, the bone–cement interface, which, like any mechanical bond under cyclic loading, has a finite life expectancy. This life expectancy is subject to a number of elements: the quality and consistency of the cement mantle, the magnitude of stress imposed, and the number of cycles. Some of the early elbow designs, which were either hinges or highly constrained articulations, ultimately failed due to the high stress levels at the cement interfaces (i.e., cement–bone and cement–implant). However, as a result of moving away from highly constrained articulations, the longevity of cemented elbow replacements has increased considerably. Cement has proven to be a consistent and reliable fixation method in implants such as the Iowa State Elbow. As a result, TER systems that are still in development, such as the Sirius Elbow, are utilizing the benefits of a cemented interface.

Over time, every cemented implant will loosen due to fatigue at the implant–cement interface; however, depending on the implant design, this could be in months or well beyond the life expectancy of the patient.

Biological fixation

A biologically fixed implant must reach a number of "checkpoints" postoperatively in order to create a bone–implant interface capable of lasting the life of the patient. Biological fixation is dependent on the implant itself remaining stable (<40 μm of motion) (Bragdon et al. 1996) in the first postoperative stage, 0–8 weeks, for osteointegration to occur. During the first 8 weeks, the implant is stabilized through the press-fit or interference fit created during insertion of the implant or by screw fixation. In the canine recovery phase, normal activities will typically begin during this stage, so the implant stabilizers must resist normal physiological loads. Studies have shown that excessive micromotion will disrupt the stroma, resulting in a fibrous encapsulation of the implant. In order to sufficiently stabilize the implant in the first stage, different techniques are currently being explored for canine elbow replacements, such as screw fixation (e.g., Kyon) and press-fit (e.g., TATE Elbow, CUE). In the canine elbow, which typically experiences some load immediately after surgery, achieving the level of stability required for osseointegration can be challenging. The second postoperative stage, 8 weeks to 1 year, results in an adaptation of the bone to the new distribution of loads through the bone–implant interface. The interface will continue to strengthen through bone ingrowth and remodeling until it is proportionally equal to the interfacial stresses to which it is subjected. Ultimately, a balance of bone remodeling, at approximately 1 year, is achieved where there is no change to the structure and density of the periprosthetic bone. The final stage, around 1 year, should see no change to the surrounding bone and any remodeling would be indicative of excessive stress shielding or implant instability (Schiller et al. 1993).

The long-term success of a biologically fixed implant is dependent upon a number of factors: the implant design (e.g., implant surface finish, material, coatings); the surgical technique; and the host (e.g., available bone stock, age).

The implant design, from the articular surfaces to the surface finishes and material of the implant, greatly affect the potential for biological fixation. If the articulation is too constrained and the bone–implant interface is absorbing too much of the transarticular stabilizing forces, a fibrous union may result as a consequence of excessive motion in the first stage, or late failure due to insufficient osseointegration. The second generation of the TATE, released in 2010, has a modified polyethylene articular surface in an attempt to reduce the transmission of transarticular stabilizing forces to the bone–implant interface of the radioulnar component. This modified polyethylene surface improves the possibility for bone ingrowth into the radioulnar component, but it also increases the potential for implant wear due to reduced articular surface contact.

The location and the variety of implant surfaces and coatings that create the bone–implant interface are critical for long-term success. A smooth surface can achieve bone apposition, but will result in a weak bond capable of resisting minimal shear forces. An irregular surface, such as a titanium plasma coating or machined divots, will lead to a mechanical bond due to interdigitation of the bone with the implant surface, resulting in an interface with greater shear strength than a smooth surface. Porous surfaces, which allow for bone ingrowth into the implant, are capable of resisting even higher shear and tensile strengths than smooth or irregular surfaces. Therefore, not only the use of these finishes and coatings but also their location on an implant can greatly affect the longevity and strength of an osseointegrated implant.

The surgical technique of osseointegrative-dependent implants is a critical factor that can greatly influence the success of the implant. The optimal design will result in compression, or minimal gap (<1 mm), between the surfaces of the implant prepared for biological fixation and the bone. Any gap exceeding 1 mm might result in a fibrous union, as the bone cannot "bridge" the gap prior to the primary stabilizers (e.g., screws) failing.

Osseointegrative implants are fundamentally dependent upon the regenerative capabilities of the host. Biologically fixed implants have a provisional method for achieving the postoperative stability necessary to create an environment favorable to bone ingrowth. These methods include the interference fit, or press-fit, between the posts and the bone as with the TATE Elbow, or by screw fixation in the radioulnar component as with the Sirius Elbow. Because these techniques are not designed to sustain the stabilizing loads for the life of the patient, they need to be reinforced, or off-loaded, through bone ingrowth. Therefore, biologically fixed implants are better suited for younger and healthier hosts capable of superior regeneration when compared with geriatric patients.

Hybrid fixation

Clearly, there are benefits to both cement fixation and biological fixation when considering an elbow replacement. Cement offers immediate postoperative stability that is critical for the success of any implant. However, biological fixation, with sufficient bone ingrowth, should provide a dependable interface for the life of the patient. Therefore, in an attempt to adopt the benefits of both methods of fixation, the Iowa and the TATE have both created what could be described as a "hybrid" fixation method. In the most recent generation of the Iowa, sintered beads were added to the medial and lateral surfaces of the humeral component. Ideally, this would allow for bone ingrowth and slightly off-load the cement mantle. Similarly, the TATE Elbow was modified to have hollow, slotted posts instead of solid posts. This provides the surgeon with the intraoperative option of injecting a highly viscous cement (i.e., PMMA, calcium phosphate, etc.) into the posts and substantially improving a less than adequate press-fit. This "hybrid" adaptation to the TATE facilitates the stabilization of the implant during the critical first postoperative stage.

Varus angle abnormality

The progression of elbow OA leads to substantial bone and soft tissue remodeling, resulting in large osteophytic growth and extensive changes to the kinematics of the joint. Early on, these changes tend to be isolated to the medial compartment due to a number of potential dysplastic abnormalities. Ultimately, as a result of medial articular cartilage erosion, there is a resulting increase in the naturally occurring varus angle. This varus increase compounds the osteoarthritic changes in the medial compartment simultaneously off-loading the lateral compartment, forcing the trochlea to function like a fulcrum. This "snapshot" of the progression of elbow OA is what is now commonly referred to as MCD. As the disease progresses to end-stage elbow OA (Figure 11.11), there is a "dramatic medial collapse and a laterally

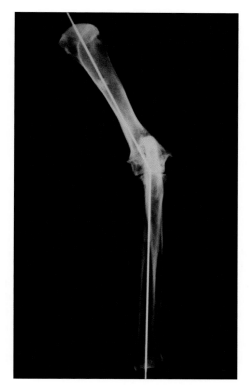

Figure 11.11 This radiograph depicts an elbow that has undergone substantial medial compartment collapse resulting in a significant varus deformity. (Courtesy of Dr. Susan A Cannon from the work of Dr. Ralph H Lewis)

displaced elbow."[15] This is very similar to what occurs in human knees afflicted with severe OA, and as a result, the angular deformity must be corrected intraoperatively through soft tissue release and ligament balancing to restore the mechanical axes of the limb (Insall et al. 1985). This is done not only to achieve the optimal biomechanics of the joint, but it is also critical to the function and longevity of the implant. In cases of severe canine elbow OA where excessive varus deformity has occurred, it would seem logical that the correction of this abnormal angulation would be necessary for optimal limb function.

The two commercially available elbow systems, the Iowa and the TATE, addressed this notion from different perspectives. The Iowa's humeral articular surface is perpendicular to the long axis of the implant stem, resulting in an articulation that is normal to the anatomical axis (i.e., the axis of the diaphysis) of the humerus. This results in a straight elbow without the previously described MAD. In order to achieve this, the periarticular soft tissues must be released and ligaments adjusted in order to balance the articulation. Because the TATE is a resurfacing implant, it is not dictated by the medullary cavities and therefore has no preset angle that must be established, straight or otherwise. The TATE allows for correction of the varus deformity intraoperatively through realignment of the limb to the desired varus angle prior to removal of the articular surfaces.

Stress shielding

The material properties (i.e., tensile strength, modulus of elasticity, etc.) of alloys commonly used in joint replacements (e.g., Ti6Al4V and CoCrMo) are substantially greater than that of bone. As a result, the natural load distribution through the surrounding bone is reduced, which, according to Wolff's law, leads to periprosthetic bone resorption, or osteolysis. Depending on the implant design, this can lead to fracture of the surrounding bone or implant loosening as the bone atrophies to a state unable to endure the required loads.

A degree of stress shielding has been found to occur with both the Iowa and TATE implants, as it is nearly unavoidable with current implant technology. The cemented stems of the Iowa State Elbow are understandably reliant on a substantial cement mantle for implant stability; however, this results in a higher potential for stress shielding of the distal humerus. Therefore, the fifth generation of this implant resulted in the addition of porous surfaces to the medial and lateral surfaces of the humeral component. Ideally, if bone ingrowth is achieved at these interfaces, it will off-load the cement mantle surrounding the stem and increase the stress in the distal humerus, reducing the potential bone resorption. The TATE, which is reliant on bone ingrowth for stability, also has potential for stress shielding (Déjardin and Guillou 2011). A biological implant interface will only be as strong as the stresses it is subjected to. Therefore, the semicircular humeral component has high potential for shielding the subchondral bone where bone ingrowth has not occurred. Another location of potential stress shielding with the TATE implant is the bone surrounding the caudal post of the radioulnar component. Stress shielding is not a new phenomenon; for the most part, we know how and why it occurs. Therefore, implants can theoretically be designed to transfer stress to optimal locations, reducing the negative impacts of stress shielding.

Supratrochlear foramen

The supratrochlear foramen of the distal humerus creates a unique challenge for implant design. The combination of large, concentric, articular surfaces and a considerable ROM result in the biological need for the supratrochlear foramen and thus the two bony columns supporting the humeral condyle. From an implant design perspective, this obstacle has been dealt with by two different techniques. The Iowa State Elbow uses a medullary stem that effectively fills the supratrochlear foramen. However, in order to still retain a complete ROM, the caudal aspect of the humeral component has what resembles a supratrochlear fossa and the radioulnar component has a substantially abbreviated articular surface compared with the natural joint surface (Conzemius et al. 2003). This is an effective method for retaining a full ROM, but does come with potential complications. Due to the removal of the anconeal process, one of the joint's primary stabilizers, there is an increased potential for joint luxations. The TATE, being a resurfacing implant, does not fill the supratrochlear foramen and therefore has a radioulnar component that utilizes the biological foramen. Although the anconeal process is still removed, the radioulnar component articular surface approximates a substantial amount of the natural joint surface; thus, it does not jeopardize joint stability. The primary drawbacks to this design approach are primarily confronted in the surgical technique. For the implant to achieve a full ROM, it must collaborate with the natural bony structures, specifically the supratrochlear foramen. Therefore, accurate placement of the components must be achieved to avoid caudal impingements when articulated into extension. Impingements that are not dealt with intraoperatively can lead to either wear of the bone or, in the case of polyethylene contact, implant wear and potential osteolysis due to third-body wear.

Conclusions

Although much remains to be learned, there have been great strides made in establishing a better understanding of elbow kinematics in recent years. With these advances will come a more suitable foundation for the development of prosthetic implants designed to manage not only end-stage OA but early OA (i.e., MCD) as well.

Implant designs, up until the last few years, were clearly based upon a limited collective knowledge of the biomechanics and kinematics of the elbow. As a result, prosthetic implants were designed to achieve no more than basic function (i.e., flexion and extension) and, at best, possibly "salvage" a limb. However, the addition of recent kinematic studies and future research will lead to an implant design and surgical technique capable of restoring all levels of function to the canine patient.

Ultimately, the ideal elbow implant may not be a single implant but a system designed to treat the dramatically different stages of OA. Due to the way in which the elbow isolates the disease to the medial compartment early on, a manner of intervention at this juncture would be welcome.

As mentioned above, there are currently groups pursuing implant designs that would ideally replace the medial compartment and retard the progression of OA throughout the rest of the joint. Whether this method of retardation would work for the life of the dog will need further study, but early clinical results show promise. As the disease progresses out of the medial aspect and into the lateral compartment, the resulting arthritic changes dictate the need for a TER capable of restoring complete function back to the joint.

Regardless of implant design and arthritic application, the ideal TER system would fundamentally need to embody a number of features that would optimize the life expectancy of the implant and restore the natural kinematics of the joint. The implant should be designed to facilitate a simple surgical technique that accurately allows for implantation, replication of the axis of rotation, no detrimental effect to joint stability, and the capacity to achieve the kinematics necessary for normal life. In an effort to minimize potential bone–implant interface stresses, utilization of the natural joint stabilizers, intrinsic and extrinsic, is critical; therefore, any ligamentous structures essential to joint stability that have been compromised must be accurately and anatomically repaired.

Endnotes

1. Sidebotham C. Personal communication, September 4, 2011.
2. Lewis RH. Development of elbow arthroplasty (canine) clinical trials. In: *Proceedings of the 6th Annual ACVS Symposium*. San Francisco, CA, 1996.
3. Conzemius MG. Total elbow replacement in the dog—Development and evaluation. PhD dissertation, Iowa State University, 2000.
4. Cook JL, Lower J. Elbow arthroplasty system. Patent US007419507B2. USA, The Curators of the University of Missouri, Columbia, MO, 2008.
5. Acker R, Van Der Meulen G. Resurfacing arthroplasty of the canine elbow. In: *Proceedings of the 34th Annual Veterinary Orthopedic Society Conference*. Sun Valley, ID, 2007, p. 55.
6. Innes J. Personal communication, August 10, 2011.
7. Schulz KS, Cook JL, Karnes J. Canine unicompartmental elbow arthroplasty system. In: *Proceedings of the Annual ACVS Symposium*. Chicago, IL, November 1–5, 2011.

8. Wendelburg K. Personal communication, November 4, 2011.
9. Guillou RP, Déjardin LM, McDonald C, et al. Three dimensional kinematics of the normal canine elbow at the walk and trot. In: *Proceedings of the 39th Annual Veterinary Orthopedic Society Conference.* Crested Butte, CO, March 3–10, 2012.
10. Lewis RH. Elbow arthroplasty replacement course notebook. Elbow Course, Diagnostic Osteonecrosis Center and Research Foundation, Lakeport, CA, 2003.
11. Wood MC, Fox DB, Tomlinson JL, et al. Determination of the mechanical axes and joint orientation lines in the canine humerus: A radiographic cadaveric study. In: *Proceedings of the 38th Annual Veterinary Orthopedic Society Conference.* Snowmass, CO, March 5–12, 2011.
12. Fasanella FJ, Tomlinson JL, Welihozkiy A, et al. Radiographic measurements of the axes and joint angles of the canine radius and ulna. In: *Proceedings of the 37th Annual Veterinary Orthopedic Society Conference.* Breckenridge, CO, March 4–9, 2010.
13. Saviori CM, Fox DB, Flynn P. Determination of the thoracic limb mechanical axis in the dog: A cadaveric radiographic study in the frontal plane. In: *Proceedings of the 36th Annual Veterinary Orthopedic Society Conference.* Steamboat, CO, March 1–6, 2009.
14. Déjardin LM, Guillou RP. Total elbow replacement continues to produce good results. Internal Michigan State University Publication, 2010, VTH Messenger, 5(4).
15. Conzemius M. Iowa State TER. Results and complications. In: *Proceedings of the 3rd WVOC and 15th ESVOT Congress.* Bologna, Italy, 2010.

References

Armstrong AD, King GJW, Yamaguchi K. Total elbow arthroplasty design. In: *Shoulder and Elbow Arthroplasty*, vol. 1, Williams GR, Yamaguchi K, Ramsey ML, et al. (eds.). Philadelphia: Lippincott Williams & Wilkins, 2005, pp. 297–312.

Bragdon CR, Burke D, Lowenstein JD, et al. Differences in stiffness of the interface between a cementless porous implant and cancellous bone *in vivo* in dogs due to varying amounts of implant motion. J Arthroplasty 1996;11:945–951.

Conzemius MG, Aper RL. Development and evaluation of semiconstrained arthroplasty for the treatment of elbow osteoarthritis in the dog. Vet Comp Orthop Traumatol 1998;11:54A.

Conzemius MG, Aper RL, Hill CM. Evaluation of a canine total-elbow arthroplasty system: A preliminary study in normal dogs. Vet Surg 2001;30:11–20.

Conzemius MG, Aper RL, Corti LB. Short-term outcome after total elbow arthroplasty in dogs with severe, naturally occurring osteoarthritis. Vet Surg 2003;32: 545–552.

Dee R. Total replacement arthroplasty of the elbow for rheumatoid arthritis. J Bone Joint Surg Br 1972;54(1): 88–95.

Déjardin LM, Guillou RP. Total elbow replacement in dogs in veterinary surgery. In: *Small Animal Surgery*, Tobias KM, Spencer JA (eds.). St. Louis, MO: Saunders, 2011, pp. 752–759.

Evans HE. The skeleton. In: *Miller's Anatomy of the Dog*, 3rd ed., Evans HE (ed.). Philadelphia: Saunders, 1993, pp. 122–218.

Insall JN, Binazzi R, Soudy M, et al. Total knee arthroplasty. Clin Orthop Relat Res. 1985;192:13–22.

Jaegger G, Marcellin-Little DJ, Levine D. Reliability of goniometry in Labrador retrievers. Am J Vet Res 2002;63:979–986.

Mason DR, Schulz KS, Fujita Y, et al. *In vitro* force mapping of normal canine humeroradial and humeroulnar joints. Am J Vet Res 2005;66:135–135.

Morrey BF, Chao EY. Passive motion of the elbow joint. J Bone Joint Surg Am 1976;58:501.

Newton CD, Nunamaker DM. Appendix B: Normal joint range of motion in the dog and cat. In: *Textbook of Small Animal Orthopaedics*, 1st ed., Newton CD, Nunamaker DM (eds.). Philadelphia: Lippincott Williams & Wilkins, 1985.

Nielsen C, Stover S, Schulz KS, et al. Two-dimensional link-segment model of the forelimb of dogs at a walk. Am J Vet Res 2003;64:5.

Pfaeffle HJ, Fischer KJ, Manson TT, et al. Role of the forearm interosseous ligament: Is it more than just longitudinal load transfer? J Hand Surg 2000;25A: 683–688.

Schiller TD, DeYoung DJ, Schiller RA, et al. Quantitative ingrowth analysis of a porous-coated acetabular component in a canine model. Vet Surg 1993;22:276–280.

Talcott KW, Schulz KS, Kass PH, et al. *In vitro* biomechanical study of rotational stabilizers of the canine elbow joint. Am J Vet Res 2002;63:1520–1526.

12 Clinical Application of Total Elbow Replacement in Dogs

Loïc M. Déjardin, Reunan P. Guillou, and Michael Conzemius

History of canine total elbow replacement

The last two decades have seen a growing interest in total elbow replacement (TER) as a salvage treatment of intractable, end-stage canine elbow osteoarthritis (OA). Early prostheses were designed as pure cemented hinges in the late 1980s and early 1990s (see Chapter 11).[1,2] The poor clinical outcome associated with the use of these linked, fully constrained systems rapidly led to their demise and to a paradigm shift toward unlinked TER designs (Armstrong et al. 2005). Following unacceptable postoperative morbidity, most early unlinked designs by Vasseur,[3] Lewis,[2] Cook,[4] and Conzemius (Conzemius and Aper 1998; Conzemius et al. 2001)[5] were abandoned. Iterations of an earlier design by Conzemius led to encouraging results in research dogs initially and later in dogs affected with end-stage OA (Conzemius et al. 2001, 2003). The fifth generation of the Iowa State Elbow became available in 2005 (Iowa State University [ISU] Elbow, BioMedtrix, Boonton, NJ; Figure 12.1A).

In 2008, Acker and Van Der Meulen proposed a novel TER system (TATE Elbow system, BioMedtrix). Although unlinked and semiconstrained, the TATE design is, unlike previous conventional cemented and stemmed systems, a cementless implant designed to use a new resurfacing concept with less aggressive bone removal and without the need for elbow luxation for surgical exposure.[6,7] Short-term satisfactory results in dogs affected with end-stage OA led to the clinical use of this and a second-generation design in approximately 200 patients worldwide (Figure 12.1B).[8] In an effort to preserve the kinematics of the elbow, particularly with regard to radioulnar (RU) pronation and supination, this group is currently investigating a three-component TER (Figure 12.2D).

More recently, Innes devised a hybrid system that combines resurfacing of the humeral and RU components with cementing of the stemmed humeral component. Unlike the TATE system, the RU component is screwed into the radius and the ulna (Figure 12.1C). At the time of this writing, the prosthesis has been implanted in two clinical cases beginning in December 2011. Short-term subjective feedback (10 weeks) showed no complications and very good function.[9]

Finally, new research efforts have been geared toward addressing early stages of OA with medial hemiarthroplasty systems developed by Tepic and Wendelburg,[10] as well as Acker and Van Der

Advances in Small Animal Total Joint Replacement, First Edition. Edited by Jeffrey N. Peck and Denis J. Marcellin-Little.
© 2013 John Wiley & Sons, Inc. Published 2013 by John Wiley & Sons, Inc.

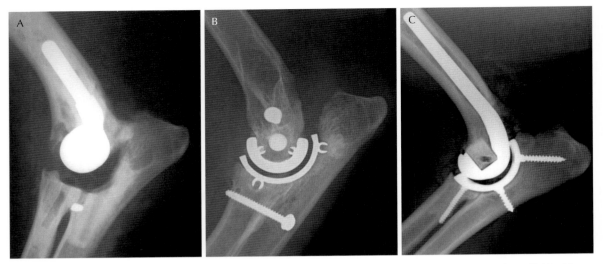

Figure 12.1   Postoperative lateral radiographs of the three unlinked, semiconstrained TER systems currently available. The Iowa State University Elbow (Conzemius; A) and TATE (Acker/Van Der Meulen; B) have been used clinically since 2005 and 2007, respectively. The Sirius system (Innes; C) has been implanted experimentally in two dogs since December 2011. The current Iowa State prosthesis is a cemented hybrid design that allows bone ingrowth at the level of the lateral and medial condylar surfaces. The TATE prosthesis is designed as a resurfacing cementless cartridge unit. The Sirius system combines a cemented and stemmed design with resurfacing components. (Courtesy of Chris Preston, Animal Surgery Center, Sydney, NSW [A]; and John Innes, University of Liverpool, School of Veterinary Medicine, United Kingdom [C])

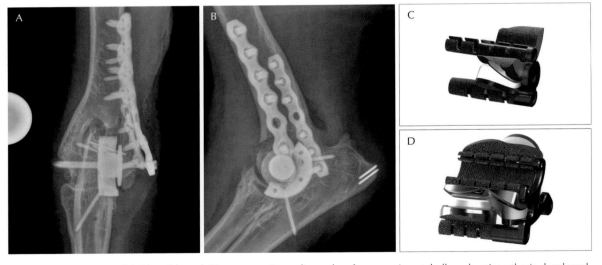

Figure 12.2   Craniocaudal (A) and lateral (B) postoperative radiographs of an experimental elbow hemiprosthesis developed by Tepic and Wendelburg. Computer-assisted designs of a TATE hemi- (C) and three-component (D) prostheses currently under development (C). Hemiprostheses are designed to address early stages of elbow dysplasia when osteoarthritis is limited to the medial compartment of the joint. Three-component prostheses feature a separate radial head component designed to allow radioulnar pronation and supination. (Courtesy of Kirk Wendelburg, Animal Specialty Group, Los Angeles, CA [A and B]; and Greg Van Der Meulen, BioMedtrix, Boonton, NJ [C and D])

Meulen. At the time of writing, the Tepic–Wendelburg prosthesis has been implanted in one live dog (Figure 12.2A,B), while the Acker–Van Der Meulen prosthesis is in a design and development phase (Figure 12.2C).

This chapter will focus on currently commercially available prostheses (i.e., the fifth-generation ISU and the TATE elbow systems).

Evolution rationale of the ISU Elbow

The maturation of the ISU TER components and system has been described in the veterinary literature and this historical documentation provides a unique opportunity to "witness" the development of design rationale. The initial report of the ISU Elbow in 1998 depicted two semiconstrained (snap-fit) components (humeral and radio-ulnar [RU]) that were implanted via transection of the lateral collateral ligament (Conzemius and Aper 1998). The components and cutting guide system were developed from morphometric data of the humerus, radius, and ulna of normal dogs, tested in plastic and cadaver bones and piloted in an *in vivo* study in six, normal greyhounds. The

components were machined from ultrahigh-molecular-weight polyethylene (UHMWPE) for this short-term (4-month) study (Figures 12.3 and 12.4).

At the conclusion of the 1998 study, only two of six dogs had ground reaction forces that were more than 80% of their preoperative normal limb function (Figure 12.5). Findings suggested that failure was common, the RU design would require

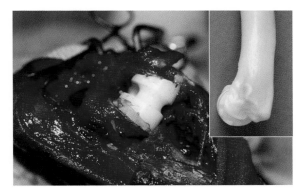

Figure 12.3 Intraoperative photograph of the humeral component cemented into the humerus (*left*), and a photograph of a lateral view of the humeral component in the humerus of a cadaveric bone (*inset*).

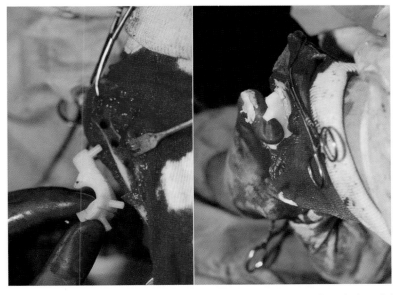

Figure 12.4 Intraoperative photograph of the radioulnar component of the initial ISU Elbow before (*left*) and after (*right*) placement and cementing of the component.

several key changes, and the cutting guide system was unacceptably bulky. However, it also demonstrated that success was possible and several aspects of the humeral component worked well. Ultimately, the 1998 study provided key data that helped explain both failures and successes. For example, early failure at the cement–bone interface of the RU component was identified via computed tomography (CT) and gross pathology in four dogs (Figure 12.6). The short pegs of the RU component and the semiconstrained nature of the articulation likely contributed to this by placing too much strain at the cement–bone interface, resulting in early loosening. Thus, two immediate design changes were made in order to reduce this strain. The design changes included switching to a nonconstrained (unlinked) articulation between the humeral and RU components and lengthening the pegs of the RU component. This study also found that (1) the proximal ulnar osteotomy resulted in an ulna that was too unstable and that a distal ulnar osteotomy was sufficient; (2) a screw between the radius and ulna to encourage

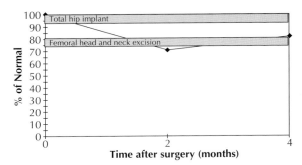

Figure 12.5 Peak vertical force of the operated leg of the two dogs that did not have premature loosening of their semiconstrained total elbow implants. The shaded areas represent previous reports of limb function in normal greyhounds 4 months after research surgeries. Note: % of Normal = Peak vertical force (%BW) presurgery/Peak vertical force (%BW) postsurgery. (Reproduced from Conzemius et al. [2001], with permission from Wiley-Blackwell)

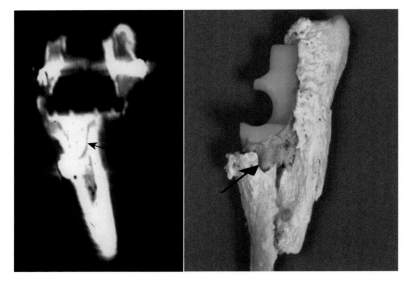

Figure 12.6 A CT image (*left*) of a dog 2 months after elbow replacement (ISU initial study). Note the lucency (dark line) around the cement of the radioulnar component (arrow). The same elbow is shown as a cadaver specimen on the right. The space between the cement and bone is again identified with a black arrow.

synostosis (initially thought to be necessary because the implant bridged the two bones) may have been unnecessary, as an autogenous cancellous bone graft placed between the two bones was sufficient to produce synostosis without the screw; and (3) the humeral component was exceptionally stable and that screws to secure it to the humerus were not required.

Translation to the next phase of development required reengineering of each component and the cutting guides, as well as modifying the surgical technique. Retesting was necessary prior to clinical application of the second-generation prosthesis and technique. Thus, the purpose of the second *in vivo* study was to test long-term function of a modified TER system in six large-breed dogs (Conzemius et al. 2001). The second-generation instrumentation and implants were used and prostheses were implanted as with the first-generation implants (Figure 12.7). Due to either osteomyelitis or ulnar fracture, three of six dogs did not reach the planned 1-year termination of the study. The three dogs that remained in the study had limb function on the side of TER that was similar to the unoperated, normal limb (Figure 12.8).

The study evaluating the second-generation prosthesis also identified factors that helped explain both success and failure. First, the humeral and RU components remained stable, confirming that a nonconstrained articulation and the lengthening of the RU pegs were beneficial design changes. Second, the cutting guides used (Conzemius et al. 2001) were adequate, although they remained bulky, to correctly position each component. Since the components were positioned independently of each other, it was possible to position each component in a different center of rotation, potentially resulting in malalignment. A cutting guide system that allowed the implants to be positioned on the same center of rotation needed to be developed. Third, while the articulation was semiconstrained, it still had corners with a small radius that could result in the metal component cutting into the UHMWPE and leading to rapid polyethylene wear. The articulation needed softer corners. Fourth, the caudal aspect of the RU component had a nearly 90-degree corner that could function as a fulcrum and predispose to ulnar fracture. The corner needed to be eliminated. Fifth, an RU

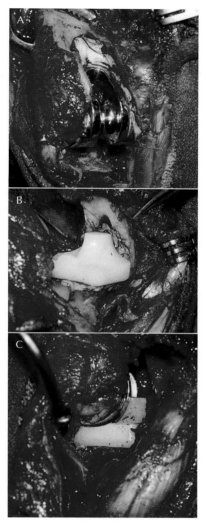

Figure 12.7 Intraoperative photograph of the humeral (A) and the radioulnar (B) components cemented into position. An intraoperative photograph of the implants after reduction (C) is also shown.

synostosis successfully formed in each case with only the placement of an autogenous cancellous bone graft (from the excised humeral condyle) placed between the radius and the ulna. These and several other factors led to a design that could be used in a controlled clinical case series.

A prospective clinical case series for the treatment of 20 canine patients with severe, naturally occurring OA using TER was reported in 2003 (Conzemius et al. 2003). Inclusion criteria for this

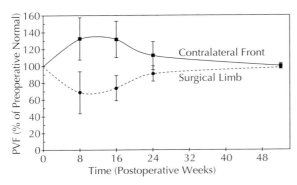

Figure 12.8   The mean peak vertical force of each front limb of dogs studied is expressed as a percent of the force recorded before surgery. Standard deviation bars are shown. (Reproduced from Conzemius et al. [2001], Figure 8, with permission from Wiley-Blackwell)

investigation required that dogs have forelimb lameness and pain from elbow OA that was unresponsive to nonsurgical management. Informed owner consent was required, but sponsored funding allowed for no financial burden to the pet owner. The primary outcome measure for this study was force platform gait analysis, with success defined as an improvement in ground reaction forces. Radiographic evaluation and gait analysis was performed before surgery and at 3, 6, and 12 months after surgery. The components used for this case series were modified based on the studies reported above. The major changes included (1) removal of the 90-degree corner on the caudal aspect of the RU component, (2) removal of the hole (supratrochlear foramen) in the humeral component, and (3) larger radii to the surfaces of articulation of both components (Conzemius et al. 2003). The outcome of this prospective study and interpretation of the findings are reported in a subsequent paragraph in this chapter.

Current systems: Design rationale summary

The ISU Elbow is a hybrid system featuring a symmetrical cobalt-chromium (CoCr) humeral stem component and a side-specific, 120-degree-arc UHMWPE RU component with asymmetrical

posts. Primary fixation is achieved via cementing the humeral stem and RU posts. Porous-coated lateral and medial humeral surfaces provide additional long-term fixation via osseointegration. The humeral and RU components are implanted individually in sequence following preparation of the respective bones.

The design rationale for the TATE Elbow was discussed in Chapter 11. The TATE Elbow system (second generation) is a cementless resurfacing design consisting of a CoCr humeral component and a 175-degree-arc UHMWPE RU component supported by a CoCr backing (Figure 12.9). Using an approach via osteotomy of the mdial humeral epicondyle, the side-specific prosthetic components are inserted simultaneously as a "cartridge implant" within a milled articular groove. Primary and secondary fixations are respectively achieved via mechanical interlock of mediolateral hollow posts and bone ingrowth onto porous surfaces coated with hydroxyapatite (HA).

Contrary to linked systems, the stability of unlinked prostheses is provided by the surrounding soft tissues and by the geometry of the prosthetic articulating surfaces (Armstrong et al. 2005). Specifically, varus and valgus disruptive forces are counteracted by collateral ligaments, while internal/external rotation and mediolateral translation are controlled by the geometry of the articular surfaces of both the humeral and the RU components. To replicate normal elbow kinematics and optimize long-term stability, TER prostheses would require a complex three-component system (Figure 12.2D). Nonetheless, both current TER systems were eventually designed with a single RU component that constrains RU motion as a compromise between optimal joint kinematics, as well as decreased prosthetic complexity and related risk of implant failure. In either system, the surgical procedure includes an RU synostosis to reduce bone/RU component interfacial motion.

Indications and contraindications

The primary indication for TER is severe, intractable degenerative joint disease that is not responsive or is poorly responsive to medical management. Although elbow OA is most commonly associated with elbow dysplasia, it can also result from

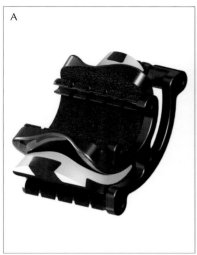 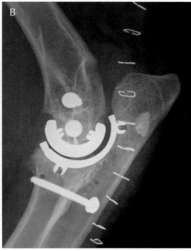 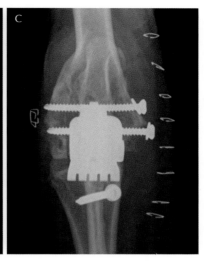

Figure 12.9   Computer-assisted drawing (A) and postoperative radiographs (B and C) of a TATE second generation. Note the presence of new hollow slotted posts used for primary fixation. Compared with the original design, the TATE second generation features porous HA-coated humeral and RU components and less congruent articular profiles. These later modifications, along with the use of radioulnar synostosis via lag screw fixation, were implemented to optimize secondary fixation through improved bone ingrowth and reduced interfacial shear stresses. (Courtesy of Greg Van Der Meulen, BioMedtrix, Boonton, NJ [A])

articular fracture, elbow luxation, or angular limb deformities with subsequent elbow incongruity. Because of the potential complications and/or limited long-term follow-up available for the currently available systems, TER should be restricted to older dogs with a clearly decreased quality of life on a day-to-day basis, which cannot be satisfactorily managed with medical treatment. As for any total joint replacement, systemic or local infections (e.g., local pyoderma, bacterial cystitis, otitis externa, periodontal disease) increase the risk of postoperative infection and should be identified and addressed prior to surgery. Chronic elbow luxation is a relative contraindication to TER. The compromised periarticular soft tissue envelope may increase the risk of postoperative luxation with the currently available, unlinked, systems. However, successful use of the ISU Elbow system after chronic elbow luxation has been reported (Conzemius et al. 2003). Finally, severe malunion may preclude the use of the resurfacing TATE Elbow system. Cases with severe malunion may be successfully addressed using the ISU Elbow (Conzemius et al. 2003). Severe malunion may preclude the use of the resurfacing TATE Elbow system. Neurological dysfunction and

skeletal immaturity represent other potential contraindications.

Preoperative evaluation and planning

Comprehensive physical, orthopedic (including goniometry), and neurological examinations are mandatory to fully assess functional alterations in the affected elbow joint in order to rule out other possible causes of thoracic limb lameness and to document concurrent abnormalities.

Well-positioned standard mediolateral and craniocaudal views are essential for accurate templating. Accordingly, radiographs should be obtained under heavy sedation or general anesthesia. The use of a calibration marker (spherical or linear) is mandatory in order to use appropriately magnified templates (acetate template overlays), or to calibrate the radiograph (digital templating; Figure 12.10).

Although not absolutely necessary, CT scan of the elbow is highly recommended when extensive osteophytosis is present. Comprehensive three-dimensional understanding of the size and distribution of the osteophytes is invaluable during the

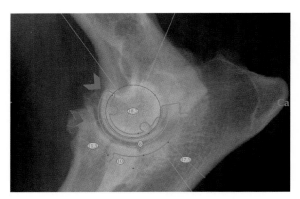

Figure 12.10 Digital templating for a TATE prosthesis using the OrthoView Veterinary Orthopaedic Digital Planning software (www.orthoview.com). The size of the prosthesis (19 mm in this case) should be equal or greater than the diameter of the humeral trochlea (18.5 mm; purple circle). Ideal implant position requires that (1) the cranial aspects of the humeral and RU components are respectively aligned with the osteochondral junction (green arrow) and with the native radial head (red arrow); (2) the radial post approximately bisects the radial head (11.5 and 10 mm in this case); and (3) the width of the ulnar bridge behind the prosthesis (17.5 mm) is no less than the width of the prosthesis (8 mm).

implantation procedure, as poor identification of anatomical landmarks can result in an improperly aligned implant, and adversely affect the outcome.

ISU Elbow preoperative planning

Preoperative lateral and craniocaudal radiographs can be used to estimate component size; however, final decisions for sizing are made intraoperatively. Four ISU total elbow sizes are available for medium-, large-, and giant-breed dogs with an approximate range of body weight of 25–65 kg.

TATE Elbow preoperative planning

The humeral trochlear diameter is measured (in millimeters) from the mediolateral radiograph. Current TATE prostheses are described based on the diameter of the humeral component and are currently available from 15 mm to 21 mm in 2-mm increments. Selection of the implant size is such that it is equal to or slightly greater than the measured trochlear diameter. As an example, if the

humeral trochlear diameter is 17 mm, the 17-mm implant will be chosen; if the diameter of the trochlea is 18 mm, then the 19-mm implant will be chosen. The template of the elected implant is then placed at the planned location, and several criteria are verified (Figure 12.10). First, the cranial aspect of the RU component is aligned with the cranial aspect of the native radial head. As a redundant feature, the radial post should then be approximately at the center of the radial head. It is important to estimate where the native radial head is and not align the prosthesis with osteophytes that are often prominent at this location in chronically arthritic elbows. Second, the milling path should equally remove the subchondral bone on all three articular surfaces. Lastly, the surgeon should ensure that enough bone stock will remain after the milling process in the proximal portion of the ulna. This step is particularly important when a relatively oversized implant is to be used and/or when the caudal aspect of the ulna has a concave profile. Although important, templating of the humeral component is less critical as a slight positioning error will be more forgiving. Conversely, templating errors of the RU component can significantly affect postimplantation range of motion, implant stability, and risk of fracture after surgery. Digital templating is recommended as it may be more accurate and allows independent templating of the humeral and RU components, irrespective of the elbow flexion angle.

Surgical techniques

ISU Elbow

This replacement system requires transection of the lateral collateral ligament; lateral luxation of the elbow; removal of a wedge-shaped portion of the humeral condyle that includes the articular surface; removal of the articular portion of the proximal radius and ulna; and securing the components with a combination of bone cement, locking screws, and press-fit mechanisms.

Humeral preparation

The current surgical technique involves positioning the patient in lateral recumbency and a caudal lateral approach to the elbow via transection of the lateral collateral ligament. After inducing lateral luxation of the elbow, the humerus is prepared. Humeral preparation involves drilling a 5- to 9-mm-diameter hole from the supratrochlear foramen into the medullary canal. A cutting guide is introduced into the medullary canal and used to remove a wedge-shaped piece of humerus that includes the majority of the humeral articular surface. Great care is taken to preserve bone stock proximally so that fracture of the condyle is avoided. A larger cut can be made later if the original cutting guide used was too small. The drill guide and the ostectomized bone are removed.

RU preparation

The anconeal process of the ulna is excised and the elbow is reduced. With the elbow reduced, a circular mounting bracket is placed laterally onto the drill bit that extends from the humerus and the humeral trial component. The RU cutting guide is then placed onto the mounting bracket. Linking the RU cutting guide to the humeral component helps to ensure congruity of the prosthesis. The RU cutting guide has drill bit guide holes; two 3.2-mm drill bits are used. One bit is drilled into the radius and one into the ulna. These steps secure the RU cutting guide onto the radius and ulna on the same center of rotation as the humeral component. The mounting bracket is removed and the elbow is luxated laterally. The RU cutting guide is then used to remove the articular portion of the radius and the ulna using the circular cutting saw that fits into the cutting guide. After this step is completed, the cutting guide and ostectomized bone are removed. A hole is then drilled from proximal to distal down the medullary canal of the radius; the size of the hole is dependent on the implant size.

Implant positioning and fixation

Following humeral preparation, a humeral trial component is positioned. The humeral trial component has a hole that accepts a 3.5-mm drill bit. A long 3.2- or 3.5-mm drill bit is used to drill from the origin of the lateral collateral ligament, through the hole in the trial component to the medial collateral ligament. This hole ensures proper placement of the humeral component.

Similarly, at the conclusion of the RU preparation, a trial RU component is placed and the elbow is reduced to ensure that the two trial components articulate correctly. If they do articulate correctly, the elbow is luxated and a hole for the locking screw is made by drilling through the caudal hole in the RU component. Again, the size of this hole is dependent on component size.

The trial components are removed, the surgical field flushed, and the final components are positioned and secured (bone cement for the stem of the humerus; press-fit for the radial stem; and a locking screw for the RU body). The elbow is reduced and a final check is performed to confirm proper placement of the components.

Surgical closure

Before closing, a distal ulnar osteotomy is performed and autogenous bone graft (from the excised bone) is placed between the radius and ulna. Closure is mainly focused on reconstruction of the lateral collateral ligament.

TATE Elbow

Preoperative preparation

After routine preparation for aseptic surgery, the dog is temporarily placed in dorsal recumbency in the operating room (OR). To facilitate unrestricted movement of the surgical team, anesthesia personnel and equipment are located at the rear end of the dog. The uppermost, nonoperated thoracic limb is pulled caudally and secured to the surgery table. After routine four-corner draping, the dog is positioned in lateral recumbency with the operated limb down, such that the vertical post of a dedicated bracket secured to the table is located at the level of the axillary fold. Layered draping is then completed routinely using cloth and impervious paper drapes as well as stockinette around the forelimb. Superficial, adherent antimicrobial surgical incise drapes are strongly recommended (Figure 12.11).

Surgical approach to the elbow joint

The elbow joint is approached through a medial incision. The ulnar nerve is carefully dissected and

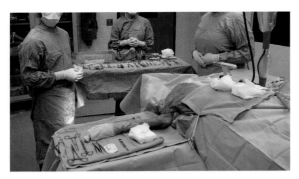

Figure 12.11 Typical operating room setup for a TATE prosthesis at Michigan State University. General (*far center*), prosthesis-specific (*left*), and milling (*right*) instrumentations are kept on two separated tables and a Mayo stand. With the dog in lateral recumbency, the operated limb is abducted over an additional dedicated Mayo stand to expose the medial aspect of the elbow. The entire dog and limb is covered with several layers of sterile impervious drapes. These include a stockinette and plastic iodine-impregnated adhesive drape over the operated limb.

retracted cranially. Transection of caudal branches of the ulnar nerve innervating the joint capsule and the flexor carpi ulnaris muscle allow appropriate mobilization and protection of the ulnar nerve during the remainder of the surgery. The cranial and caudal aspects of the humeral condyle are exposed in order to identify the medial osteochondral junction cranially and the edge of the medial epicondyle caudally. In severely arthritic joints, thorough osteophyte debridement is imperative for accurate identification of proper anatomical landmarks.

A medial epicondylar osteotomy is performed using an oscillating saw, starting at the caudal edge of the medial epicondyle, aiming at the osteochondral junction cranially. Prior to completion of the osteotomy, the epicondyle is prepared for later lag screw fixation. The osteotomy is completed with a proximal chevron cut and the epicondylar bone flap is retracted distally. Access to the caudal joint space is permitted by the release of tendon of origin of the deep digital flexor muscle followed by an oblique ostectomy of the caudodistal corner of the medial epicondyle. The elbow joint is slightly subluxated to allow for an ostectomy of the anconeal process.

Identification of the elbow axis of rotation and joint positioning

A dedicated trochlear clamp is used to identify the axis of rotation (AOR) of the elbow, which closely corresponds to the mediolateral axis of the humeral trochlea. A datum pin, inserted along the AOR, serves as a reference throughout the remainder of the procedure (Figure 12.12A). A sterile positioning system is then attached, over the draping, to the previously mentioned bracket. The datum pin is secured to the positioning device, thus immobilizing the humerus. A dedicated alignment plate, loaded over the datum pin, is rotated until the cranial humeral osteochondral junction is aligned with a corresponding laser mark on the plate. The plate is secured to the humerus using one or two cortical bone screws. The elbow is then flexed until the cranial aspect of the radial head is aligned with a second laser mark on the plate). This typically brings the elbow to 85–95 degrees of flexion. Proper joint congruity is ascertained and adjusted, if needed, with the positioning system. The alignment plate is fixed to the radius (one screw) and the ulna (two screws), which effectively secures the elbow in the desired position before articular surface preparation (Figure 12.13A).

Articular resurfacing and implant impaction

A drilling guide is then loaded onto the alignment plate and used to drill four transverse holes (two in the humerus, one in the radius, and one in the ulna) that will accommodate the mediolateral primary fixation posts in the matching prosthetic components. Using a custom end mill, the proximal (humeral) and distal (RU) articular surfaces are simultaneously removed along a 200-degree arc concentric to the AOR (Figures 12.12A,B and 12.13B). A plastic trial prosthesis is used to confirm proper milling depth. A final "cartridge" implant is then gradually impacted into the open joint space (Figures 12.13C and 12.14). The set plate used to link the components during impaction and the alignment plate are sequentially removed to allow assessment of the elbow range of motion. If cranial or caudal impingements are present, osteophytes are debrided using rongeurs or a high-speed bur.

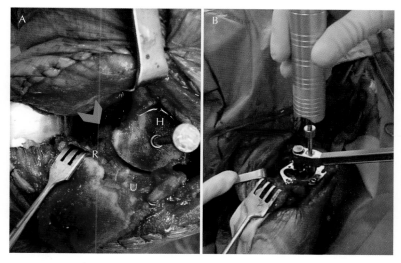

Figure 12.12   Intraoperative views of a TATE implantation procedure. The joint is exposed via an osteotomy of the medial epicondyle and the elbow axis of rotation is identified (A). To optimize postoperative range of motion and avoid impingement, the RU component must be aligned with the radial head, which requires meticulous debridement of osteophyte(s) cranial to the radial head (blue arrow). A milling bit is used to simultaneously remove the articular surfaces of the humerus, radius, and ulna (resurfacing) along an arc centered on the joint axis of rotation (B). H: humerus; U: ulna (coronoid process); R: radial head.

Surgical closure

A proximal RU synostosis is performed immediately below the level of the radial fixation post using an appropriately sized lag screw loaded on a washer. The medial aspect of the RU joint is roughened with a high-speed bur and a generous autogenous cancellous bone graft from the previous milling is packed at that location. The medial epicondyle is reduced and fixed with trans- and epicondylar lag screws or a bone plate (Figure 12.13D). Routine closure in layers concludes the procedure.

Different characteristics of the ISU and TATE procedures are summarized in Table 12.1.

Postoperative evaluation and management

True mediolateral and craniocaudal elbow radiographic views are obtained to assess proper implant alignment and positioning as well as ostectomy reduction and fixation.

ISU Elbow

Implant alignment, positioning, cementing technique, as well as bone/cement/implant interfaces are evaluated on orthogonal radiographic views. Regular follow-up radiographs are recommended to evaluate implant stability, implant failure, and aseptic loosening. Postoperatively, the joint can be supported with a spica splint until suture removal at 2 weeks.[11] Implementation of a physical rehabilitation program is advocated following an initial 6-week period of restricted activity. Postoperative antibiotic therapy is left to the discretion of the surgeon.

TATE Elbow system

Particular attention is paid to the position of the cranial aspect of the radial component, which should be flush with the native radial head, and to the radial post, which should bisect the radial head (mediolateral views). To avoid postoperative

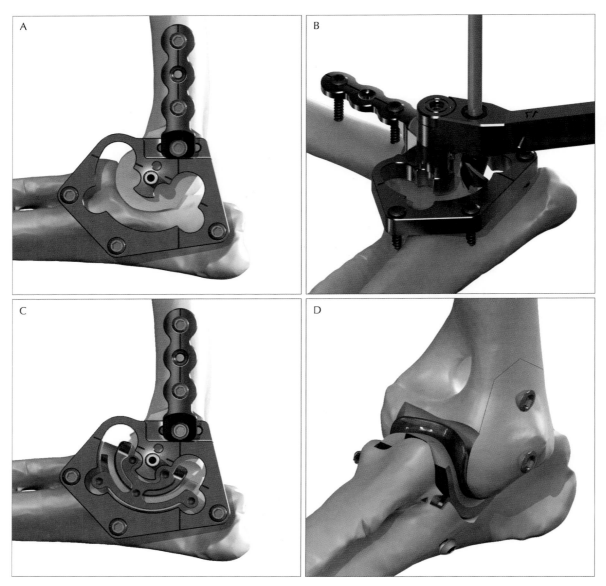

Figure 12.13 Schematics of the four key steps of the TATE implantation procedure. With the elbow is flexed at ~85–95 degrees, an alignment plate centered on the axis of rotation of the joint is affixed to the humerus, radius, and ulna (A). A circular groove is milled along the joint articular surface (B) prior to impaction of the TATE cartridge (C). A blue X-shaped set plate maintains the prosthetic components aligned during simultaneous impaction. Following removal of the alignment and set plates, the joint range of motion is evaluated for possible impingement. A radioulnar synostosis is performed using an autogenous cancellous bone graft and a lag screw immediately below the prosthesis RU component (D). Finally, the medial epicondyle is reduced and stabilized using two lag screws, one of which is applied through the joint axis of rotation. (Courtesy of Greg Van Der Meulen, BioMedtrix, Boonton, NJ)

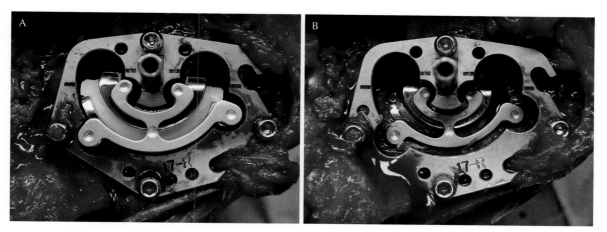

Figure 12.14 Intraoperative photographs illustrating the placement of a TATE prosthesis within the resurfaced milling path (A). Once fully impacted, the medial surface of the prosthesis should be flushed with the plane of the medial epicondyle osteotomy (B). The X-shaped set plate links the humeral and RU component, thus facilitating their simultaneous implantation.

Table 12.1 Characteristics of the ISU and TATE prostheses

	ISU Elbow system	TATE Elbow system
Surgical approach	Lateral collateral ligament (LCL) desmotomy Elbow luxation	Medial epicondyle osteotomy No elbow luxation
Bone preparation	Sequential ostectomies (condylar wedge [humerus]—semicircular [RU])	Simultaneous humeral and RU articular resurfacing Limited bone resection
Implantation	Sequential—individual humeral and RU components	Simultaneous—cartridge implant design
Primary fixation	Bone cement	Press-fit—four fixation posts
Secondary fixation	Bone ingrowth (mediolateral humeral component interfaces)	Bone ingrowth onto HA-coated porous surfaces

impingement, the ulnar component should be centered over the ulna on craniocaudal views. Of critical importance is the evaluation the bone–implant interfaces, which requires that the X-ray beam be precisely tangent to the interface of interest. Ideally, intimate contact between each prosthetic component and corresponding bone should be present, although a thin (less than 1 mm wide) interfacial gap may be acceptable. Subsequent radiographic evaluations are recommended at 6, 12, 24, and 52 weeks and yearly thereafter to assess bone ingrowth and implant stability (e.g., aseptic loosening).

Postoperatively, a soft-padded bandage is applied for a few days to control local swelling. Dogs are typically released within 48 hours after surgery. Restricted in-house activity and limited leash walks are recommended for approximately 4–6 weeks. During that period, passive range of motion exercises as well as distal to proximal massages are advocated as often as possible. Following the first satisfactory radiographic and clinical recheck (6 weeks), intense physical rehabilitation is strongly encouraged. Typical exercises may include underwater treadmill, swimming, as well as below and above Cavaletti rails.

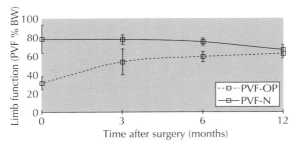

Figure 12.15 Peak vertical force of the unoperated (N) and operated (OP) front limbs of the 16 dogs with successful outcomes. (Reproduced from Conzemius et al. [2003], with permission from Wiley-Blackwell)

Clinical outcome: Complications

To date, except for two peer-reviewed publications addressing the ISU Elbow replacement, objective information on the clinical outcome after TER is scarce. Prospective clinical and experimental studies on the TATE system are ongoing and should lead to peer-reviewed data in the future. However, information presented on the outcomes of the TATE system presented here is based on the authors' (LMD and RPG) experience and on personal communications.

ISU Elbow

The overall success rate of a prospective clinical trial was 80% (Figure 12.15; Conzemius et al. 2003). This study was performed prior to many of the previously noted changes in prosthesis design.

Force plate analysis

The average dog with a successful outcome had ground reaction forces on the operated leg that increased by more than 25% over presurgical levels. Certainly, some of this improvement was the result of case selection. This clinical trial only accepted dogs that were severely affected and were ideal candidates for an experimental intervention. However, it is important to note that even with the improvement, limb function in the operated leg did not reach that of the opposite, unoperated leg that in many cases also had elbow OA.

Complications

Regardless of functional outcome, the study found that elbow replacement was a viable treatment option and confirmed that many of the design and operative changes that had been instituted were effective in decreasing the complication rate and improving efficacy. The four dogs with failed outcomes had either osteomyelitis (one case), fracture of the humeral condyle (one case), or lateral luxation (two cases) (Figure 12.16). There will always be a risk of infection with joint replacement. The fracture was associated with surgeon error, as the humeral component was impacted into place and the wedge shape of the component split the remaining portion of the condyle.

Lateral luxation represented 10% of all cases; a complication rate that alerted the investigators that additional work was required. While the exact cause for lateral luxation was not identified, the primary concerns were that the lateral collateral ligament was transected during the approach to the joint and that the cutting guide system still had the components inserted independent of each other and thus did not ensure that the components had the same center of rotation. Different centers of rotation will allow for binding and/or twisting of the components during a range of motion. Since stability of the lateral aspect of the joint is much lower than normal during the recovery period, the combination of instability and malalignment could explain lateral luxation. Empirically, this hypothesis is supported by the fact that nearly all luxations occur in the first 2–3 months following surgery. Thus, if the components remained stable until the lateral collateral ligament healed, luxation was essentially eliminated. Since correct positioning of the implants was dependent on surgeon experience, a relatively high incidence of lateral luxation was anticipated with wider distribution of this elbow replacement system. Several solutions to this problem have been reported. First, buttressing the primary suture repair of the lateral collateral ligament with suture anchors appeared to contribute to the lateral stability (Conzemius and Vandervoort 2005). Second, a cutting guide system where placement of the cutting guide for the RU component is dependent on the center of rotation of the humeral trial component has been described (Conzemius 2009). This system ensures

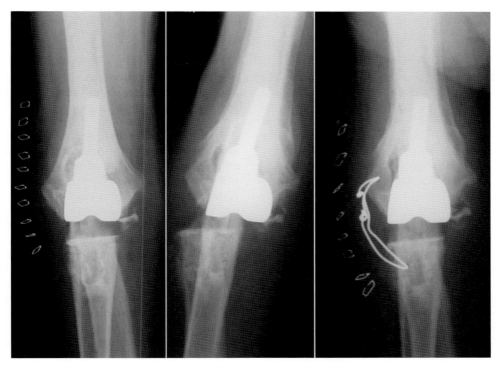

Figure 12.16   An immediate postoperative radiograph (*left*) of a clinical case after total elbow replacement. At an 8-week recheck (*middle*), lateral luxation of the radioulnar component is noted. This was treated with cerclage wires (*right*) and exercise restriction for 8 weeks.

a more congruous placement of the humeral and RU components. In addition, this system is more "user friendly" than the first- and second-generation systems and seemed reduce, but not eliminate, the frequency of lateral luxation. Finally, a change in the articulation of the components to create greater resistance to lateral luxation has been shown, in an *in vitro* experimental study, to be very effective (Rose et al. 2012). The primary modification of the components involved increasing the size of the lateral aspect of the humeral condyle and reducing the size of the medial aspect of the humeral condyle while maintaining the same center of rotation. Changes were made to the RU component to match the changes to the articular surface of the humeral component. These modified components use the identical cutting guide system as the components described above but are up to seven times more resistant to lateral luxation when shear forces or torsional forces are applied at the articulation. The other major changes were made to the RU component in an effort to make

the surgical procedure technically simpler. These included (1) removal of the ulnar stem, (2) creation of a hole in the caudal aspect of the RU component for placement of a locking screw into the ulna, and (3) creation of a metal backing for the RU component with a porous ingrowth surface. The clinical ramifications of these changes remain to be investigated in a clinical setting.

Recently, Innes described the results of 13 dogs implanted with an Iowa State prosthesis between 2004 and 2009 in the United Kingdom.[12] In the 10 dogs (11 elbows—therefore percentage is greater than 100) that survived to follow-up examination, outcomes were described as "good" (60%), "moderate" (20%), or "poor" (30%). Major complications occurred in 60% of 10 dogs that survived to a follow-up examination and included four ulnar fractures and two subluxations. Based on this experience, Innes stated that "the [ISU Elbow] remains the 'standard of care' until other systems are shown to have better efficacy/safety profiles." To date, the most common complications reported for the ISU Elbow are luxation and ulnar fracture.[11]

TATE Elbow

The lack of objective data on the TATE system results, in part, from the recent release of this prosthesis and from the desire to present longer-term follow-up periods (>1 year). The information contained in the next three paragraphs represents a synthesis of *subjective* data from fellow surgeons who performed at least five TER procedures with the TATE system. We emphasize that since this information is anecdotal in nature and has not been subject to peer review to date, it should be assessed cautiously.

It is estimated that, since July 2007, the TATE prosthesis has been implanted in ~180–200 cases worldwide over a 4.5-year period at the time of this writing. This total is based on the number of prostheses (281) sold by BioMedtrix as of January 2012, minus 30%–35% to account for unused implants. Purchased and returned implants (114) are not included.

In 2009 (~34 months follow-up), we reported subjective data on 43 procedures performed in 42 dogs.[13] Severe complications had occurred within 5 weeks postoperatively in 7% of the patients (two humeral fractures and one implant loosening associated with secondary infection [two cases] and ulnar fracture [one case]). Two dogs were euthanized without reevaluation by the primary surgeon and one was amputated due to concomitant deep infection. Other complications, consisting of pin migration, screw loosening and fracture of the medial epicondylar fragment, were seen in three dogs (7%) and were successfully treated.

Since that report, 39 more TATE prostheses were implanted in 37 dogs by the same groups of surgeons. The following is an update on these 39 cases, of which 14 were evaluated prospectively (LMD and RPG) and 25 were evaluated retrospectively (Acker).

Prospective study

Between April 2008 and October 2011, our group implanted 14 TATE prostheses in 13 dogs affected with intractable foreleg lameness attributed to elbow OA. The mean (± standard deviation [SD]) patient age at implantation was 9 ± 3 years and average weight was $35 \pm 10 \, \text{kg}$.

Force plate analysis (FPA) was conducted prior to and up to 2 years following surgery on seven dogs. Postoperative FPAs were performed at 6 and 12 weeks ($n = 7$), then at 24 weeks ($n = 5$), 52 weeks ($n = 3$), and 104 weeks ($n = 2$). Based on the ongoing evaluation, gradual improvement of the peak vertical ground reaction force (PVGRF) was evident over time, albeit after an initial worsening of the lameness at 6 weeks. Conversely, the PVGRF of the contralateral limb significantly decreased over time. By approximately 1 year postoperatively, the PVGRF of the operated limb exceeded that of the contralateral limb. In the two cases with available long-term data, that trend continued until 2 years postoperatively. The PVGRF ultimately reached the normal range previously reported by Lascelles et al. (2006) (Figure 12.17).

Clinical evaluation consisted of assessment of gait and range of motion (veterinarian evaluation) as well as pain level and quality of life (owner evaluation). While subtle lameness was occasionally reported, in the absence of complications, improvement in limb function subjectively mirrored objective FPA in all dogs. Similarly, dogs

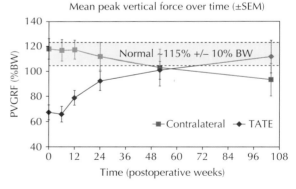

Figure 12.17   Mean (± standard error of the mean [SEM]) front limbs peak vertical ground reaction force (PVGRF) at the trot of dogs implanted with a TATE prosthesis over 2 years. The shaded bar represents the PVGRF in normal dogs at the trot (115% ± 10% BW; Lascelles et al. [2006]). The PVGRF of the operated limb significantly improved over time and exceeded that of the contralateral limb by approximately 1 year after surgery. By 2 years postoperatively, the PVGRF of the implanted front limb had returned to normal.

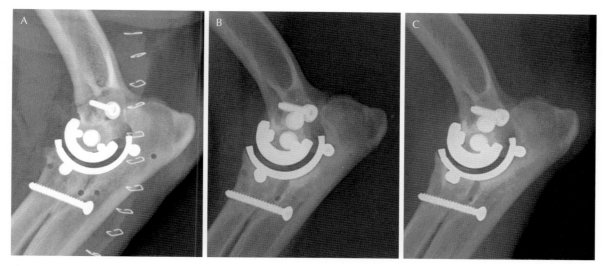

Figure 12.18 Typical radiographic appearance of a (first-generation) TATE prosthesis/bone interfaces immediately after surgery (A), then at 1 year (B) and 2 years (C) postoperatively. In most cases, there was no evidence of periprosthetic bone resorption over time. Occasionally, mild early widening of the RU component/bone interface was seen around the ulnar post. This, however, did not seem to progress beyond the postoperative 12-week time point. Unlike the smooth solid posts of the TATE first generation, the second-generation prosthesis features porous HA-coated hollow, slotted posts, as seen in Figure 12.1B, to optimize local bone ingrowth.

showed improvement and pain-free range of motion, mainly in extension, and were more active.

Radiographic evaluation revealed quiescent bone/implant interfaces over time (Figure 12.18). Occasionally, however, some limited bone resorption occurred near the ulnar post. In one case, extensive RU periprosthetic osteolysis progressed up to 36 weeks postoperatively.

Minor complications included superficial wound dehiscence ($n = 1$). The wound was successfully treated with local wound care and systemic antibiotics for 3 weeks.

Major complications (i.e., any complication requiring additional surgery) consisted of epicondylar screw loosening ($n = 1$) and a humeral fracture ($n = 1$) with secondary infection (noted above) that led to amputation of the limb 2 weeks postoperatively. The loose screw was successfully treated using an additional screw implanted percutaneously under fluoroscopic guidance. The case of extensive, self-limiting periprosthetic osteolysis described above is included as a potential severe complication, although catastrophic failure has not occurred at this point. Both complications were attributed to surgical errors associated with suboptimal milling technique and subsequent excessive gap at the bone–RU component interface.

Retrospective study

Twenty-five TATE prostheses were implanted in 24 dogs since July 2007. Signalment was similar to the prospective study described above. Subjective clinical evaluation was conducted by the lead surgeon and by client assessment. Functional improvement beyond preoperative levels, consistent elimination of pain, and improved quality of life were reported in most cases. Based on client assessment, overall outcome was very good in 84% of the cases (return to normal activity), fair in 12% of the cases (improvement compared with preoperative activity level), and poor in 4% (no improvement compared with preoperative activity).

Complications were reported as intraoperative, as well as minor and major. Iatrogenic, intraoperative complications consisted of a transection of the ulnar nerve without clinically evident consequence ($n = 1$) and of a trochlear fracture that was stabilized at the time of surgery ($n = 1$). A minor

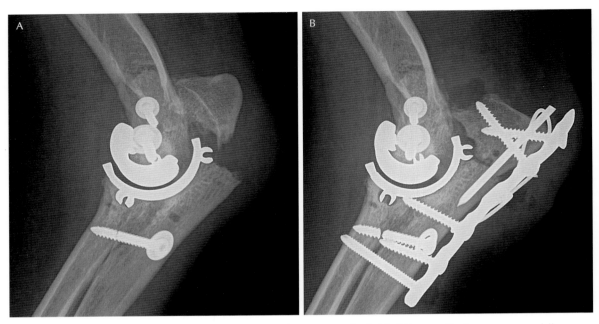

Figure 12.19   Ulnar fracture 2 months after implantation of a TATE prosthesis (A). This complication was successfully revised using a combination of tension band and plate fixation (B). Functional recovery continued until the death of the animal 18 months postoperatively for reasons unrelated to this procedure. (Courtesy of Randy Acker, Sun Valley Animal Center, Ketchum, ID)

postoperative complication (epicondylar pin migration) was successfully treated by removal of the migrating implant. One major complication occurred 2 months postoperatively. This ulnar fracture was successfully revised using a pin/tension band combined with a caudal locking compression plate (Figure 12.19).

Clinical summary (prospective and retrospective studies)

In this limited series of 39 cases, long-term objective and subjective evaluations seem to agree on the following points: (1) functional recovery steadily improves over time; however, return to normal function is slow and may take between 6 months and 1 year; (2) the procedure seems effective in controlling pain and improving quality of life; (3) minor complications occurred in less than 8% of the cases; (4) some major complications may be revised successfully; (5) with nearly 4 years follow-up, the rate of major complications is approximately 8% prior to revision and 5% after revision; and finally, (6) complications occurred

fairly early after surgery. There were no instances of elbow luxation or primary ulnar fracture. Similarly, explantation or arthrodesis has not been necessary. Forequarter amputation, however, particularly in cases of deep infection, may be a valid revision option if the contralateral elbow is sound.

Needed and ongoing studies

An important aspect of long-term evaluation of any prosthesis is retrieval analysis. This information is currently lacking with either system. At the time of writing, one TATE has been evaluated for osseointegration 6 months postoperatively after the dog had died of an unrelated cause. While limb function had subjectively improved compared with preoperative evaluation, high-resolution radiographs suggested limited bone ingrowth at the bone/implant interfaces despite the fact that both implant components appeared grossly stable.

Design modifications have been recently devised for both systems in response to their perceived respective shortcomings, whether documented (e.g., elbow luxation in the ISU Elbow) or potential (e.g., incomplete osseointegration of the TATE Elbow components). Modifications aimed at improving resistance to luxation with the ISU Elbow are described above. In an effort to optimize bone ingrowth, a second-generation TATE system was released early 2010. Design changes included hollow primary fixation posts and HA coating. In addition, reduced prosthetic constraint in rotation and mediolateral translation was achieved through modification of the RU articular profile.[14,15]

Limitations of TER

Regardless of design, a major limitation of TER is the absence of satisfactory options for revision in the event of failure. The bilateral nature of end-stage elbow OA precludes amputation in most cases, and thus arthrodesis remains the most valid alternative. Although some fractures or luxations may be successfully revised, others may require explantation and arthrodesis. Infection remains the most challenging complication, as antibiotic therapy is unlikely to be effective in the presence of the prosthesis. Accordingly, explantation with subsequent arthrodesis may be the only viable revision. Alteration of limb function, or even quality of life, following arthrodesis should be carefully considered, particularly if painful contralateral ankylosis is present. With unilateral arthrodesis, however, limb function may be acceptable despite continuous limb circumduction. Conversely, amputation might represent an acceptable alternative in dogs affected by unilateral end-stage OA. Considering these limitations, owner education is critical and must be thorough and objective. A fair disclosure of alternative treatments and realistic expectations, particularly with regard to complications and revisions should be presented to clients contemplating TER.

Conclusions

Thanks to forward-thinking surgeons and engineers, an enormous amount of work has been performed in the field of canine TER in recent years. Nonetheless, the ideal prosthetic design and surgical procedure remains elusive. Numerous questions regarding optimal articular surface constraint as well as long-term periprosthetic osteolysis or osseointegration have yet to be answered. Similarly, long-term prospective, objective clinical trials, and retrieval analyses are desperately needed. Imperfect revision options will continue to constitute one of the most serious hurdles to overcome for the foreseeable future and may limit the widespread acceptance of TER as a reliable treatment option for end-stage canine elbow OA. Novel ideas, along with promising, although imperfect, clinical results, will likely continue to generate interest and much needed research in the open and challenging field of elbow replacement surgery.

Endnotes

1. Chancrin J. Personal communication, December 2008.
2. Lewis RH. Development of elbow arthroplasty (canine) clinical trials. In: *ACVS Symposium*. 1996, p. 110.
3. Sidebotham CG. Personal communication, February 2008.
4. Cook JL, Lower J. Elbow arthroplasty system. Patent US007419507B2. USA, 2008.
5. Conzemius MG. Total elbow replacement in the dog—Development and evaluation. Thesis, Iowa State University, Ames, 2000.
6. Acker RL, Van Der Meulen GT. Joint prosthesis and method of implanting same. Patent US20070073408A1. USA, 2007.
7. Acker RL, Van Der Meulen GT. Joint prosthesis. Patent US20080154384A1. USA, 2008.
8. Acker R, Van Der Meulen GT. Tate elbow preliminary trials. In: *35th VOS Annual Conference*. 2008.
9. Innes J. Personal communication, January 2012.
10. Wendelburg K. Personal communication, January 2012.
11. Conzemius MG. Total elbow replacement: facts, fiction and opinions. In: *ACVS Veterinary Symposium*. 2007, p. 440.
12. Innes J. Total elbow replacement—The UK experience. In: *BVOA Salvage Surgery Joint Replacement and Arthrodesis*. 2009, p. 19.
13. Déjardin LM, Guillou RP. Total elbow replacement in dogs—Recent design evolution and early results with the TATE system. In: *18th Annual Scientific*

Meeting, European College of Veterinary Surgeons. 2009. [CD-ROM]

14. Déjardin LM, Guillou RP, Sawyer MJ, et al. Effect of articular design on rotational constraint of two unlinked canine total elbow prostheses. Presented at the *3rd World Veterinary Orthopedic Congress (WVOC)*. Bologna, Italy, September 5–18, 2010. [CD-ROM]

15. Guillou RP, Demianiuk R, Déjardin LM, et al. Effect of articular design on mediolateral constraint and stability of two unlinked canine total elbow prostheses. Presented at the *38th Annual Meeting of the Veterinary Orthopedic Society (VOS)*. Snowmass, CO, March 5–12, 2011. [CD-ROM]

References

Armstrong AD, King GJW, Yamaguchi K. Total elbow arthroplasty design. In: *Shoulder and Elbow Arthroplasty*, Williams GR, Yamaguchi K, Ramsey ML, Galatz LM (eds.). Philadelphia: Lippincott Williams & Wilkins, 2005, p. 297.

Conzemius MG. Nonconstrained elbow replacement in dogs. Vet Surg 2009;38:279.

Conzemius MG, Aper RL. Development and evaluation of semiconstrained arthroplasty for the treatment of elbow osteoarthritis in the dog. Vet Comp Orthop Traumatol 1998;11:54.

Conzemius MG, Vandervoort J. Total joint replacement in the dog. Vet Clin North Am Small Anim Pract 2005;35(5):1213–1231.

Conzemius MG, Aper RL, Hill CM. Evaluation of a canine total-elbow arthroplasty system: A preliminary study in normal dogs. Vet Surg 2001;30:11–20.

Conzemius MG, Aper RL, Corti LB. Short-term outcome after total elbow arthroplasty in dogs with severe, naturally occurring osteoarthritis. Vet Surg 2003;32: 545–552.

Lascelles BD, Roe SC, Smith E, et al. Evaluation of a pressure walkway system for measurement of vertical limb forces in clinically normal dogs. Am J Vet Res 2006;67:277–282.

Rose ND, Freeman A, Conzemius MG. Resistance to lateral luxation of two canine total elbow replacement systems under variable mechanical loads. Vet Surg 2012; in press.

13

Emerging Arthroplasties

Jeffrey N. Peck

Total joint arthroplasty for the elbow, hip, and stifle has been described in previous chapters. These are the three joints for which commercially produced joint replacements are available for dogs and cats. Total joint arthroplasty or hemiarthroplasty is commercially available for other joints in human surgery and several of these have potential application in veterinary surgery. The purpose of this chapter is to collate information from the human and veterinary literature regarding joint arthroplasties that may have veterinary applications, but for which prostheses are not yet available. Certainly, the development of a commercially available and efficacious prosthesis requires years of development and investment. The veterinary caseload for a particular joint prosthesis may not be adequate to garner commercial attention in many cases. However, the information in this chapter could also be utilized as a springboard for the development of custom prostheses for individual patients.

Total disc arthroplasty

Total disc arthroplasty (TDA) is a relatively new procedure, emerging in the late 1980s and early 1990s. There were no Food and Drug Administration (FDA)-approved TDA devices in the United States until 2004 (Le et al. 2004). The development and use of lumbar disc arthroplasty preceded cervical disc arthroplasty. People who undergo either lumbar or cervical spinal fusion surgery are at increased risk of developing adjacent site degeneration, compared with patients managed without fusion. Approximately 3% of patients need to undergo second site surgery each year following either lumbar or cervical disc fusion. Roughly 25% of patients have had second site surgery by 10 years after their original surgery (Le et al. 2004; Harrop et al. 2008). In one study (Goffin et al. 2004), 92% of patients with anterior cervical disc fusion (ACDF) developed radiographic changes, although not necessarily clinical signs, consistent with degenerative disc disease. Similar numbers are reported in the veterinary literature following decompression, with or without stabilization, for caudal cervical spodylomyelopathy (CCSM) (da Costa 2010). While it is tempting to extrapolate results from lumbar or lumbosacral fusion in people, reports of adjacent site degeneration are not available for lumbosacral stabilization in veterinary patients. Therefore, this discussion will focus more on cervical disc replacement than on lumbar disc replacement.

Advances in Small Animal Total Joint Replacement, First Edition. Edited by Jeffrey N. Peck and Denis J. Marcellin-Little.
© 2013 John Wiley & Sons, Inc. Published 2013 by John Wiley & Sons, Inc.

In general, the primary justification for the development of TDA has been to maintain the range of motion at the site of decompression. As with veterinary patients, human patients that have had ACDF are at higher risk of developing adjacent site disc disease, often described as a "domino lesion." It is theorized that spinal fusion results in a transfer of load to adjacent disc spaces and articular facets (Pickett et al. 2005; Chang et al. 2007a). A second theory for the development of adjacent site disc degeneration is that it is the natural progression of degenerative disc disease (Le et al. 2004).

In vitro spinal fusion models have documented increased intradiscal pressure, increased range of motion and increased articular facet joint loads at sites adjacent to the fused segment (McAfee et al. 2003; Chang et al. 2007a). The increase in intradiscal pressure will, theoretically, prevent the transport of nutrients into the disc, resulting in chondrocyte death and disc degeneration. Increases in range of motion and facet joint loads can result in ligamentous and synovial hypertrophy.

While there are several studies that document preservation of range of motion at the operated site following TDA (McAfee et al. 2003; Pickett et al. 2005; Chang et al. 2007a,b; Snyder et al. 2007; Barrey et al. 2009), there is only one study that has evaluated the incidence of adjacent site disc degeneration following TDA (Harrop et al. 2008). That study was a systematic review of the literature evaluating the incidence of adjacent site lumbar disc degeneration (radiographic or symptomatic) following either arthrodesis (fusion) or TDA. Based on logistic regression analysis, patient age and time to follow-up were significant factors in the incidence of adjacent site degeneration; however, 14% of arthrodesis patients (1732 patients) and 1% of arthroplasty patients (758 patients) developed adjacent site degeneration. The difference was statistically significant.

The three main indications for TDA in humans are (1) radiculopathy secondary to disc herniation or foraminal stenosis; (2) myelopathy secondary to disc herniation; and (3) any combination of radiculopathy and myelopathy (Pracyk and Traynelis 2005). Total disc replacement (TDR) is not indicated in cases of vertebral canal stenosis or compression secondary to articular facet hypertrophy or synovial hypertrophy.

The general requirements for TDA are similar to the requirements for other forms of arthroplasty. The materials must be biocompatible, implants should have long-term stability, and implantation should relieve pain and restore function. Additionally, if TDR is to be successful in the prevention of adjacent site degeneration, as well as relieve clinical signs at the affected site, it must fulfill several additional requirements. It must provide distraction, if necessary, in order to relieve foraminal stenosis. The range of motion of the prosthesis should be similar to the range of motion of the normal, natural joint. Range of motion and distraction must be preserved in the long term (i.e., the implantation procedure must not predispose to future ankylosis, with its associated loss of range of motion). The center of rotation of the prosthesis should mimic the natural location of the center of rotation (Le et al. 2004).

As with other joint prostheses, titanium (or titanium alloy), stainless steel, and cobalt-chromium (CoCr) have each been used to manufacture of TDA implants. Metal-on-metal, metal-on-plastic (polyethylene, ultrahigh-molecular-weight polyethylene), ceramic-on-ceramic, and ceramic-on-plastic implants have been described (Hofstetter et al. 2009). In addition, the full range of constraint (constrained, semiconstrained, and unconstrained) has been utilized, although classification of constraint has not been consistent throughout the literature, even for a particular prosthesis (Le et al. 2004; Bertagnoli et al. 2005a,b; Chang et al. 2007a; Barrey et al. 2009). For constrained prostheses, the center of rotation is fixed during motion. There are three degrees of freedom of motion with a constrained prosthesis: bending, flexion/extension, and rotation. Constrained prostheses require more precise implantation in order to mimic the axes of rotation.(Barrey et al. 2009) Unconstrained prostheses allow the above mentioned motions, in addition to translation, resulting in six degrees of freedom of motion (Pickett et al. 2005; Hofstetter et al. 2009; Figure 13.1). Further, the description of intervertebral motion must also include coupled motion, which should be matched by the prosthesis (Le et al. 2004). Coupled motion is the motion in a plane that is secondary to the plane of primary motion. For example, when lateral bending force

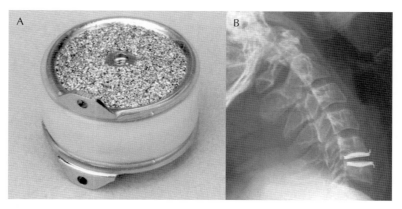

Figure 13.1 (A) The Bryan total disc prosthesis (Medtronic, Minneapolis, MN). (Reproduced from Goffin et al. [2002], with permission from Lippincott, Williams & Wilkins) (B) Mediolateral cervical radiograph of an implanted Bryan prosthesis. Note the offset of the metallic endplates (arrows), indicating translation, which is consistent with the unconstrained nature of this prosthesis. (Reproduced from Goffin et al. [2002], with permission from Lippincott, Williams & Wilkins)

(the primary motion) is applied to the cervical spine, the coupled motion of axial rotation occurs in the same direction as the lateral bending.

When reviewing reported range of motion, it is important to be aware of how the data are reported. For example, some researchers will report left lateral and right lateral bending separately, while others will report only a total from right to left (Chang et al. 2007a; Barrey et al. 2009). At C5–C6, in the intact human spine, range of motion in flexion/extension is roughly 10 degrees, lateral bending is roughly 6 degrees, and axial rotation is roughly 5 degrees (Pickett et al. 2005; Chang et al. 2007a,b; Barrey et al. 2009). The coupled axial motion that occurs during lateral bending is approximately 34% of the primary motion. With a primary axial motion, the coupled motion for lateral bending is approximately 56% of the primary motion (Barrey et al. 2009). An additional value that is considered in implant design is the neutral zone (NZ), or the arc of movement with no applied load. The NZ is a descriptor of laxity. The NZ of the intact human spine is roughly 6, 3, and 4.5 degrees in flexion/extension, lateral bending, and axial rotation, respectively (Wilke et al. 1998).

Cervical disc replacement implants with most peer-reviewed data include the following: (1) Discoserv (Scient'x, Voisins-le-Bretonneux, France); (2) Prestige (Medtronic, Minneapolis, MN); (3) ProDisc-C (Synthes, Solothurn, Switzerland),

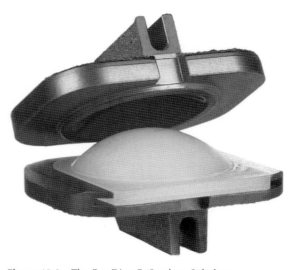

Figure 13.2 The Pro-Disc C (Synthes, Solothurn, Switzerland) prosthesis, a semiconstrained, ball-and-socket design. (Reproduced from Pracyk and Traynelis [2005], with permission from Wolters Kluwer Health)

which is the cervical disc version of the ProDisc (Synthes) lumbar prosthesis; (4) PCM prosthesis (Cervitech, Rockaway, NY); and (5) Bryan prosthesis (Medtronic). Constrained (Discoserv) and semiconstrained (Prestige, ProDisc-C, Discoserv) are ball-and-socket type designs (Figure 13.2) and allow minimal translation. The PCM is not described as ball-and-socket, but its appearance suggests otherwise, and it is reportedly minimally constrained (McAfee et al. 2003). The Bryan prosthesis is unconstrained. It is implanted as a single unit and has titanium endplates connected by a flexible polyethylene membrane that surrounds the polyurethane-filled nucleus (Figure 13.1; Pickett et al. 2005). A cohort study of patients receiving the Bryan prosthesis and patients with ACDF with plating found that the Bryan prosthesis was associated with a significantly lower incidence of adjacent site ossification 2 and 4 years after surgery (Garrito et al. 2011).

Regardless of the form of constraint, kinematic evaluation of each of the implants mentioned above suggest that they each closely mimic the range of motion of the intact, normal spinal segment. In a study comparing the ProDisc-C and Prestige prostheses, implantation of either prosthesis resulted in increased range of motion at the implanted site and decreased range of motion at adjacent sites (Chang et al. 2007b). This is actually the reverse of the changes that occur following ACDF. One may, therefore, suspect that adjacent sites would consequently be protected from degeneration. However, increased motion at the implanted site could have deleterious effects on the posterior (dorsal in the dog) compartment of the joint. For example, increased range of motion could results in synovial hypertrophy surrounding the articular facets. Additionally, one study reported that constrained implants result in a decrease in articular facet loading (Barrey et al. 2009), while another found the opposite (Chung et al. 2009). Variation in experimental methodologies has yielded opposing results and the long-term clinical implications of cervical TDA remain to be seen.

The PCM prosthesis is unique in that it is available with or without anterior screw fixation (Figure 13.3). In the study by McAfee et al. (2003), the authors concluded that screw fixation is indicated when removal of the posterior longitudinal ligament (PLL) is a necessary component of the surgery. They hypothesized that an intact PLL maintains the prosthesis within the disc space. PLL removal may be necessary when disc material is lodged within the spinal canal. The prosthesis without screw anchorage is described as low profile, with the advantage of minimizing the potential for mechanical irritation from the pres

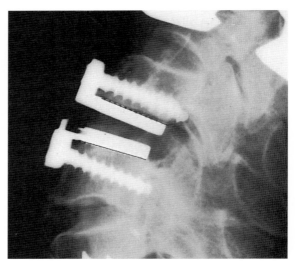

Figure 13.3   The PCM (Cervitech, Rockaway, NY) prosthesis with screw fixation for cases in which there is dissection of the posterior longitudinal ligament. Screw fixation prevents posterior migration. (Reproduced from McAfee et al. [2003], with permission from Wolters Kluwer Health)

ence of a portion of the implant anterior to the disc space. Other authors have not expressed concern regarding incision or thinning (using a high-speed bur) of the PLL in order to retrieve disc material from the spinal canal (Chang et al. 2007a).

Simulator testing, as well as prosthesis retrievals from 11 Bryan prostheses (of over 5500 implanted) and 3 Prestige prostheses (of over 300 implanted) suggest wear characteristics that would support a 40-year fatigue life of the implants (Anderson et al. 2004). The wear predicted by simulator testing was 5–10 times greater than the wear seen in retrieved specimens and the surrounding soft tissues did not demonstrate the inflammatory response typically seen surrounding failed diarthrodial joints.

Several complications of TDA have been reported. These complications include, but are not limited to, ankylosis of adjacent vertebrae, lordosis, kyphosis, heterotopic ossification (HO), facet pain, expansion of osteophytes, implant loosening, and implant migration.

Fibrosis, as well as ligamentous and synovial hypertrophy, can result in loss of range of motion over time. This can occur as a consequence of excessive range of motion (i.e., instability) or increased articular facet loading (Barrey et al. 2009; Chung et al. 2009). Facet loading may be increased by the position of the implant within the disc space. In people, the center of rotation of the spinal segment is located in the posterior half of the disc space, although, due to translation, it is not fixed. Additionally, the center of rotation is less posterior in the more distal cervical vertebral segments (Pickett et al. 2005). If the center of motion of the prosthesis is in the anterior portion of the disc space, facet loads will be increased (Dooris et al. 2001; Chung et al. 2009).

Implant sizing must be appropriate for maintenance of range of motion, independent of implant design. An undersized implant can result in instability with secondary fibrosis and capsular and ligamentous hypertrophy, ultimately resulting in a decrease in the range of motion at the surgical site (Buchowski et al. 2009; Roberto et al. 2010). An oversized implant causes a diminished range of motion and increases stress at adjacent disc sites. Unfortunately, oversizing of implants is occasionally utilized by surgeons in order to improve foraminal decompression (Roberto et al. 2010).

Osteophytes reportedly atrophy following ACDF, but can grow following cervical disc arthroplasty (Roberto et al. 2010). Growth of osteophytes may be a response to increased range of motion or instability. Development of foraminal osteophytes may result in recurrence of radiculopathy and the need for additional surgery. Roberto et al. found that there was no significant increase in instability following progressive foraminotomies and PLL resection in prosthesis-implanted cadavers. They concluded that the PLL could be safely resected and bilateral foraminotomies performed in cases of recurrent radiculopathy following TDA.

In addition to implant design and placement, the implantation procedure must minimize the risk of future ankylosis as well as loss of disc space width (subsidence). The risk of ankylosis is minimized by maintenance of normal range of motion. When implantation of the prosthesis leaves exposed subchondral bone at the endplates, the disc space may be prone to ankylosis (Buchowski et al. 2009). Subchondral bone exposure may occur when the uncinate process (not present in dogs) needs to be removed to provide foraminal

decompression in people. Subchondral bone exposure may also occur as a result of excessive bone removal at the endplate.

Lordosis can occur at the surgical site as a result of incomplete seating of the implant. Incomplete seating can be a consequence of surgical error or from partial ankylosis, which does not allow complete seating. Conversely, segmental kyphosis can develop following TDA and can be associated with prosthesis migration (Gwynedd et al. 2006). A finite element analysis (FEA) model of TDA predicted that the altered stresses produced by various implants, as well as the elastic modulus mismatch between the vertebral endplate and the prosthesis, will result in vertebral body destruction with subsequent subsidence and loosening of the prosthesis (Chung et al. 2009). While the prediction of the FEA study is supported by a few case reports, subsidence and loosening appear to be uncommon (van Ooij et al. 2003).

Articular facet pain has been reported as a consequence of malposition of ball-and-socket types of prosthesis. This is a consequence of asymmetrical loading (Pickett et al. 2005).

HO is one of the more commonly reported complications following TDA. However, while some reports consider this to be of minimal clinical significance (Tu et al. 2011), others report the development of ankylosis as a consequence of the presence of HO (Gwynedd et al. 2006). In the study that found no clinical implication for the development of HO, the incidence of HO was found to be 48%, based on computed tomography (CT) scan findings (Tu et al. 2011). The pathogenesis of HO is unclear. It appears to be prevented by nonsteroidal anti-inflammatory drug (NSAID) use and possibly by the intraoperative application of bone wax (Gwynedd et al. 2006; Barbagallo et al. 2010; Tu et al. 2011). The location of HO is generally at the anterolateral surface of the vertebral bodies (Barbagallo et al. 2010).

Findings from several studies suggest that short-term and long-term (>2 years) outcomes are similar for TDA and ACDF (Bertagnoli et al. 2005a; Buchowski et al. 2009; Roberto et al. 2010). TDA will have a significant advantage over ACDF if future studies corroborate the lower incidence of adjacent site degeneration shown in the study that evaluated the Bryan prosthesis.

Disc arthroplasty in small animals

The primary indication for TDA in veterinary patients would likely be disc-associated Wobbler's syndrome and, possibly, dorsal longitudinal ligament hypertrophy.

Hofstetter et al. (2009) evaluated range of motion of the canine C4–C5 cervical spine segment. The mean range of motion was roughly 8, 7, and 1 degrees for flexion/extension, lateral bending, and axial rotation, respectively. Interestingly, Hofstetter et al. found that coupled motion for lateral bending (primary motion of axial rotation) was 172% of the primary motion and coupled motion for axial rotation (primary motion of lateral bending) was 356% of the primary motion and no coupled motion with flexion/extension. This suggests that dogs have a much greater coupled motion than humans. However, the authors of the canine study acknowledged that variation measurement methods for their study, compared with the human study, may have substantially altered the results. Additional evaluation of coupled motion in the canine cervical spine is warranted. The NZ for the canine cervical spine, as evaluated by Hofstetter et al., was 1.4, 0.7, and 1.3 degrees for flexion/extension, lateral bending, and axial rotation, respectively.

When designing an implant for the canine spine, one must also consider morphological differences compared with humans. The morphological differences at least partially explain differences in range of motion. Hofstetter et al. found that larger dogs had relatively wider disc spaces than smaller dogs and that the ventrodorsal width of the cranial endplate, disc thickness, and horizontal width of the caudal endplate had a negative correlation with range of motion in flexion/extension. Additionally, dogs have proportionally smaller endplates than humans, allowing greater range of motion (Breit and Kunzel 2002).

Three-dimensional motion and morphometry of the canine lumbar spine, from L4 through S1, has also been evaluated (Benninger et al. 2006). However, the intent of that study was not an investigation into the feasibility of lumbar or lumbosacral disc replacement. Rather, the intent was to evaluate the dog as a model for degenerative disc disease in people. Range of motion was not evaluated as described above for the cervical spine, and additional studies are necessary for use in the development of designs of lumbar or lumbosacral disc prostheses for dogs.

An *in vitro* pilot study for the first TDA for veterinary use was published recently (Adamo et al. 2007). The prosthesis is a stainless steel, metal-on-metal ball-and-socket design. It is semiconstrained (unconstrained in rotation) and allows 30 degrees of motion in flexion/extension, as well as in lateral bending. This range is substantially greater than the range reported for the intact canine cervical spine (Hofstetter et al. 2009). In this study, the range of motion of the TDA implanted site and adjacent sites was compared with ventral slot, as well as pins and polymethylmethacrylate (PMMA). While the disc replacement prosthesis was more similar to intact spine than either ventral slot or pins and PMMA, there was decreased range of motion in flexion/extension and in lateral bending compared with the intact spine at the implanted site. Torsional range of motion was similar to the intact spine. There was a decrease in the range of motion at the disc space caudal to the implanted site. The study did not evaluate coupled motion.

If the development of TDA prostheses yields protection against adjacent site degeneration in dogs with disc-associated Wobbler's syndrome, a veterinary market for such prostheses likely exists. The prosthesis developed by Adamo (2011) has been implanted in two clinical cases (Figure 13.4).

Clinical signs of myelopathy and nerve root compression resolved following surgery. However, vertebral segment range of motion was not preserved on one case and was preserved only temporarily in the other case. Therefore, although clinical signs of adjacent site disease did not occur in these two cases during the study, this TDA cannot be considered as an effective means to prevent adjacent site degeneration. It appears that the prosthesis had an effect similar to an interbody methylmethacrylate plug. As can be expected, additional studies are necessary to optimize implants and techniques and to evaluate the safety and efficacy of TDA prostheses for veterinary use.

Shoulder arthroplasty

Total shoulder arthroplasty (TSA) was first performed by Péan in 1893, 25 years before the first

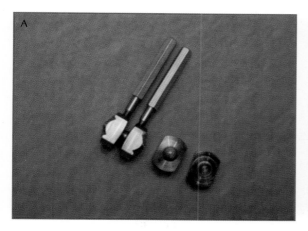

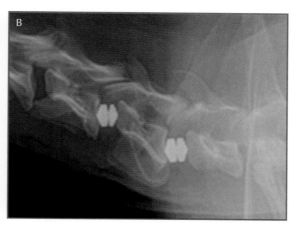

Figure 13.4 (A) The canine cervical disc prosthesis. (B) Mediolateral radiograph of two-level implantation of the canine cervical disc prosthesis. (Adamo artificial disc prosthesis [Patent #US2008/0306597])

reported total hip arthroplasty (Wirth and Rockwood 1996). However, widespread clinical application of TSA, using commercial implants began in the 1970s.

Indications for implantation of TSA, or hemiarthroplasty, include shoulder disability secondary to rotator cuff arthropathy, primary osteoarthritis, traumatic osteoarthritis, rheumatoid arthritis, and tumor resection (Wirth and Rockwood 1996; Hasan et al. 2002; Fox et al. 2009).

Since TSA was initially performed primarily for shoulder instability secondary to rotator cuff insufficiency, prostheses aimed to provide a maximally stable joint. This was achieved with various forms of constrained prostheses (Wirth and Rockwood 1996). Implant developers felt that a fully constrained prosthesis was necessary due to the ineffective rotator cuff and kinematic studies were not utilized in prosthesis development. This resulted in a nonanatomical prosthesis. The constrained implants were fixed-fulcrum or semifulcrum concentric ball-and-socket components. Fixed-fulcrum resulted in maximal constraint with coupling of humeral and scapular motion, whereas semifulcrum designs more closely mimic typical THA components. Constraint was likely the cause of most of the complications with early prostheses. Constrained prostheses met with limited success, with reported complication rates of 100% and revision rates of up to 54% in case series with the longest follow-up (Wirth and Rockwood 1996). The top three factors associated

with complications with constrained prostheses were mechanical loosening, instability, and implant failure. Post et al. published reports based on the same patient cohort in both 1979 and 1983 and reported implant failure rates of 33% and 48%, respectively. (Post et al. 1979; Post and Jablon 1983) Clearly, longer follow-up led to higher failure rates. With the exception of a few forms of salvage procedures, constrained TSA prostheses have, for the most part, been abandoned.

Based on the unacceptably high failure rates of constrained prostheses, kinematic studies were performed in an attempt to improve prosthetic design. It was determined that semiconstrained prostheses would result in less shear stress on the implants, the glenoid component in particular, and improve prosthesis survival (Wirth and Rockwood 1996). Additionally, one surprising finding was that shoulder joint reaction forces approximate body weight when elevating the arm above the level of the shoulder (Wirth et al. 2001).

Unconstrained prostheses have had greater success than constrained prostheses. In unconstrained prostheses, mismatch between the diameter of the humeral head and the diameter of the glenoid fossa allows glenohumeral translation and, therefore, unconstrained motion. The Neer prosthesis, and its subsequent generations, are the most commonly encountered in the human literature (Brenner et al. 1989; Sperling et al. 2004; Fox et al. 2009). However, the complication rate remains relatively high and several aspects of their design are continuing to evolve, particularly for the glenoid component. The largest systematic review of the TSA literature included 41 case series from 1975 to 1993 (Wirth and Rockwood 1996). The complications associated with unconstrained prostheses, in decreasing order of frequency, were component loosening (nearly always the glenoid component), glenohumeral instability, rotator cuff tear, periprosthetic fracture, infection, implant failure, and deltoid dysfunction. Recent advances have led some authors to comment that complication rates are clearly decreasing and, with recent changes in prosthesis design, the types of complications have changed. A 2006 study (Chin et al. 2006) did not include glenoid component loosening in the top three complications seen and listed an overall major complication rate of 7.4%.

Lucency surrounding the glenoid component has been reported in up to 90% of cases (Neer et al. 1982; Wirth and Rockwood 1996; Wirth et al. 2001; Groh 2010; Figure 13.5); however, Neer, who developed the prosthesis, reported that this finding is rarely of clinical significance (Neer et al. 1982). Others have found that the lucency was frequently associated with diminished function and pain (Hasan et al. 2002). In two case series that included the same cases at different time points,

first at 2–6 years follow-up, then again at an average of 12 years after surgery, lucency was seen, but was not clinical, in 84% of cases at 4 years. At the later follow-up, 44% of cases had definite loosening, including shifting of the glenoid component (Cofield 1984; Torchia et al. 1997).

Virtually all TSA components have a metallic humeral head that articulates with a polyethylene glenoid surface. The glenoid component can be metal backed or all polyethylene (Chin et al. 2006; Pelletier et al. 2008; Fox et al. 2009). Both cemented and press-fit components have been described for both the humerus and the glenoid.

Since the greatest source of complications with TSA, including both constrained and unconstrained prostheses, is glenoid component loosening (Wirth and Rockwood 1996; Chin et al. 2006; Fox et al. 2009), much attention has been given to developing and comparing complication rates between different forms of glenoid prostheses. Three glenoid considerations have been given the most attention: keeled versus peg anchorage, metal backed versus all polyethylene, and cemented versus cementless (Figure 13.5).

Beginning with the Neer I total shoulder replacement, keeled glenoid designs have been the standard. Both cemented and press-fit designs have

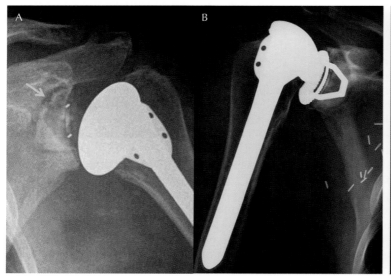
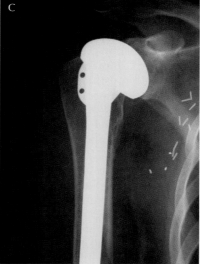

Figure 13.5   (A) Loosening of a keeled glenoid prosthesis. Note the lucent line surrounding the glenoid component (arrow). (Reproduced from Gartsman et al. [2005], with permission from Elsevier) (B and C) Conversion of a loose glenoid component to a hemiarthroplasty. (Reproduced from Sperling et al. [2007], with permission from Elsevier)

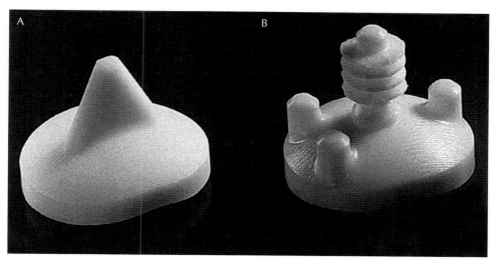

Figure 13.6   Keeled (A) and peg (B) glenoid components used in a canine study. While the peg implant is described as cementless, the peripheral, smooth pegs are cemented. (Reproduced from Wirth et al. [2001], with permission from Elsevier)

been utilized. More recently, designs have included a central peg, either press-fit or cemented, with two or three peripheral stabilizing pegs (Wirth et al. 2001; Groh 2010; Figure 13.6). In a study using a weight-bearing, canine model, an uncemented peg prosthesis was compared with a cemented, keeled prosthesis (Wirth et al. 2001). The central peg of the peg prosthesis had circumferential fins or flanges, providing space for bone ingrowth for long-term stability. Although the peg prosthesis was referred to as uncemented, the three peripheral pegs, but not the central peg, were cemented. The peripheral pegs were shorter and did not have flanges. Twenty-eight dogs were included in this study, half assigned to the keeled group, half to the peg. Half of the dogs in each group were sacrificed at 3 months and half at 6 months. After euthanasia, an implant was placed in the opposite shoulder to allow a time 0 evaluation. The mean initial pullout strengths were $165.5 \pm 84\,N$ for keeled implants and $102.7 \pm 33\,N$ for pegged implants. From time 0 to 6 months, the pullout strength of keeled implants decreased by more than 90%, while the pullout strength of pegged implants increased by over 300%. Failure of keeled implants occurred at the cement–keel interface and failure of pegged implants was at the peg–glenoid interface (i.e., failure of the implant rather than failure of fixation). Radiographically

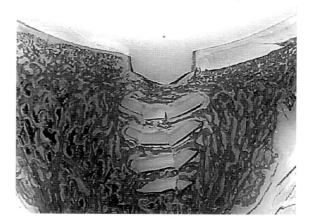

Figure 13.7   Histological appearance of bone ingrowth into the central, fluted peg of the glenoid prosthesis from Figure 13.6. (Reproduced from Wirth et al. [2001], with permission from Elsevier)

and histologically, bony ingrowth was evident between flanges in the peg design and lucent lines were seen at 3 and 6 months in the keeled design (Figure 13.7).

In a study using a similar design to the canine model above, no periprosthetic lucency was evident at 2-year radiographic follow-up in a series of 83 TSAs (Groh 2010). Based on the studies performed to date, it appears that pegged glenoid prostheses have less radiolucency than keeled designs. However, follow-up time available for the newer pegged prostheses is more limited and long-term follow-up is necessary before a clear determination of superiority can be made (Gartsman et al. 2005).

Glenoid prostheses that are all polyethylene result in greater load transfer to trabecular bone, whereas metal-backed prostheses have greater load transfer to cortical bone (Boileau et al. 2002; Pelletier et al. 2008). It is unknown which form of load transfer is more physiological or longer lasting; however, in studies comparing survival of metal-backed glenoid prostheses with that of all-polyethylene glenoid prostheses, the all-polyethylene components fare consistently better. Unfortunately, there is inconsistency in metal-backed versus all-polyethylene comparisons. For example, one study compared an uncemented, keeled, metal-backed component with a cemented, pegged component (Pelletier et al. 2008). Certainly, in that study, it is difficult to distinguish the effect of cemented versus cementless, keeled versus pegged, and metal backed versus all polyethylene. Fox et al. reported that metal-backed glenoid prostheses have a significantly higher failure rate than all-polyethylene designs (Fox et al. 2009). The all-polyethylene designs evaluated in this study were cemented. The authors described three reasons for this increased complication rate with metal-backed glenoid components: (1) increased generation of wear debris (both metallic and polyethylene); (2) increased incidence of component loosening, likely secondary to the increase in wear debris, as well as increased polyethylene stress in a metal-backed prosthesis; and (3) higher incidence of glenohumeral instability associated with asymmetrical polyethylene wear, as well as development of Bankart-like lesions (Fox et al. 2009). Bankart lesions are labral tears of the glenoid that are associated with trauma and cause instability. Additional risk factors for glenoid component loosening identified in the Fox study included TSA for avascular necrosis or for posttraumatic arthritis, as well as being a male.

Although cemented and uncemented glenoid, as well as humeral, prostheses have been described, and are in clinical use, there has not been a clear comparison made between similar glenoid implant designs used in both cemented and uncemented fashion. A recent study compared cemented versus uncemented humeral prostheses for TSA. The randomized, prospective, double-blinded study found that cemented humeral implants resulted in better function, comfort, and strength over a 2-year follow-up period (Litchfield et al. 2011).

Several other modifications and surgical techniques have been implemented in order to increase survival of the glenoid component. Mismatch of the diameter of the glenoid and the humeral head, with a greater radius of curvature for the glenoid, decreases glenoid rim contact with the humeral head during translation. The decreased contact decreases loading of the glenoid rim and, consequently, decreases polyethylene deformation and subsequent loosening. Preservation of the subchondral bone of the glenoid has also led to improved glenoid component fixation and diminished subsidence (Wirth et al. 2001). The use of concentric reaming techniques, improved bone ingrowth materials, and plasma spraying of prostheses have also been described as methods to improve fixation of the glenoid component (Cofield and Daly 1992; Wirth et al. 2001).

Glenohumeral instability is the second most common complication of TSA, with a reported incidence of 29%. The normal passive constraints that aid in shoulder stability are disrupted by TSA. The passive constraints include the architecture of the joint surface, fixed joint volume, and the adhesive/cohesive properties of the joint fluid (Wirth and Rockwood 1995, 1996; Sidaway et al. 2004). The deltoid muscles and the rotator cuff, as well as the joint capsule and bony architecture, which balance moderate and large loads, respectively, are also disrupted by TSA. Glenohumeral instability can be described in four different directions: anterior, posterior, superior, or inferior. Anterior instability is typically the result of poor surgical technique and complete luxation cannot occur without a torn subscapularis tendon. Subscapularis tendon tears can result for poor suturing technique or use of oversized implants that stress the subscapularis suture line (Wirth and Rockwood 1996; Wirth et al. 2001). Poor implant positioning, specifically decreased retroversion of the humeral head, can also lead to anterior instability. Superior (proximal) instability is typically a consequence of the combination of a strong deltoid muscle and a weak rotator cuff. Superior instability may not be associated with pain, but often leads to eccentric glenoid loading and subsequent glenoid loosening (Collins et al. 1992). Posterior instability is less frequently reported, but can be a consequence of excessive (>20 degrees) retroversion of the glenoid component or excessive retroversion (>45 degrees) of the humeral component (Brewer et al. 1986). Posterior instability can also result from posterior glenoid erosion, which can lead the surgeon to place the glenoid component in excessive retroversion. Bone graft of the posterior glenoid has been recommended in cases of severe posterior glenoid erosion (Neer and Morrison 1988). Inferior instability is usually a complication associated with the use of TSA for the treatment of proximal humeral fractures or rheumatoid arthritis. These conditions can result in collapse or shortening of the proximal humerus and cause a decrease in resting deltoid and rotator cuff tension (Wirth and Rockwood 1996).

Rotator cuff tears are the third most common complication of TSA, comprising approximately 2% of TSA cases. Unfortunately, revision is typically of limited benefit and recurrence of tears is likely (Wall et al. 2007). Salvage revisions for cases with rotator cuff tears include reverse arthroplasty, to be discussed later.

Periprosthetic fractures, including intraoperative and postoperative fractures, are the fourth most common TSA complication. However, one case series found them to be the most common complication (Chin et al. 2006). Most fractures are of the humerus and occur at the time of surgery. They are often secondary to intraoperative errors, such as reaming errors, aggressive impaction, and manipulation of the upper extremity during exposure of the glenoid (Wirth and Rockwood 1996; Chin et al. 2006). When postoperative fractures occur, they are most common in older patients with osteoporotic or osteopenic bone or rheumatoid arthritis. Open reduction and stabilization is typically required (Groh et al. 2008).

Infection rates with TSA are similar to other joint arthroplasties, at a reported rate of 0.5%–3.9% (Fox et al. 2009). The risk of infection is increased in patients with diabetes mellitus, rheumatoid arthritis, systemic lupus erythematosus, distant infection, and patients using immunosuppressive drugs. The most common management choice after infection is resection arthroplasty (Wirth and Rockwood 1996).

Nerve injury is another reported complication of TSA. This typically involves neurapraxia of the axillary nerve, but can also affect the median, ulnar, and musculocutaneous nerves, as well as generalized brachial plexus injury. The neurapraxia is typically self-limiting (Wirth and Rockwood 1996). Interestingly, suprascapular nerve injury was not described. Axillary nerve injury can cause deltoid muscle dysfunction, which can lead to glenohumeral instability.

Complications related to implant failure are infrequent, but several are described. These include displacement of the polyethylene insert from the glenoid tray, fracture of the glenoid keel, screw fracture (for glenoid with screw fixation), and disassociation of a modular humeral component at the Morse taper (Woolson and Pottorff 1990; Wirth and Rockwood 1996).

Hemiarthroplasty with a humeral component, but no glenoid prosthesis, is commonly used in patients with proximal humeral fractures and a normal glenoid (Matsen et al. 2005). Hemiarthroplasty has also been utilized in an attempt to avoid complications associated with glenoid prosthesis loosening, as well as a salvage or revision procedure in cases with a failed glenoid component (Figure 13.5; Wirth and Rockwood 1996; Sperling et al. 2004, 2007; Matsen et al. 2005). Findings from studies comparing outcomes of TSA versus hemiarthroplasty have varied. Studies have not noted significant differences in pain relief or range of motion (Hasan et al. 2002; Sperling et al. 2007). While several reports have described higher revision rates and higher unsatisfactory outcome rates with hemiarthroplasty than with TSA, the differences have not usually been statistically significant. One study did find an increased incidence of radiolucency surrounding the humeral component in the TSA group, compared with the hemiarthroplasty group. The same study concluded, however, that TSA was a better choice than hemiarthroplasty for patients under 50 years of age (Sperling et al. 2004). The most common complications reported with hemiarthroplasty are posterior glenoid erosion and painful glenoid arthrosis (Hasan et al. 2002; Sperling et al. 2004, 2007; Matsen et al. 2005).

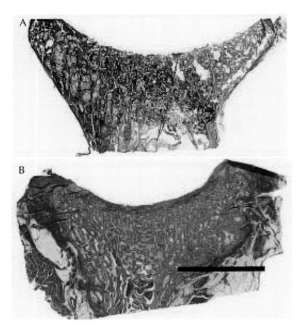

Figure 13.8   Hemiarthroplasty with concentric reaming of the canine glenoid at time 0 (A) and 24 weeks (B). Note the smooth, concave, fibrous tissue lined cavity at 24 weeks. Bar: 10 mm. (Reproduced from Matsen et al. [2005], with permission from Wiley-Blackwell)

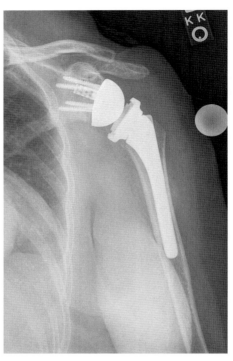

Figure 13.9   Reverse total shoulder arthroplasty. Note that the hemispherical component is on the scapular side, rather than the humeral side. Reverse TSA is performed primarily in rotator cuff-deficient shoulders. (Radiograph courtesy of Jewett Orthopedic Clinic, Winter Park, FL)

Since posterior glenoid erosion is a major factor in either failure or unsatisfactory outcomes with hemiarthroplasty, Matsen et al. performed a hemiarthroplasty study using concentric reaming in a canine model (Matsen et al. 2005). The authors hypothesized that concentric, spherical reaming would result in improved load transfer and improved stability of the glenohumeral articulation. The study included 12 dogs with a mean body weight of approximately 50 lb. Based on radiographic and histological evaluation at 10 weeks (six dogs) and 24 weeks (six dogs), the authors concluded that concentric, spherical glenoid reaming resulted in consistent healing of the glenoid, lines with living fibrocartilage with a congruent curvature that matched the prosthetic humeral head (Figure 13.8).

Reverse TSA was first described by Grammont in 1987 and utilizes a polyethylene humeral cup with a cemented or uncemented stem, and a metallic, hemispherical glenoid component (Wall et al. 2007). Reverse TSA is typically a more constrained, full-hinge type of prosthesis, which

maximizes stability but limits function; however, recent modifications allow for more degrees of freedom of motion (Figure 13.9). The reverse TSA has primarily been used for cases with rotator cuff arthropathy, but has also been used for revisions and following tumor resections, as well as cases where glenoid deformity precludes anchorage of a keeled or peg component. In general, the reverse TSA is used in patients with the expectation of "limited goals rehabilitation" (Wall et al. 2007). The best results, considering the limited expectations, are seen in patients with rotator cuff tears; however, the revision rate is fairly high (20%–70%) and appears to depend on case selection.

Arthroplasty of the shoulder in small animals

The two studies utilizing canine models, discussed earlier in this section, provide useful information for the future development of a canine TSA or hemiarthroplasty procedure/prosthesis. Both the TSA and the hemiarthroplasty studies utilized a lateral approach and required an osteotomy of the greater tubercle. The TSA study also incorporated an osteotomy of the lesser tubercle, as pilot studies indicated that primary repair of a subscapularis tenotomy consistently failed (Wirth et al. 2001). Osteotomies were repaired using either Kirschner wires and a figure-of-eight tension band, or with Dacron suture. The subscapularis insertion was protected in the hemiarthroplasty study and, therefore, did not require tenotomy (Matsen et al. 2005). In the TSA study, the authors found it imperative to avoid disruption of the biceps tendon for postoperative stability; however, in the hemiarthroplasty study, the biceps was freed from the intertubercular groove by transection of the transverse humeral ligament that was repaired at the conclusion of surgery. In a study by Sidaway et al., the authors found that the canine biceps tendon contributes to passive shoulder stability, especially in neutral and flexed positions, and contributes to medial stability during shoulder flexion. The Sidaway study also found that complete luxation of the canine shoulder will not occur without transection of the medial glenohumeral ligament (Sidaway et al. 2004). In neither arthroplasty study was the tendon of origin of the biceps disrupted. Each of the studies placed subjects in a Velpeau sling for 1–2 weeks after surgery. The reader is encouraged to refer to each of the canine shoulder arthroplasty studies for a detailed description of the surgical approach and procedure.

Each of the studies using canine models utilized medium- to large-breed dogs and implant dimensions were taken from measurements on cadavers. For the TSA study, the dimensions of the articulating component of the glenoid prosthesis were the same for both the keeled and peg implants. The glenoid was oval, with dimensions of 20.3 mm × 22.9 mm, a radius of curvature of 14.5 mm, and a thickness of 2.5 mm. For the peg implant, the central peg length was 12.6 mm, with a core diameter of 3.6 mm and four circumferential fins having an outside diameter of 7.6 mm and a thickness of 0.6 mm. Each of the fins was 1.3 mm apart. The three peripheral pegs were each 5.6 mm long and had diameters of 3.9 mm. The keeled component had a keel that was 3 mm thick and

9.9 mm long, with a 13.1-mm base (Wirth et al. 2001).

In the canine hemiarthroplasty study, following its curettage, the glenoid was reamed with a 15-mm hemispherical reamer and extended through the subchondral plate. The metallic humeral head had a 14-mm radius of curvature and the stem was press-fit; however, stem loosening was common, although not specifically evaluated, and stem design was not described (Matsen et al. 2005).

Arthroplasty of the carpus

The first attempt at total wrist arthroplasty (TWA) was performed by Gluck in Berlin in 1890 and utilized an ivory prosthesis. The outcome was unsuccessful and TWA did not begin to gain acceptance until Swanson introduced a silicone prosthesis in 1967 (Taljanovic et al. 2003; Cavaliere and Chung 2008a; Gupta 2008).

The most common indication for TWA is rheumatoid arthritis (Taljanovic et al. 2003). However, some authors believe that, as advances in prostheses are seen, TWA, rather than arthrodesis or partial arthrodesis, will be used in more posttraumatic arthritis (Gupta 2008). Several studies have compared outcomes between TWA and arthrodesis (Palmer et al. 1985; Taljanovic et al. 2003; Cavaliere and Chung 2008a,b, 2010). While TWA generally offers improved function, revision, residual pain, and complication rates are higher with TWA than with arthrodesis. Maintenance of range of motion is an important potential advantage of TWA over arthrodesis. Reported angles for functional range of motion are inconsistent; however, angles reported by Palmer et al. (1985) are commonly referenced. Palmer reported functional angles as follows: 5 degrees flexion, 30 degrees extension, 10 degrees radial deviation (i.e., varus motion), and 10 degrees ulnar deviation (i.e., valgus motion). By comparison, with straight extension considered as 180 degrees, normal carpal extension and flexion angles of dogs at a walk have been recently reported between 200 and 239 degrees and 128 and 130 degrees, respectively (Feeney et al. 2007; Holler et al. 2010).

There are several contraindications for TWA. These include sensory or motor neurological dysfunction, infection, poor bone quality, chronic or severe volar (palmar) and ulnar subluxation, and probably the most relevant contraindication with regard to a possible veterinary prosthesis, the need for weight bearing across the joint. In people, weight bearing would be necessary in patients that utilize a cane or a walker (Taljanovic et al. 2003).

The silicone Swanson prosthesis, developed in 1967, was a double-stemmed, flexible hinge that was ultimately stabilized by scar tissue. It had a very high complication rate, with silicone disintegration and an associated inflammatory response. In the 1970s, ball-and-socket prostheses were introduced. These prostheses were meant to be unconstrained, but impingement rendered them functionally constrained (Taljanovic et al. 2003). Modifications of the ball-and-socket led to the development of semiconstrained prostheses with ellipsoid articulating surfaces and range of motion similar to the normal wrist. However, loosening of the distal (i.e., carpal) component remained a significant problem. The Swanson prosthesis, as well as the ball-and-socket prostheses, was progressively abandoned due to high failure rates. However, forms of the silicone prostheses are used, to some extent, in interphalangeal joints.

In the 1980s and 1990s the Biaxial (DePuy, Warsaw, IN; Figure 13.10) and Universal prostheses (Integra Lifesciences, Plainsboro, NJ; Figure 13.11) were developed, respectively.

These are the prostheses most currently in use that have a body of literature describing outcomes. Both of these prostheses are cobalt-chromium alloys. The Biaxial TWA is an unconstrained prosthesis with a rounded articular face and the radial component of the prosthesis was shifted to a more volar (palmar) position to diminish impingement seen with other prostheses. The polyethylene surface is on the radial side (Cobb and Beckenbaugh 1996). In a study with a mean follow-up time of 52 months, there was a 26% clinical failure rate. Functional range of motion was achieved in fewer than 50% of patients; however, this has much to do with the preexisting severity of bone destruction (Takwale et al. 2002). Additionally, many patients with a range of motion below what is considered functional still feel that the range of

motion that is preserved is of value for quality of life. This may be an important consideration in the design of a veterinary prosthesis. The Biaxial implants can be used as press-fit or cemented, but a higher failure rate has been seen in patients with severe bone loss receiving uncemented prostheses, including patients with advanced rheumatoid arthritis. In 2008, one author commented that the Biaxial prosthesis was discontinued (Gupta 2008); however, the DePuy website still lists the prosthesis at the time of this writing.

The Universal 2 TWA (Integra Lifesciences) differs from the Biaxial prosthesis in that the polyethylene is on the carpal side. The articulating surfaces are ellipsoid. The carpal component is stabilized using a cemented central peg in the scaphoid and two peripheral screws. Luxation is the most common complication with the Universal 2 prosthesis (Menon 1998).

Two additional TWA prostheses are now available: Maestro (Biomet, Warsaw, IN) and ReMotion (Small Bone Innovations, Morrisville, PA). Both have limited or no published follow-up. However, the ReMotion has an interesting modification. The polyethylene, which is on the carpal component, can pivot approximately 10 degrees in either direction on the carpal plate. This is meant to diminish torque transmission to the carpal component and is somewhat similar to the "mobile bearing" type of implant discussed in the "Total Ankle Arthroplasty" section. It will be important to monitor the development of wear debris on long-term follow-up. In one case series, authored by the inventor of the prosthesis, no significant complications were reported (Gupta 2008). In another, however, 4 out of 20 wrists had a fair or poor outcome (Herzberg 2011). In one study (Cavaliere and Chung 2008a), third-generation TWA prostheses had no better rate of satisfactory results than first-generation prostheses. To date, the superiority of TWA over arthrodesis has not been established and arthrodesis remains much more broadly accepted than TWA.

Arthroplasty of the carpus for small animals

It has been recommended that a TWA should be able to withstand a load of 200 N during daily activities (Youm and Flatt 1984). However, it is not

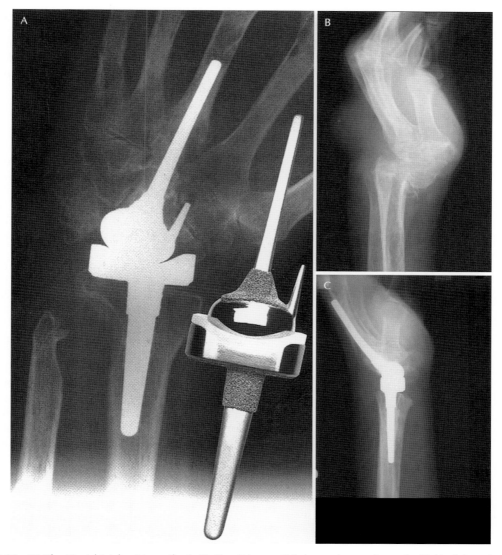

Figure 13.10   (A) The Biaxial total wrist prosthesis (DePuy, Warsaw, IN) dorsopalmar radiograph. (B) Mediolateral radiograph of a patient with rheumatoid arthritis affecting the wrist. (C) Mediolateral radiograph of the Biaxial total wrist prosthesis. (Reproduced from Rizzo and Beckenbaugh [2003], with permission from Elsevier)

clear from which direction the load is to be applied. In most recent veterinary reports, the ground reaction forces of a limb using force plate or pressure-sensitive walkway analysis are expressed, in a normalized fashion, as a percent of body weight (Lascelles et al. 2006; Voss et al. 2010). However, in one study, for a group of dogs with a mean body weight of 40 kg, the mean peak vertical force (PVF) at a trot for the forelimb was 437 N (Voss et al. 2010). Another study found PVF of the forelimb, at a trot, to be between 105% and 115% of body weight (Lascelles et al. 2006). Certainly, these parameters, in addition to the joint angles through which the force is applied, must be considered in the design of a prosthesis for veterinary use.

In addition to range of motion and the load requirements of TWA prostheses, intact triangular fibrocartilage (i.e., palmar fibrocartilage) is

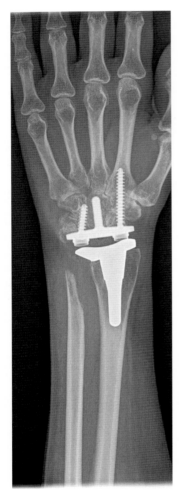

Figure 13.11   The Universal total wrist arthroplasty. (Radiograph courtesy of Jewett Orthopedic Clinic, Winter Park, FL)

necessary for support in patients with TWA (Gupta 2008). The palmar fibrocartilage is typically damaged or nonfunctional in veterinary patients with carpal hyperextension injury.

The most common veterinary indications for a TWA are likely to be hyperextension injury, comminuted articular fractures, erosive arthritis/polyarthritis, and limb sparing. Unfortunately, weight bearing across the joint is critical for veterinary patients and current design rationale for human TWA prostheses will need to be substantially altered for a veterinary prosthesis. Regardless, an overview of the progression and

development of designs for human TWA prostheses is of value.

There are no published reports of the use of small animals as a model for TWA. There are also no reports of a custom TWA used in companion animals.

Total ankle arthroplasty

Total ankle arthroplasty (TAA) has been performed since the 1970s. Early prostheses were cemented and highly constrained and suffered failure rates in excess of 70% (Kitaoka et al. 1994; Gougoulias et al. 2009). This history is similar to that described for both shoulder and wrist arthroplasties above.

The most common indications for TAA are posttraumatic arthritis and inflammatory (e.g., rheumatoid) arthritis (Gougoulias et al. 2009, 2010). As with TWA, substantial controversy exists regarding the advantages and disadvantages of TAA versus arthrodesis. The loss of tibiotalar motion with arthrodesis is associated with development of adjacent joint arthritis, specifically, stifle arthritis and subtalar (intertarsal) arthritis (Gougoulias et al. 2009; Saltzman et al. 2009; Krause et al. 2011). Prevention of adjacent joint arthritis is one of the primary justifications for TAA. Successful TAA should result in normal or near normal kinematics of the hip and knee (Doets et al. 2007). However, restoration of normal tarsal range of motion is not an expectation with TAA. In fact, the goal is to preserve, or slightly improve, existing range of motion. Various studies report an improvement in the dorsoplantar range of motion of 4–14 degrees (Hvid et al. 1985). An overall dorsoplantar range of motion of 23–27 degrees is considered adequate for walking. In patients with chronic restriction of motion, lengthening of the Achilles tendon may be necessary to permit an adequate range of motion (Wood and Deakin 2003).

In addition to arthritis of adjacent joints, nonunion, persistent pain, wound complications, and malalignment are common complications following arthrodesis (Gougoulias et al. 2009; Saltzman et al. 2009; Krause et al. 2011). A systematic review comparing outcomes with arthrodesis with outcomes with TAA reported revision rates of 9% and 7%, respectively, and fair to poor outcomes in 26%

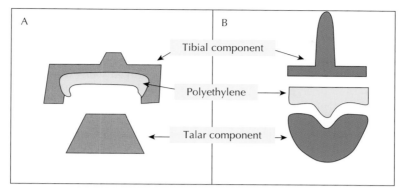

Figure 13.12   Schematic rendering of two-component (A) and three-component (B) ankle replacements. Note that the polyethylene component in panel B is independent of both the tibial and talar components.

and 29%, respectively (Haddad et al. 2007). Most arthrodesis revisions were for nonunion. Despite a higher complication rate, patient satisfaction has reportedly been higher after TAA than after arthrodesis.

Absolute contraindications for TAA include acute and chronic infection, neurological deficits, severe angular deformities, Charcot's arthropathy (joint changes secondary to loss of sensation), and avascular necrosis of the talus (Gougoulias et al. 2009). There have been a few case reports of talus replacement combined with TAA in patients with talar destruction or avascular necrosis of the talus (Tsukamoto et al. 2010); therefore, avascular necrosis of the talus may be a relative contraindication.

Relative contraindications for TAA, based on reported outcomes to date, are younger age, obesity, and physically demanding work (Gougoulias et al. 2009). In addition, if the patient has ipsilateral knee arthritis, it is recommended to correct the stifle pathology first.

Very few of the first-generation TAA implants are still in use. One of the more popular early TAA designs, the Mayo Ankle, had a greater-than-40% failure rate after 10 years. In a long-term study conducted at the Mayo Clinic, the study authors did not advise its use, especially in patients under 57 years of age (Kitaoka et al. 1994). The Mayo Ankle is no longer in use.

The tibial component of early designs was all polyethylene. Current designs generally consist of a metal-backed tibial component with both the tibial and talar components uncemented. In second-generation prostheses, the polyethylene is on the tibial side (Gougoulias et al. 2009). Further, the trend has clearly been toward minimal constraint designs (Wood and Deakin 2003; Doets et al. 2006; Espinosa et al. 2010; Krause et al. 2011). As with other joints, more constrained prostheses led to implant loosening, secondary to increased implant–bone or cement–bone interface stresses.

An additional trend in TAA prosthesis design is the use of a three-component, rather than two-component, prosthesis (Figure 13.12). Two-component designs are generally polyethylene-on-metal articulations, with the polyethylene component fixed to the tibial component. Three-component designs are also referred to as mobile-bearing designs, with the polyethylene component able to move independent of both the tibial and talar components, acting as a meniscus (Gougoulias et al. 2009; Saltzman et al. 2009; Krause et al. 2011).

In recent years, two-component designs have primarily been used in the United States, and three-component designs have been used in Europe. No three-component design prostheses were approved by the FDA until 2009. In fact, some European three-component prostheses were modified as two-component prostheses for the U.S. market (Stengel and Bauwens 2005; Krause et al. 2011). Three-component prostheses have reportedly had superior initial results. It has been hypothesized that the freedom of motion of the polyethylene meniscus would dampen both the contact stresses applied to the polyethylene, as well as the shear stresses applied to the implant–bone interface. These improvements should, in turn, decrease polyethylene wear and mechanical loosening, respectively.

As noted above, no current TAA implants utilize cement fixation. The method of fixation of the components is either press-fit or screw fixation, or both. Tibial anchorage is accomplished using one of the following: stem, flange, pegs, or screws. Talar anchorage utilizes either keel or peg. Fixation by means other than screws is by press-fit (Gougoulias et al. 2009). The human talus is approximately 40% stronger in compression that is the distal tibia. At a distance of 1–1.5 cm from the joint, tibial bone is mostly loose, fatty bone and does not provide stable fixation. Therefore, minimal bone resection (<4 mm) is advised in order to minimize the risk of subsidence (Hvid et al. 1985). Implants that incorporate a long tibial stem risk excessive load transmission to the relatively weak anterior tibial cortex. Talar component loosening is less frequent than tibial component loosening because of this difference in bone strength (Kofoed and Saltzman 2004).

There are several common complications following TAA, including delayed wound healing, deep infection, malleolar fracture, aseptic loosening, misalignment, edge loading, and gutter impingement. Gutter impingement occurs when the talar component impact the malleoli with either varus or valgus stress (Wood and Deakin 2003; Gougoulias et al. 2009).

While wound healing is consistently among the most common complications, most authors comment that it is also the complication that most consistently decreases in frequency with greater experience. Similarly, deep infection, which generally results in implant loosening and either revision or explantation, generally decreases in incidence with operator experience (Wood and Deakin 2003; Espinosa et al. 2010).

Fracture of either the medial or lateral malleolus can occur either during or after surgery. Malleolar fractures have been associated with excessive bone resection, gutter impingement, and the use of oversized talar implants. Malleolar fractures that occur after surgery are often managed conservatively.

Aseptic loosening is frequently associated with excessive shear stress applied to either the polyethylene or the implant–bone interface with

prostheses that have excessive constraint (Wood and Deakin 2003; Doets et al. 2006; Gougoulias et al. 2009). Excessive polyethylene loading, as well as edge (asymmetrical) loading, also results in greater polyethylene wear and subsequent loosening. Excessive polyethylene loading and edge loading are typically a consequence of either failure to recognize or correct preexisting limb deviation or due to implant misalignment during surgery. Preoperative ankle alignment can be affected by traumatic osteoarthritis, in which case the deviation is typically varus. Immune-mediated arthritis can also affect alignment, and typically results in valgus deviation (Wood and Deakin 2003). Some authors consider a preoperative ankle malalignment of greater than 10–15 degrees a relative contraindication for TAA and require corrective osteotomy prior to TAA (Wood and Deakin 2003; Doets et al. 2006).

Espinosa et al. evaluated the effect of malalignment on polyethylene wear (Espinosa et al. 2010). They found that the yield stress of polyethylene (18–20 MPa) is exceeded when the tibial or talar components are implanted at greater than 5 degrees of eversion (Figure 13.13). That study also found that the lower kinematic constraint of three-component designs results in a more even pressure distribution than two-component designs. Furthermore, the study noted that, even with appropriate implant placement, two-component prostheses exceeded polyethylene yield stress. The long-term effect of the independent movement of the polyethylene meniscus in three-component prostheses on the development of polyethylene wear debris is unknown.

An additional reported contributor to the incidence of aseptic loosening is the type of implant coating. Nearly all current prostheses are cobalt-chrome alloys. The incidence of aseptic loosening decreased when the type of coating of implants changed from a single-layer hydroxyapatite coating to a dual coating of plasma-sprayed titanium and calcium phosphate. This change was common to a variety of prostheses in the late 1990s (Wood and Deakin 2003).

Various two-component prostheses designs are in use, including Agility, INBONE (Inbone Technologies, Boulder, CO), Salto (Tornier, St. Ismier, France), and Eclipse (Kineticos Medical, Carlsbad, CA). The most commonly used two-component

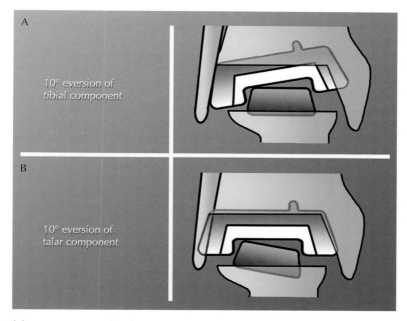

Figure 13.13   (A) Malalignment associated with eversion of tibial component. (B) Malalignment associated with eversion of the talar component. (Image by Derek Fox)

prosthesis is the Agility Total Ankle Replacement (DePuy; Figure 13.14), which was the only FDA-approved TAA until 2007 (Knecht et al. 2004; Gougoulias et al. 2009; Espinosa et al. 2010). The Agility prosthesis is semiconstrained. A space between the medial and lateral sides of the talar component and the malleoli allow the talus to slide side-to-side. In addition to application of the TAA implants, the Agility prosthesis required creation of a tibiofibular syndesmosis via screw fixation (Figure 13.14). Delayed syndesmosis is one of the more common complications with the Agility prosthesis and is often associated with lysis surrounding the tibial component (Knecht et al. 2004; Alvine and Conti 2006; Gougoulias et al. 2009). Delayed syndesmosis is reported in approximately 10% of cases. A specialized radiographic projection, termed the mortise view, is used to evaluate the syndesmosis (Knecht et al. 2004). Reported complication rates, revision rates, and failure rates vary widely. Failure rates reportedly range from 6% to 31% (Pyevich et al. 1998; Knecht et al. 2004; Alvine and Conti 2006). The first three-component TAA design was the Low-Contact-Stress, or LCS, prosthesis. The LCS design evolved into the Buechel–Pappas, or BP (Endotec, Orange, NJ;

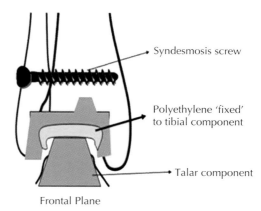

Figure 13.14   The Agility (DePuy, Warsaw, IN) total ankle. Note the screw placed for tibiofibular syndemosis. (Reproduced from Gougoulias et al. [2009], with permission from Oxford University Press)

Figure 13.15), prosthesis (Gougoulias et al. 2009). The BP, Salto, Scandinavian Total Ankle Replacement (STAR, Waldemar Link, Hamburg, Germany; Figure 13.16), and Mobility prostheses are the most commonly encountered in the literature. The Salto Talaris (Tornier, Bloomington, MN) was developed as a three-component prosthesis in Europe, but

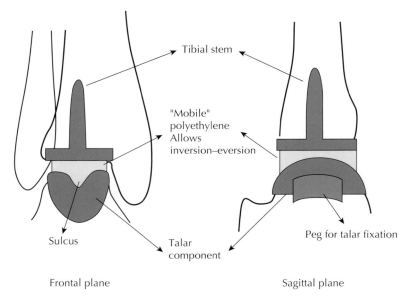

Figure 13.15 The Buechel–Pappas (BP) (Endotec, Orange, NJ) total ankle, a three-component system with a tibial fixation peg. (Reproduced from Gougoulias et al. [2009], with permission from Oxford University Press)

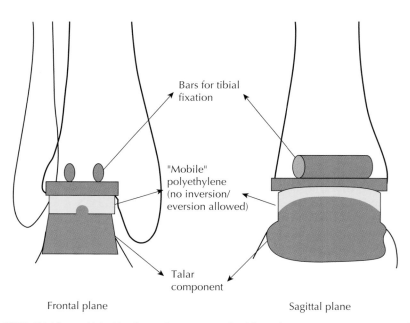

Figure 13.16 The STAR (Waldemar Link, Hamburg, Germany) total ankle, a three-component system with cylindrical bars for tibial fixation. (Reproduced from Gougoulias et al. [2009], with permission from Oxford University Press)

modified as a two-component prosthesis in the United States due to FDA restrictions. The BP prosthesis is an unconstrained design with a flat upper (tibial) surface allowing inversion (pronation) and eversion (supination). The distal meniscal surface has a sulcus, making it congruent with the talar component. This meniscal design is described as having a flat upper surface and a congruent distal surface. The tibial component is anchored with a stem, which has been a concern due to the previously described weak distal tibia (Doets et al. 2006). Studies evaluating the most recent generation of BP prostheses report a 90% 12-year prosthesis survival rate. Of the TAA prostheses mentioned in this chapter, only the BP prosthesis is titanium. The other TAA prostheses are CoCr, although many have plasma-sprayed Ti coating.

The STAR prosthesis is the first three-component TAA to receive FDA approval. The meniscal design is similar to the BP prosthesis. The tibial component is anchored with two bars (Wood and Deakin 2003). Success rates for the STAR prosthesis are similar to those described for the BP prosthesis.

Tarsal arthroplasty in small animals

Likely indications for tarsal arthroplasty in veterinary patients include traumatic arthritis, degenerative joint disease secondary to developmental abnormalities (e.g., talar ridge osteochondritis dissecans [OCD]), and erosive immune-mediated polyarthritis. Two canine studies have helped establish normal range of motion angles in flexion/extension and external/internal rotation. Through a swing–stance cycle, the tarsal joint angle traverses a dorsoplantar range from approximately 115 through 140 degrees and an internal/external range from approximately −5 to −15 degrees (Kim et al. 2008; Fu et al. 2010). As noted in the section on TWA, hyperextension injury of the canine carpus typically disrupts the palmar fibrocartilage in addition to the palmar carpal ligaments. Trauma affecting the tibiotarsal joint in small animals does not have a similar issue. However, TAA does require intact collateral ligaments and ligamentous reconstruction and appropriate healing would likely be necessary prior to performing TAA. Alternatively, as has been reported in some forms of TAA in people (Gougoulias et al. 2009), a transarticular external fixator may be applied during healing from a TAA.

References

Adamo PF. Cervical arthroplasty in two dogs with disc-associated cervical spondylomyelopathy. J Am Vet Med Assoc 2011;239:808–817.

Adamo PF, Kobayashi H, Markel M, Vanderby R Jr. *In vitro* biomechanical comparison of cervical disk arthroplasty, ventral slot procedure, and smooth pins with polymethylmethacrylate fixation at treated and adjacent canine cervical motion units. Vet Surg 2007;36(8):729–741.

Alvine FG, Conti SF. The AGILITY ankle: Mid- and long-term results. Orthopaede 2006;35(5):521–526.

Anderson PA, Rouleau JP, Toth JM, et al. A comparison of simulator-tested and retrieved cervical disc prostheses: Invited submission from the joint section meeting on disorders of the spine and peripheral nerves. J Neurosurg Spine 2004;1(2):202–210.

Barbagallo GM, Corbino LA, Olindo G, Albanese V. Heterotopic ossification in cervical disc arthroplasty: Is it clinically relevant? Evid Based Spinal Care J 2010;1(1):15–20.

Barrey C, Mosnier T, Jund J, et al. *In vitro* evaluation of a ball-and-socket cervical disc prosthesis with cranial geometric center. J Neurosurg Spine 2009;11(5):538–549.

Benninger MI, Seiler GS, Robinson LE, et al. Effects of anatomic conformation on three-dimensional motion of the caudal lumbar and lumbosacral portions of the vertebral column of dogs. Am J Vet Res 2006;67(1):43–50.

Bertagnoli R, Yue JJ, Pfeiffer F, et al. Early results after ProDisc-C cervical disc replacement. J Neurosurg Spine 2005a;2(4):403–410.

Bertagnoli R, Yue JJ, Shah RV, et al. The treatment of disabling single-level lumbar discogenic low back pain with total disc arthroplasty utilizing the prodisc prosthesis. Spine 2005b;30(19):2230–2236.

Boileau P, Avidor C, Krishnan SG, et al. Cemented polyethylene versus uncemented metal-backed glenoid components in total shoulder arthroplasty: A prospective, double-blind, randomized study. J Shoulder Elbow Surg 2002;11(4):351–359.

Breit S, Kunzel W. Shape and orientation of articular facets of cervical vertebrae C3-C7 in dogs denoting axial rotational ability: An osteological study. Eur J Morphol 2002;40:43–51.

Brenner BC, Ferlic DC, Clayton ML, Dennis DA. Survivorship of unconstrained total shoulder arthroplasty. J Bone Joint Surg Am 1989;71(9):1289–1296.

Brewer BJ, Wubben RC, Carrera GF. Excessive retroversion of the glenoid cavity: A cause of non-traumatic posterior instability of the shoulder. J Bone Joint Surg Am 1986;68(5):724–731.

Buchowski JM, Anderson PA, Sekhon L, Riew KD. Cervical disc arthroplasty compared with arthrodesis for treatment of myelopathy: Surgical technique. J Bone Joint Surg Am 2009;91(2):223–232.

Cavaliere. CM and Chung KC. A systematic review of total wrist arthroplasty compared with total wrist arthrodesis for rheumatoid arthritis. Plast Reconstr Surg 2008a; 122(3):813–825.

Cavaliere CM, Chung KC. Total wrist arthroplasty and total wrist arthrodesis in rheumatoid arthritis: A decision analysis from the hand surgeon's perspective. J Hand Surgery 2008b;33(10):1699–1674.

Cavaliere. CM and Chung KC. A cost-utility analysis of non-surgical management, total wrist arthroplasty and total wrist arthrodesis in rheumatoid arthritis. J Hand Surg 2010; 35(3):379–391.

Chang U-K, Kim DH, Lee MC, et al. Changes in adjacent-level disc pressure and facet joint force after cervical arthroplasty compared with cervical discectomy and fusion. J Neurosurg Spine 2007a;7(1):33–39.

Chang U-K, Kim DH, Lee MC, et al. Range of motion change after cervical arthroplasty with ProDisc-C and Prestige artificial discs compared with anterior cervical discectomy and fusion. J Neurosurg Spine 2007b;7(1):40–46.

Chin PYK, Sperling JW, Cofield RH, et al. Complications of total shoulder arthroplasty: Are they fewer or different? J Shoulder Elbow Surg 2006;15(1):19–22.

Chung SK, Kim YE, Wang KC. Biomechanical effect of constraint in lumbar total disc replacement: A study with finite element analysis. Spine 2009;34(12):1281–1286.

Cobb TK, Beckenbaugh RD. Biaxial total-wrist arthroplasty. J Hand Surg Am 1996;21(6):1011–1021.

Cofield RH. Total shoulder arthroplasty with the Neer prosthesis. J Bone Joint Surg Am 1984;66(6):899–906.

Cofield RH, Daly PJ. Total shoulder arthroplasty with a tissue-ingrowth glenoid component. J Shoulder Elbow Surg 1992;1(2):77–85.

Collins D, Tencer A, Sidles J, Matsen F. Edge displacement and deformation of glenoid components in response to eccentric loading. The effect of preparation of the glenoid bone. J Bone Joint Surg Am 1992;74(7):501–507.

da Costa RC. Cervical spondylomyelopathy (Wobbler's) in dogs. Vet Clin N Am Sm Anim Pract (Small Animal) 2010;40(5):881–913.

Doets HC, Brand R, Nelissen RG. Total ankle arthroplasty in inflammatory joint disease with use of two mobile-bearing designs. J Bone Joint Surg Am 2006;88(6):1272–1283.

Doets HC, van Middelkoop M, Houdijk H, et al. Gait analysis after successful mobile bearing total ankle replacement. Foot Ankle Int 2007;28(3):313–322.

Dooris AP, Goel VK, Grosland NM, et al. Load-sharing between anterior and posterior elements in a lumbar motion segment implanted with an artificial disc. Spine 2001;26(6):E122–E129.

Espinosa N, Walti M, Favre P, Snedeker JG. Misalignment of total ankle components can induce high joint contact pressures. J Bone Joint Surg Am 2010;92(5):1179–1187.

Feeney LC, Cheng-Feng L, Marcellin-Little DJ, et al. Validation of two-dimensional kinematic analysis of walk and sit-to-stand motion in dogs. Am J Vet Res 2007;68(3):277–282.

Fox TJ, Cil A, Sperling JW, et al. Survival of the glenoid component in shoulder arthroplasty. J Shoulder Elbow Surg 2009;18(6):859–863.

Fu YC, Torres BT, Budsberg SC. Evaluation of a three-dimensional kinematic model for canine gait analysis. Am J Vet Res 2010;71(10):1118–1122.

Garrito BJ, Wilhite J, Nakano M, et al. Adjacent-level cervical ossification after Bryan cervical disc arthroplasty compared with anterior cervical discectomy and fusion. J Bone Joint Surg Am 2011;93(13):1185–1189.

Gartsman G, Elkousy H, Warnock K, Edwards T, Connor D. Radiographic comparison of pegged and keeled glenoid components. J Shoulder Elbow Surg 2005;14(3):252–257.

Goffin J, Casey A, Kehr P, et al. Preliminary experience with the Bryan cervical disc prosthesis. Neurosurgery 2002;51(3):840–847.

Goffin J, Geusens E, Vantomme N, et al. Long-term follow-up after interbody fusion of the cervical spine. J Spinal Disord Tech 2004;17(2):79–85.

Gougoulias N, Khanna A, Maffulli N. History and evolution in total ankle arthroplasty. British Med Bull 2009;89(1):111–151.

Gougoulias NE, Khanna A, Maffulli N. How successful are current ankle replacements: A systematic review of the literature. Clin Orthop Relat Res 2010;468(1):199–208.

Groh GI. Survival and radiographic analysis of a glenoid component with a cementless fluted central peg. J Shoulder Elbow Surg 2010;19(8):1265–1268.

Groh GI, Heckman MM, Curtis RJ, et al. Treatment of fractures adjacent to humeral prosthesis. J Shoulder Elbow Surg 2008;17(1):85–89.

Gupta A. Total wrist arthroplasty. Am J Orthop 2008;8(Suppl.):12–16.

Gwynedd PE, Sekhon LH, Sears WR, Duggal N. Complications with cervical disc arthroplasty. J Neurosurg Spine 2006;4(2):98–105.

Haddad SL, Coetzee JC, Estok R, et al. Intermediate and long-term outcomes of total ankle arthroplasty and ankle arthrodesis: A systematic review of the literature. J Bone Joint Surg Am 2007;89(9):1899–1905.

Harrop JS, Youssef JA, Maltenfort M, et al. Lumbar adjacent segment degeneration and disease after arthrodesis and total disc arthroplasty. Spine 2008;33(15):1701–1707.

Hasan SS, Leith JM, Campbell B, et al. Characteristics of unsatisfactory shoulder arthroplasties. J Shoulder Elbow Surg 2002;11(5):431–441.

Herzberg G. Prospective study of a new total wrist arthroplasty: Short-term results. Chirurgie de la main 2011;30(1):20–25.

Hofstetter M, Gédet P, Doherr M, et al. Biomechanical analysis of the three-dimensional motion pattern of the canine cervical spine segment C4-C5. Vet Surg 2009;38(1):49–58.

Holler PJ, Brazda V, Dal-Bianco B, et al. Kinematic motion analysis of the joints of the forelimbs and hind limbs of dogs during walking exercise regimens. Am J Vet Res 2010;71(7):734–740.

Hvid I, Rasmussen O, Jensen NC, Nielsen S. Trabecular bone strength profiles at the ankle joint. Clin Orthop Relat Res 1985;199:306–312.

Kim J, Rietdyk S, Breur G. Comparison of two-dimensional and three-dimensional systems for kinematic analysis of the sagittal motion of canine hindlimbs during walking. Am J Vet Res 2008;69(9):1116–1122.

Kitaoka HB, Patzer GL, Ilstrup DM, et al. Survivorship analysis of the Mayo total ankle arthroplasty. J Bone Joint Surg Am 1994;76(7):974–979.

Knecht SI, Estin M, Callaghan JJ, et al. The Agility total ankle arthroplasty. Seven to sixteen-year follow-up. J Bone Joint Surg Am 2004;86(6):1161–1171.

Kofoed H, Saltzman C. Scandinavian Total Ankle Replacement (STAR). Clin Orthop Relat Res 2004;424:73–80.

Krause FG, Windolf M, Bora B, et al. Impact of complications in total ankle replacement and arthrodesis. J Bone Joint Surg Am 2011;93(9):830–839.

Lascelles BDX, Roe SC, Smith E, et al. Evaluation of a pressure walkway system for measurement of vertical limb forces in clinically normal dogs. Am J Vet Res 2006;67(2):277–282.

Le H, Thongtrangan I, Kim DH. Historical review of cervical arthroplasty. Neurosurg Focus 2004;17(3):E1–E9.

Litchfield RB, McKee MD, Balyk R, et al. Cemented versus uncemented fixation of humeral components in total shoulder arthroplasty for osteoarthritis of the shoulder: A prospective, randomized, double-blind clinical trial-A JOINTs Canada Project. J Shoulder Elbow Surg 2011;20(4):529–536.

Matsen FA, Clark JM, Titelman RM, et al. Healing of reamed glenoid bone articulating with a metal humeral arthroplasty: A canine model. J Orthop Res 2005;23(1):18–26.

McAfee PC, Cunningham B, Dmitriev A, et al. Cervical disc replacement—porous coated motion prosthesis: A comparative biomechanical analysis showing the key role of the posterior longitudinal ligament. Spine 2003;28(20S):S176–S185.

Menon J. Universal total wrist implant: Experience with a carpal component fixed with three screws. J Arthroplasty 1998;13(5):515–523.

Neer CS, Morrison DS. Glenoid bone-grafting in total shoulder arthroplasty. J Bone Joint Surg Am 1988;70(8):1154–1162.

Neer CS, Watson KC, Stanton FJ. Recent experience in total shoulder replacement. J Bone Joint Surg Am 1982;64(3):319–337.

van Ooij A, Oner FC, Verbout AJ. Complications of artificial disc replacement: A report of 27 patients with the Charite disc. Spine 2003;28(0):369–383.

Palmer AK, Werner FW, Murphy D, Glisson R. Functional wrist motion: A biomechanical study. J Hand Surg Am 1985;10(1):39.

Pelletier MH, Langdown A, Gllies RM. Photoelastic comparison of strains in the underlying glenoid with metal-backed and all-polyethylene implants. J Shoulder Elbow Surg 2008;17(5):779–783.

Pickett GE, Rouleau JP, Duggal N. Kinematic analysis of the cervical spine following implantation of an artificial cervical disc. Spine 2005;30(17):1949–1954.

Post M, Jablon M. Constrained total shoulder arthroplasty: Long-term follow-up observations. Clin Orthop Relat Res 1983;173:109–116.

Post M, Jablon M, Miller H, Singh M. Constrained total shoulder joint replacement: A critical review. Clin Orthop Relat Res 1979;144:135–150.

Pracyk JB, Traynelis VC. Treatment of the painful motion segment: Cervical arthroplasty. Spine 2005;30(16S):S23–S32.

Pyevich MT, Saltzman CL, Callaghan JJ, Alvine FG. Total ankle arthroplasty: A unique design. Two to twelve-year follow-up. J Bone Joint Surg Am 1998;80(10):1410–1420.

Rizzo M, Beckenbaugh R. Results of biaxial total wrist arthroplasty with a modified (long) metacarpal stem. J Hand Surg 2003;28(4):577–584.

Roberto RF, McDonald T, Curtiss S, et al. Kinematics of progressive circumferential ligament resection (decompression) in conjunction with cervical disc arthroplasty in a spondylotic spine model. Spine 2010;35(18):1676–1683.

Saltzman CL, Mann RA, Ahrens J, et al. Prospective controlled trial of STAR total ankle replacement versus ankle fusion: Initial results. Foot Ankle Int 2009;30(7):579–593.

Sidaway BK, McLaughlin RM, Elder SH, et al. Role of the tendons of the biceps brachii and infraspinatus muscles and the medial glenohumeral ligament in the maintenance of passive shoulder joint stability in dogs. Am J Vet Res 2004;65(9):1216–1222.

Snyder JT, Tzermiadianos MN, Ghanayem AJ, et al. Effect of uncovertebral joint excision on the motion response of the cervical spine after total disc replacement. Spine 2007;32(26):2965–2969.

Sperling JW, Cofield RH, Rowland C. Minimum fifteen-year follow-up of Neer hemiarthroplasty and total shoulder arthroplasty in patients aged fifty years or younger. J Shoulder Elbow Surg 2004;13(6):604–613.

Sperling JW, Cofield RH, Schleck CD, et al. Total shoulder arthroplasty versus hemiarthroplasty for rheumatoid arthritis of the shoulder: Results of 303 consecutive cases. J Shoulder Elbow Surg 2007;16(6):683–690.

Stengel D, Bauwens K. Ekkernkamp A and Cramer J. Efficacy of total ankle replacement with meniscal-bearing devices: A systematic review and meta-analysis. Arch Orthop Trauma Surg 2005;125(2):109–119.

Takwale VJ, Nuttall D, Trail IA, Stanley JK. Biaxial total wrist replacement in patients with rheumatoid arthritis. J Bone Joint Surg (Br) 2002;84:692–699.

Taljanovic MS, Jones MD, Hunter TB, et al. Joint arthroplasties and prostheses. Radiographics 2003;23(5):1295–1314.

Torchia ME, Cofield RH, Settergren CR. Neer total shoulder arthroplasty: Long-term results. J Shoulder Elbow Surg 1997;6(6):495–505.

Tsukamoto S, Tanaka Y, Maegawa N, et al. Total talar replacement following the collapse of the talar body as a complication of total ankle arthroplasty. J Bone Joint Surg (Am) 2010;92(11):2115–2120.

Tu TH, Wu JC, Huang WC, et al. Heterotopic ossification after cervical total disc replacement: Determination by CT and effects on clinical outcomes. J Neurosurg Spine 2011;14(4):1–3.

Voss K, Galeandro L, Wiestner T, et al. Relationship of body weight, body size, subject velocity, and vertical ground reaction force in trotting dogs. Vet Surg 2010;39(7):863–869.

Wall B, Nove-Josserand L, O'Connor DP, et al. Reverse total shoulder arthroplasty: A review of results according to etiology. J Bone Joint Surg Am 2007;89(7):1476–1485.

Wilke HJ, Wenger K, Claes L. Testing criteria for spinal implants: Recommendations for the standardization of *in vitro* stability testing of spinal implants. Eur Spine J 1998;7(2):148–154.

Wirth MA, Rockwood CA Jr. Current concepts review—Complications of total shoulder-replacement arthroplasty. J Bone Joint Surg Am 1996;78(4):603–616.

Wirth MA, Rockwood CA Jr. Glenohumeral instability following shoulder arthroplasty. Orthop Trans 1995;19(4):459.

Wirth MA, Korvick DL, Basamania CJ, et al. Radiologic, mechanical, and histologic evaluation of 2 glenoid prosthesis designs in a canine model. J Shoulder Elbow Surg 2001;10(2):140–148.

Wood PL, Deakin S. Total ankle replacement: The results in 200 ankles. J Bone Joint Surg Br 2003;85(3):334–341.

Woolson ST, Pottorff GT. Disassembly of a modular femoral prosthesis after dislocation of the femoral component. A case report. J Bone Joint Surg Am 1990;72(4):624–625.

Youm Y, Flatt AE. Design of a total wrist prosthesis. Ann Biomed Eng 1984;12(3):247–262.

14 Custom Total Joint Arthroplasty

Denis J. Marcellin-Little and Ola L.A. Harrysson

Custom orthopedic implants are primarily used to manage complex orthopedic situations. For total joint arthroplasties, custom implants are used to manage bone loss, abnormalities in bone shape or structure, or unusual bone sizes. Custom implants may be used as part of limb-sparing procedures, to fill large bone defects, or to replace a missing bone or limb segment. The purpose of this chapter is to describe the rationale, features, fabrication, and applications of custom implants for use in companion animals.

The need for custom orthopedic implants

Custom implants are intended for the management of unusual patients or unusual situations, where conventional commercial implants cannot be used. The term "custom" refers to a process that is customized to a specific application or patient. In some instances, a custom total joint replacement refers to the use of commercially available components that are combined in a manner that is patient-specific (Sporer and Della Valle 2010). In other instances, a custom implant refers to a unique implant designed and fabricated for a specific patient and situation.

Because the design and fabrication of custom implants is time-consuming, technically demanding, and costly, commercial implants, when available, are always preferred over custom implants. Patients that receive custom implants may be particularly small or large, or may have bones of an unusual shape because of previous injury or disease or because of their breed or species. Custom implants may be used to fill large bone defects (Liska et al. 2007), where they represent an alternative to intercalary allografts, autoclaved autografts, extracorporeally irradiated autografts, vascularized autografts, or distraction osteogenesis (Kiatisevi et al. 2009).

Fabrication of custom implants

Custom metal implants are generally designed and fabricated by bioengineers within commercial or academic laboratories. Some commercial fabrication laboratories are freestanding, others are part of large medical implant companies. In veterinary medicine, several companies offer custom

Advances in Small Animal Total Joint Replacement, First Edition. Edited by Jeffrey N. Peck and Denis J. Marcellin-Little.
© 2013 John Wiley & Sons, Inc. Published 2013 by John Wiley & Sons, Inc.

Table 14.1   Implant companies offering custom orthopedic implants to veterinarians

Company[a]	BioMedtrix LLC (Boonton, NJ)	INNOPLANT (Hannover, Germany)	Synthes Vet (West Chester, PA)	Veterinary Instrumentation Limited (Sheffield, U.K.)
Custom division	BioMedtrix-Customs	INNOPLANT Medizintechnik	Surgeon Response Group (SRG)	V.I. Custom Implants
Creation date	1989	2005	2007	1985
Design capabilities	In house	In house	In house	In house
Fabrication and finishing	In house and business association with multiple human implant vendors	In house	In house or approved vendors	In house
Quality control	In house	In house	In house	In house
Products	Total joints and trauma for veterinary applications	Custom metal, plastic, or bioresorbable implants for the management of deformities, trauma, and neoplasia	Implants with FDA clearance (510K or other) Modification of almost any implant from the Synthes catalog	Plates and screws
Most common products	Total hip replacements (cemented and cementless), elbow replacements, knee replacements, and intramedullary fixator system	Custom hip prostheses for humans	Arthrodesis implants, design and production of special surgical instruments	Medial pantarsal bone plates
Particular expertise	Biomechanical analysis for the development of medical prostheses	Custom total hip prostheses	Patient-specific implants for craniomaxillofacial (CMF) applications	Custom hybrid joint arthrodesis plates

[a]Listed in alphabetical order. This is not a list of all companies providing custom implants in human and veterinary medicine.

implants, including BioMedtrix (Boonton, NJ), INNOPLANT (Hannover, Germany), Kyon Pharma (Boston, MA), Synthes Vet (West Chester, PA), and Veterinary Instrumentation (Sheffield, U.K.) (Table 14.1).

Custom implants are often based on patient imaging, usually computed tomography (CT) scan images. These images are converted into three-dimensional (3D) computer models that are then exported into modeling or computer-aided design (CAD) software (Marcellin-Little et al. 2008, 2010b). Implants are then created using CAD software (Figure 14.1). Haptic feedback devices may be used to manipulate and modify 3D computer models to create implants. These implants may have complex features and geometries. Haptic devices have been used to sculpt cranial implants and for oral implant surgery (Ai et al. 2006; Kusumoto et al. 2006). Our research group uses a haptic pen (PHANTOM Omni, SensAble Technologies, Woburn, MA) to shape freeform implants (Figure 14.2; Marcellin-Little et al. 2010b). Implants designed from 3D computer models may be manufactured by adding thin layers of material to each other. This process, described below, is named direct metal fabrication.

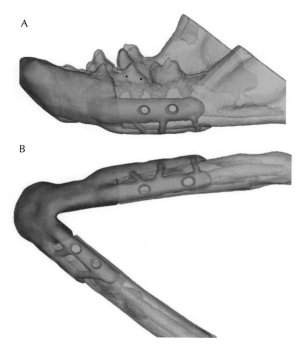

A

B

Figure 14.1   Three-dimensional computer models representing lateral (A) and ventral (B) views of the mandible of a cat with a gingival fibrosarcoma located on the labial side of the base of the third lower left incisor (tooth #303). The fibrosarcoma is not visible on the images. As part of the surgical excision of that fibrosarcoma, a rostral mandibulectomy is planned and a custom implant (in purple) has been designed to replace the missing portion of the mandible. The rostral mandibulectomy includes the removal of the lower incisors, canines, and one left lower premolar (#307). The cranial aspect of the implant is solid and the caudal aspects of the implant have flanges that extend on the ventral and labial sides of the hemimandibles. The screw holes in the implants are placed so that they do not interfere with tooth roots.

Implants intended to replace cortical bone or to sustain high mechanical loads are named structural implants. They most often have a solid metal core. Solid custom implants are most often made of titanium alloy (Ti6Al4V), but they may be made of cobalt-chromium alloy (CoCr), commercially pure (CP) titanium, or less commonly, of stainless steel. Structural implants may be machined, cast, forged, or may be made using direct metal fabrication, also know as freeform fabrication, additive manufacturing, or layered manufacturing. Direct metal fabrication relies on an electron or laser beam that repeatedly melts thin layers of metal powder to construct 3D objects (Marcellin-Little et al. 2010a). Layer thicknesses may be as thin as 50 μm. Electron beam melting (EBM) was first reported as part of Morgan Larsson's Master of Science thesis at Chalmers University (Göteborg, Sweden). Arcam AB (Mölndal, Sweden) first commercialized an EBM machine in 2003. Approximately 85 machines are in use worldwide and more than one-third of them are used for implant fabrication (Wohlers 2011). As an alternative, laser-based processes have been developed to a point where metal parts can be fabricated by lasers. These processes include selective laser melting (SLM; 3D Systems, Rock Hill, SC), laser engineered net shaping (LENS; Optomec, Albuquerque, NM), and direct metal laser sintering (DMLS; EOS GmbH, Krailling, Germany). Selective laser sintering (SLS) machines were first introduced in 1990. These machines could only be used with polymer materials. Later, the first metal applications of SLS produced porous parts that could not be used for implants. The first solid metal implants produced using the SLS/DMLS process were made in 2000. The material properties required for orthopedic implants, however, were not achieved until a few years later. Direct metal fabrication processes based on the DMLS concept are currently provided by a number of companies around the world and there are approximately 600 machines in use worldwide. Implants made by use of direct metal fabrication may have solid and porous portions that have structural and nonstructural roles. Direct metal fabrication may be used to make metal plates with shapes that match the bone surface. Our research group has, for research purposes, assessed the biocompatibility of EBM-processed titanium alloy (Haslauer et al. 2010) and has fabricated custom titanium alloy plates that fit the surfaces of the distal aspect of the femur and the proximal aspect of the tibia (Marcellin-Little et al. 2008, 2010b). These plates had acceptable mechanical properties when evaluated *in vitro*. Clinically, our group has made EBM-processed and DMLS-processed implants placed on the maxilla, the radius, the tibia, and the calcaneus of dogs and cats. The clinical performances of these implants have been satisfactory based on their proper fit and the absence of infection, inflammatory response, or mechanical failure.

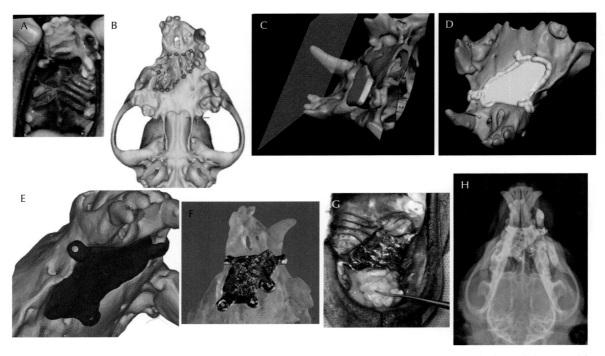

Figure 14.2   A dog presented with a large, chronic oronasal fistula secondary to head trauma (A). The bone defect is visible on a 3D rendering based on a CT scan (B), highlighted with small spheres. A haptic pen is used to create a plate into that 3D computer model (C) and position it in the defect. The haptic device software is used to extrude and sculpt the freeform plate (D) and place holes intended to secure the plate (E). The plate is made using electron beam melting and fitted on a polymer replica of the skull (F). The plate is then implanted into the patient (G). On radiographs made 3 months after surgery, the plate is stable (H).

Fabrication of structural implants

There are three main manufacturing processes used in the fabrication of commercial implants: forging, investment casting, and machining. Forging is a process where metal is "smashed" between two tool halves to form the desired shape. The development time for forging tools is measured in months. Forging is costly and is primarily used for mass production. While the forging process results in implants with the highest strength, some of the common implant metals are very hard and require very high forces during their production. This makes implant production more challenging. One disadvantage of forging is that implants cannot have any undercut geometries, which limits their design. Forged implant components usually require secondary finishing steps before they can be used.

Investment casting is a high-precision casting process that is commonly used for implant fabrication (Eufinger and Wehmoller 1998). A tool is used to create wax patterns that are placed on a casting tree. The wax tree is dipped in ceramic slurry, creating a thin shell. The tree is fired in a furnace, melting the wax and increasing the strength of the ceramic. Molten metal is cast into the ceramic shell, which is broken after the metal has solidified to retrieve the implants. The casting process can handle complex geometries, but if the wax pattern is made using a mold, then the same geometrical restrictions as forging apply. One disadvantage of the investment casting process is the reduced material properties of the implants produced, compared with wrought (forged) material. The use of additive manufacturing to produce the wax pattern would be required to make custom implants using investment casting, otherwise the cost and lead time would be too long. Secondary finishing is needed after investment casting.

Machining (manual or computer numerical control [CNC]) is a process where metal material is removed using a sharp tool that is either rotating (milling) or stationary (turning). Machining can be used to fabricate metal implants from bar stock or for the finishing process of cast or forged implants. Today, high-speed CNC machining is used to mass-produce metal implants. There are some geometrical limitations to machining processes, so the complexity of machined implants is limited. Another disadvantage of machining complex implants from bar stock is that most of the material will end up as scrap, which significantly increases costs when biocompatible metals are used. The fabrication of custom implants using machining is often easier than using forging or casting but modern CNC machines need to be programmed and the more complex the geometry is, the more difficult the programming will be. Programming costs per implant are small when implants are mass-produced, but these costs are much higher for custom implants.

Freeform fabrication, described earlier in the text, is the additive process where thin layers of material are added to each other to build structures. Titanium alloy (Ti6Al4V), cobalt-chromium, and stainless steel implants have been made using freeform fabrication. Freeform fabrication has several key advantages over other fabrication methods. It may be used to fabricate implants with complex shapes and with solid and porous portions (Harrysson et al. 2008). Freeform fabrication is less labor intensive than investment casting for custom implants. In one report, the preparation of a custom implant using EBM took 25 hours, compared with 78 hours for the preparation of an identical implant using investment casting.[1] DMLS appears better suited to the production of small implants than EBM because DMLS implants have a finer texture (i.e., lower surface roughness) that requires less finishing (Figure 14.3).[2] However, the titanium alloy powder used for DMLS fabrication is finer than the powder used for EBM fabrication. The finer powder costs approximately twice as much as the coarser powder. The EBM system constructs the implant under vacuum, while the DMLS system uses an inert gas that varies based on the alloy being used. The vacuum assists in preventing contamination and in preventing the construct from cooling down during the building process. Both EBM and DMLS processes claim to meet the American Society for Testing and Materials (ASTM) standards for chemical composition of final parts as well as mechanical properties, that have been verified by independent sources (Harrysson et al. 2008).

Fabrication of nonstructural implants

Molding (polymethylmethacrylate)

Cranial implants are used to fill skull defects resulting from traumatic injuries to the head. Since cranial defects are different for each patient, these implants are all custom-made. The conventional process for the production of implants includes the use of a polymer additive process to fabricate a model of the patient's skull based on a CT scan. A wax implant is hand-shaped, using the skull model as a base, and a silicone mold is created. Polymethylmethacrylate (PMMA) is cast into the silicone mold and sterilized before implantation. A more modern fabrication process uses a CT scan of the patient to design a cranial implant that will be printed on a polymer-based additive manufacturing process and used as master for the silicone rubber mold. This approach removes the hand-shaping step and seems to improve the accuracy of the process and reduce fabrication time. A polymer-based SLS process to fabricate cranial implants directly from PMMA powder (OXPEKK-IG OsteoFab, Oxford Performance Materials, South Windsor, CT) has recently been approved by the Food and Drug Administration (FDA). This process is expected to reduce the number of process steps, to decrease production time, and to increase accuracy.

Porous metal implants

Several types of porous metal implants are commercially available. These materials have a high porosity, ranging from 60% to 80%, and a low modulus of elasticity that resembles cancellous bone (Levine 2008). Some porous metals blur the line between cancellous and cortical bone. Regenerex (Biomet, Warsaw, IN), for example, has a reported compressive strength that is

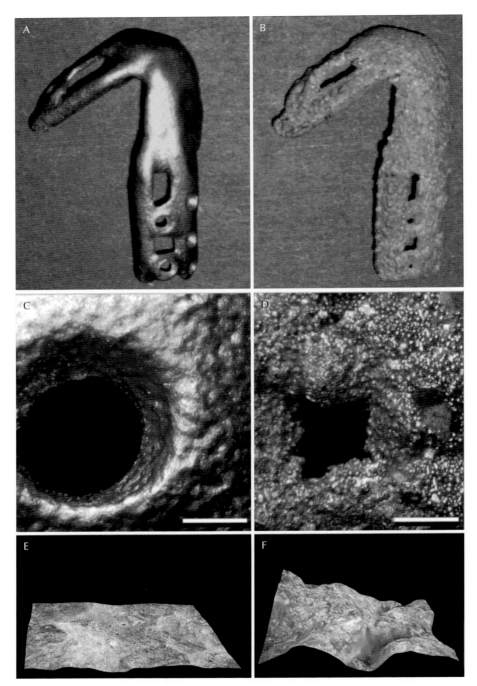

Figure 14.3 Photographs of unfinished custom implants intended for the cat in Figure 14.1. The implants were made with direct metal laser sintering (DMLS; A) or electron beam melting (EBM; B). The surface finish and hole geometry of the DMLS implant (C) is smoother and more accurate than the EBM implant (D). Magnifications bars are 1-mm long. When evaluated with a 3D microscope, the surface profile of the DMLS implant is smoother for the DMLS implant (mean surface roughness: 3 μm; E) than the EBM implant (mean surface roughness: 12 μm; F).

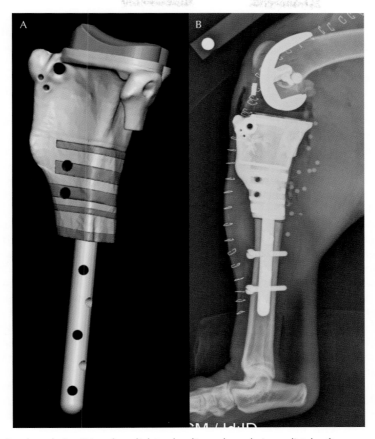

Figure 14.4   Tridimensional rendering (A) and mediolateral radiograph made immediately after surgery (B) showing a custom tibial implant designed for limb sparing in a Labrador retriever with a neoplasm affecting the proximal portion of the tibia. The tibial implant has porous portions that are visible as darker bands on the rendering and as bands with low radiopacity on the radiograph. The implant was made using electron beam melting technology. The implant has been combined with a commercial total knee implant. Thirteen plaster beads containing cisplatin have been placed on the tissue, caudal to the prosthetic tibia.

approximately 150 MPa, halfway between cortical bone (270 MPa) and cancellous bone (20 MPa) (Wirtz et al. 2000).

Porous tantalum is made by a chemical vapor infiltration process, during which pure tantalum metal is precipitated onto a reticulated vitreous carbon (RVC) skeleton, resulting in encasement of the RVC within the tantalum (Zardiackas et al. 2001). Porous titanium meshes may be made by fixing pure titanium on a polyurethane foam scaffold (later removed) to form a porous structure that resembles cancellous bone (Klika et al. 2007). Refer to Chapter 3 for additional information. For implants made by use of freeform fabrication,

porous portions are included directly on the implant (Figure 14.4; Harrysson et al. 2008). Porous portions may be used for bone ingrowth or to decrease the modulus of elasticity or weight of implants.

Applications of custom implants

Custom orthopedic implants may have a structural role of buttressing a bone or neutralizing the forces placed on that bone. Nonstructural implants are usually made of porous metal. They may be used to fill defects in bones, often in conjunction with a joint replacement or a limb-sparing procedure, after trauma or tumor removal.

Custom implants are, by definition, produced in limited numbers. They may be made in small batches, for example, for the reconstruction of the acetabulum with bone loss after aseptic loosening in humans (Sporer and Della Valle 2010). These small-batch implants may be used in areas of the body with consistent anatomical features, such as long bones. Alternatively, custom implants may be patient-specific, N-of-1 products. Patient-specific custom implants are used in areas of the body where an exact fit is deemed necessary.

Custom-designed implants have been available for decades, but modern customization started in the early 1990s, after the introduction of software packages for conversion of medical images. The most popular custom implant used in primary arthroplasty has been the prosthetic hip stem. Custom prosthetic stems were introduced in the late 1980s. These stems were based on 3D CT modeling (Robertson et al. 1987; Aldinger et al. 1988) or on a mold of the intramedullary cavity prepared during surgery (Mulier et al. 1989; Robinson and Clark 1996). Custom femoral cups and stems have been used in large patient cohorts. One report mentioned that 1123 custom hip stems were implanted between 1992 and 1994 and described 61 consecutive patients with hip dysplasia that were less than 40 years old at the time of surgery (Figure 14.5; Akbar et al. 2009). Seventy-two cementless custom cups and stems were implanted and followed for 10–16 years (mean: 14 years). Over the study period, 70 stems (97%) and 67 cups (93%) remained stable (i.e., free of loosening or revision).

The Identifit system (DePuy, Warsaw, IN) gave surgeons the ability to reproduce patient-specific femoral offset, version, and height and to achieve a high-percentage canal fill. However, the results of 53 primary Identifit prostheses were deemed disappointing, with 17% of the stems requiring revision after a mean follow-up period of only 30 months (Robinson and Clark 1996). Custom stems have been used in patients with severe skeletal deformities. In a small case series of 14 primary hip arthroplasties for nine patients with skeletal dysplasia, the mean functional hip score (Harris hip score) increased from 45 (range: 24–58) to 72 (range: 47–89) over a mean follow-up period of 3 years (Osagie et al. 2012). However, 21% of the procedures required revision at the time of follow-up. Custom stems have also been used to manage patients with bone loss after failed primary hip arthroplasty. One report described 17 patients who received custom hydroxyapatite-coated cementless stems with two 6.5-mm-diameter distal cross-locking screws (Sotereanos et al. 2006). Mean follow-up duration was 5.3 years. The mean functional hip score improved from 35 (range: 18–53) to 76 (range: 40–87) over the study period.

Structural custom implants have been used in craniomaxillofacial surgery for the reconstruction of bone defects (Singare et al. 2006). As discussed above, most cranial implants are made of PMMA. The infection rate associated with the use of PMMA cranial implants is relatively high and may require implant removal. In a series of 99 patients with warfare-related craniectomy defect reconstruction, successful reconstruction was achieved in 95% of patients (Kumar et al. 2011). The complication rate was 27% and the reoperation rate was 18%. Five implants were removed because of infections. This infection rate was low compared with the rate after placement of bone flaps from bone banks in the theater of war or the infection rate from previous reports. This lower infection rate was considered to be the result of stringent

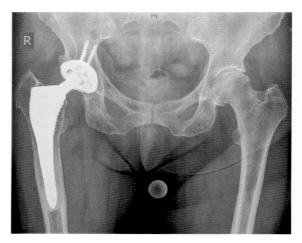

Figure 14.5 Radiograph of a 60-year-old female made 21 years after implantation of a custom prosthetic stem. Osseointegration of the stem and low cup wear are visible. (Image courtesy of Dr. Peter Aldinger, Protestant-Clinical-Center, Stuttgart, Germany, reproduced with permission)

enrollment criteria, including excellent soft tissue coverage, no preoperative clinical, biochemical (based on erythrocyte sedimentation rate), or radiographic evidence of infection (based on CT evaluation). Since metal (titanium) implants have a lower infection rate than PMMA implants, research aimed at the fabrication of cranial implants using direct metal additive manufacturing is ongoing. Because solid cranial metal implants may be heavy and may cause discomfort, titanium mesh implants have been used (Tadros and Costantino 2008). Custom implants that may be made of PMMA or titanium have also been used to fill orbitofacial defects (Scholz et al. 2007). In a case series of nine consecutive patients with orbitofacial defects, with a mean follow-up of 4.3 years (range: 6 months to 10 years), no significant complications occurred (Groth et al. 2006).

Silicone carpal bone prostheses were first implanted in the 1970s. They appear to have good subjective long-term benefits. In one report involving 32 patients, 25% of the implants were removed within 10 years and the remaining 75% were satisfactory (Vinnars et al. 2002). In another report, however, lytic bone lesions, as a result of silicone synovitis, were identified in 37 of 39 patients who had received silicone scaphoid or lunate implants, and the authors recommended not performing replacement of carpal bones with silicone implants (Egloff et al. 1993). Structural carpal lunate and scaphoid prostheses made of titanium have been used (Swanson titanium carpal lunate and carpal scaphoid implants, Wright Medical Technology, Arlington, TN; Figure 14.6). The long-term success of these implants has been satisfactory (Swanson et al. 1997).

In veterinary medicine, specialized implants that are produced in small numbers are emerging. For example, bone plates with shapes that match the surface of the proximal portion of the tibia are available from several manufacturers (Langenbach and Marcellin-Little 2010). Synthes Vet, for example, has six plates that cover the range of tibial sizes seen in companion animals (Figure 14.7). Specialized plates are also available for carpal and tarsal arthrodeses (Figure 14.8; McKee et al. 2004). These plates have mechanical advantages over conventional bone plates, including lower construct compliance, less angular

A

B

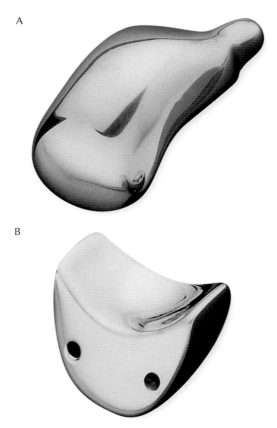

Figure 14.6 Titanium prostheses made to replace the scaphoid (A) and lunate (B) carpal bones. The prostheses are made of polished titanium. These prostheses are commercially available. (Images courtesy of Wright Medical Technology Inc., Arlington, TN, reproduced with permission)

deformation, and lower peak plate strains (Guillou et al. 2008, 2011).

A custom feline total knee implant that was also intended for use as a human metacarpophalangeal joint prosthesis was described in the early 1980s (Walker et al. 1983). A custom total knee replacement implant was implanted in a dog in June 2005 (Liska et al. 2007). The dog had a chronic, highly comminuted femoral condylar fracture resulting from a gunshot wound. A custom implant was prepared by machining a medial condylar augment in titanium alloy (Ti6Al4V) (Figure 14.9). The augment had porous proximal, distal, medial, and lateral surfaces. The augment was cemented to a conventional femoral component. The procedure

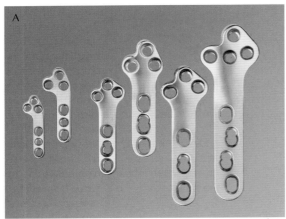

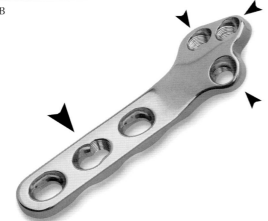

Figure 14.7 Bones plates intended for placement on the proximal portion of the tibia of companion animals. The array of plates (A) shows plates that receive screws measuring 2.0, 2.4, 2.7, or 3.5 mm. These plates have configurations for the left or right tibia. On the 3.5-mm plate (B), the contour of the proximal portion of the plate is visible. Three types of holes are seen. They are intended for nonlocking screws or for either a locking or nonlocking screw with a side-by-side configuration (large arrowhead) or a stacked configuration (small arrowheads). (Pictures courtesy of Synthes, reproduced with permission)

was clinically successful and a loss of stability of the bone–cement or cement–implant interfaces was not identified on follow-up radiographs made 4 years after surgery (Figure 14.10). Other custom total knee implants have been implanted more recently in cats and dogs in the United Kingdom, Germany, and in the United States.[3–5]

In hip replacement, a custom hip stem was used for limb sparing in a dog with osteosarcoma of the proximal portion of the femur. The long stem was fixed to an allograft of the proximal portion of the femur and to the host femoral shaft using PMMA (Liptak et al. 2005). Our research group has designed and fabricated custom hip stems for the canine femur. These porous stems with a low modulus of elasticity were designed for research purposes with the intent to create a stem that would decrease bone strain in the proximal portion of the femur when the joints are loaded (Figure 14.11; Harrysson et al. 2008; Marcellin-Little et al. 2010a). A similar concept and fabrication process could be used to make prosthetic stems for very large or small patients or for patients with femora with an abnormal shape.

Structural custom metal implants have been used in a few companion animals. In one report, a custom metal implant was used to replace a fractured central tarsal bone in a greyhound (Yocham et al. 1988). A metal block was cut from square-stock titanium alloy, machined, and hand-finished. The block was fixed with a bone screw inserted mediolaterally into the fourth tarsal bone. The dog returned to racing 14 weeks after surgery and raced successfully for 7 months afterward.

Transdermal osseointegrated implants have been placed in companion animals (Drygas et al. 2008; Fitzpatrick et al. 2011). These custom implants are designed to replace the distal portion of the thoracic or pelvic limb. Transdermal osseo-integration is an active research area in laboratory animals and clinical application in humans is expanding (Sullivan et al. 2003; Lundberg et al. 2011). Since 2005, our research group has implanted nine transdermal osseointegrated implants on the radius, tibia, or calcaneus of cats and dogs. Our implants are custom-made to match the inner or outer surfaces of the recipient bones (Figures 14.12–14.15). The initial postoperative fixation of implants may be achieved through press-fit augmented by bolts or screws. The long-term bone fixation may be achieved through bone growth into porous metal surfaces, including plasma-sprayed titanium, porous tantalum, or porous titanium. The skin–implant interface may have a locking flange used to prevent skin retraction.

The transfer of autogenous mucosal tissue has been proposed as an alternative to the simple

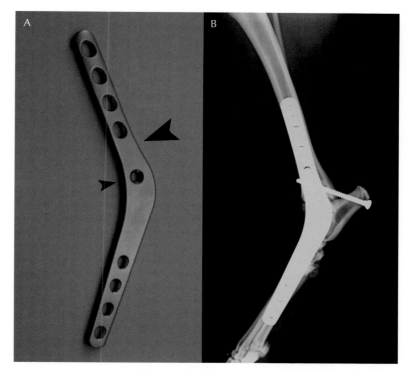

Figure 14.8 This bone plate (A), intended for pantarsal arthrodesis (B), may be placed on the medial or lateral aspects of the tibia and tarsus. The plate is shaped so that its proximal and distal portions form a 139-degree angle. The plate has 3.5-mm holes proximally and 2.7-mm holes distally. It has nine dynamic compression holes allowing interfragmentary compression, and one round hole used to place a screw in the talus (small arrowhead; A). The increased distance between screws on the distal aspect of the tibia (large arrowhead; A) allows the placement of a screw from the caudal aspect of the calcaneus to the tibia. (Adapted from McKee et al. [2004], BMJ Group, London, U.K., reproduced with permission)

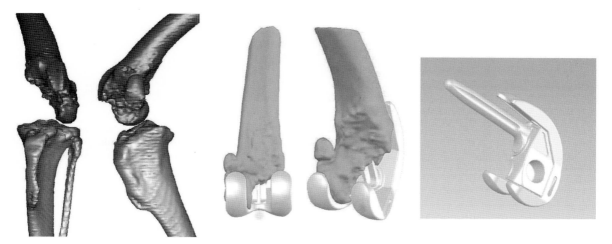

Figure 14.9 Tridimensional rendering (*left*), computer model of the bone and prosthetic component (*center*), and custom femoral component (*right*) for a canine total knee replacement in a dog with femoral condylar bone loss secondary to a gunshot wound. The customization includes a machined titanium alloy augment that is fixed to the conventional femoral component using polymethylmethacrylate. (From Liska et al. [2007], John Wiley & Sons, Malden, MA, reproduced with permission)

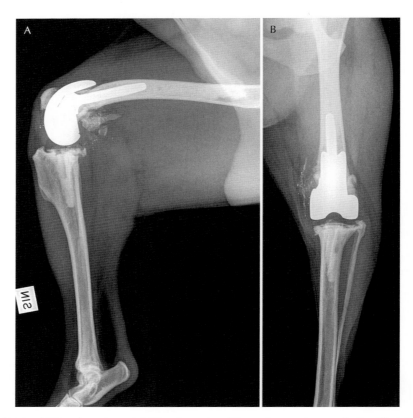

Figure 14.10 Mediolateral (A) and craniocaudal (B) radiographs of the custom canine prosthetic stifle joint in Figure 14.9 made 47 months after total knee replacement. The bone–cement and cement–implant interfaces are stable. Cortical changes along the femoral and tibial shaft are not noted, with the exception of focal cortical atrophy, present on the distal and cranial aspect of the femur. The atrophy appears unchanged, compared with the atrophy present on radiographs made 30 months earlier.

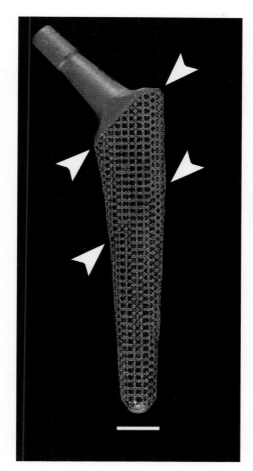

Figure 14.11 A custom prosthetic femoral stem has been made using electron beam melting. The stem is made of titanium alloy (Ti6Al4V). Its body is made of rhombic dodecahedron cells measuring approximately 1.2 × 1.6 mm. The proximal portion of the stem is 0.50 ± 0.25-mm wider than its distal portion to enable press-fit implantation, matching the shape of the commercially available BioMedtrix BFX stem. The proximal and distal aspects of that raised portion are highlighted by arrowheads. Magnification bar: 10 mm. The cell size and geometry may be adjusted to change the stiffness of the implant.

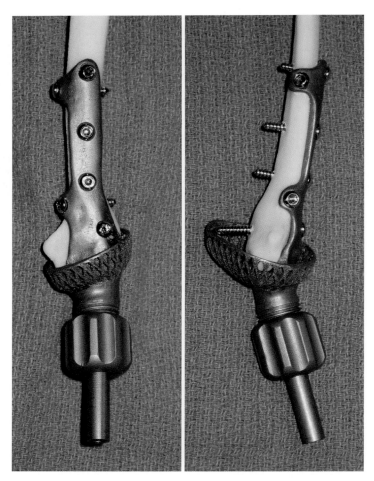

Figure 14.12 A custom implant intended for transdermal osseointegration has been made of titanium alloy using electron beam melting. The implant is contoured to the surface of the distal portion of the radius. The dog had sustained a traumatic amputation of the manus when he was a few weeks old. The implant has a contoured mesh basket used for the fixation of musculoskeletal soft tissues, subcutaneous tissues, and skin. The implant has been affixed to a polymer replica of the bone.

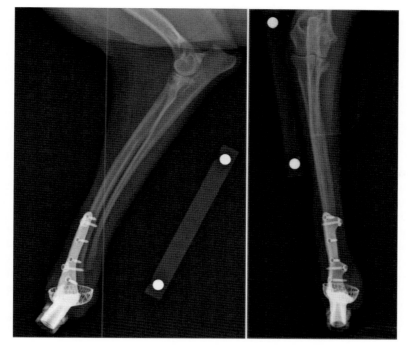

Figure 14.13 Postoperative radiographs after implantation of the transdermal osseointegrated implant shown in Figure 14.12. The soft tissues have been attached within and outside the mesh basket. A perforated titanium alloy ring has been placed on the threaded portion of the transdermal implant to hold skin sutures.

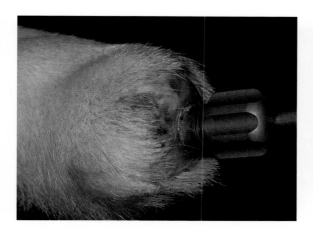

Figure 14.14 Photograph of the skin–implant interface of the dog in Figure 14.13, made 3 months after surgery. The scar tissue is associated in part with the dog's initial injuries. There is no drainage at the skin–implant interface.

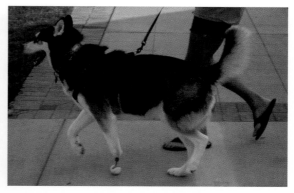

Figure 14.15 Photograph of the dog in Figures 14.13 and 14.14. The dog is walking with a training foot made using a ball filled with polyurethane.

apposition of skin to a smooth or textured metal rod.[6] The clinical results of transdermal osseointegrated implants appear promising and should be validated through a larger case series followed prospectively for a longer period of time.

For small dogs and cats, clinicians often use small commercial implants, including miniplates and 1.1 mm or 1.5 mm bone screws. Subjectively, small patients seem more vulnerable to atrophic nonunions and bone resorption that results from limb disuse, immobilization, or stress protection. The resulting bone loss greatly complicates the management of their orthopedic problems. Custom implants may be beneficial because they may allow fragment stabilization and fill bone defects. In the example illustrated below, a young Pomeranian was referred with an infected atrophic nonunion with severe radial bone loss. The dog had chronic limb disuse with loss of carpal motion. A CT scan of the forelimbs was made. The radius scan of the nonfractured forelimb was used to design a custom titanium bone plate. The plate filled the radial defect and achieved a pancarpal arthrodesis (Figure 14.16). Skull and mandibular fractures are also challenging in small dogs and cats. Human craniomaxillofacial implants have

been used to repair maxillary and mandibular fractures (Boudrieau 2004). Custom implants may be beneficial to fill voids with complex geometry (Figure 14.2).

Porous metal augments have been used to fill bone defects in humans undergoing revision arthroplasties or limb sparing. The commercially available porous metal implants include Tritanium Dimensionalized Metal™ (Stryker Orthopaedics, Mahwah, NJ), Regenerex, Stiktite (Smith & Nephew, Memphis, TN), and Trabecular Metal (Zimmer, Warsaw, IN) (Levine 2008). The most common use of porous metal implants is premanufactured metal augments used to enhance the fixation of the acetabular cup in humans with periprosthetic bone loss. These augments may be posterosuperior augments, in patients with loss of acetabular dome (i.e., the human equivalent of the dorsal rim), or anterior medial augments, in patients with segmental bone loss of the anterior or posterior columns (i.e., the human equivalent of the ilium or ischium) (Sporer and Della Valle 2010).

In veterinary medicine, a porous tantalum augment was used in a dog with radial osteosarcoma, as part of a limb-sparing procedure

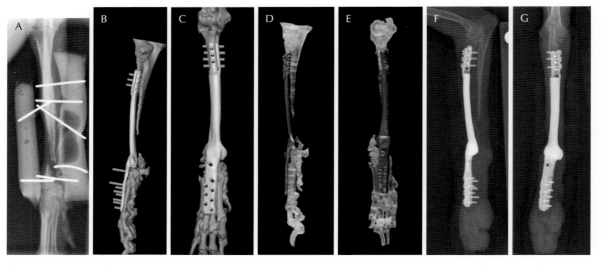

Figure 14.16 A papillon was presented with a septic atrophic nonunion after management of a radial fracture with a plate, followed by an external fixation frame (A). The radius had resorbed. A custom plate was designed (B and C) and was made using direct metal laser sintering. The plate was placed on a CT-based photopolymer replica of the antebrachium (D and E) to assess fit and then was placed on the patient (F and G). Severe osteoporosis was present after approximately 7 months of nonweight-bearing lameness.

(MacDonald and Schiller 2010). A low-grade surgical site infection was diagnosed 80 days after surgery, and it was managed conservatively. A pulmonary lesion consistent with metastatic disease was diagnosed on thoracic radiographs 248 days after surgery. The owner described the dog's quality of life as very good 332 days after surgery.

Patient-specific drill guides or osteotomy guides may also be prepared when ostectomies are planned. In an *in vitro* study involving proximal tibial leveling osteotomies in bone models, custom guides increased the accuracy of these osteotomies and increased the mechanical properties of the resulting constructs (Marcellin-Little et al. 2008). A custom osteotomy guide was used during the surgical correction of an antebrachial osteotomy in one dog (Crosse and Worth 2010). In humans, custom osteotomy guides for total knee arthroplasty are commercially available (TruMatch, DePuy). Custom osteotomy guides for segmental mandibular osteotomies, hip joint surface arthroplasty, and intra-articular distal radial malunions have also been reported (Oka et al. 2008; Raaijmaakers et al. 2010; Abou-ElFetouh et al. 2011).

Endnotes

1. Harrysson OLA, Cormier DR, Marcellin-Little DJ, et al. Direct fabrication of metal orthopedic implants using electron beam technology. In: *Proceedings of the Solid Freeform Fabrication Symposium*. Austin, TX, 2003, p. 439.
2. Cansizoglu O, Marcellin-Little D, Harrysson OLA. Comparison of direct metal fabrication technologies for production of medical implants. In: *Proceedings of the RAPID 2009 Conference and Exposition*. Schaumburg, IL, 2009.
3. Fitzpatrick N, Ash K, Meswania J, et al. Constrained total knee replacement, a novel prosthesis for salvage arthroplasty in the dog and cat. In: *Proceedings of the World Veterinary Orthopedic Conference*. Bologna, Italy, 2010, pp. 566–567.
4. Arbabian M, Berhend A. Personal communication, 2012.
5. Breed AG. Tubby tabby gets revolutionary new knee joint. Associated Press, January 27, 2012.
6. *DVM Newsmagazine*. Advancing medicine: Dr. Erick Egger talks about a successful surgery using a new prosthetic limb procedure under testing at Colorado State University. October 1, 2008.

References

Abou-ElFetouh A, Barakat A, Abdel-Ghany K. Computer-guided rapid-prototyped templates for segmental mandibular osteotomies: A preliminary report. Int J Med Robot 2011;7:187–192.

Ai Z, Evenhouse R, Leigh J, et al. New tools for sculpting cranial implants in a shared haptic augmented reality environment. Stud Health Technol Inform 2006;119:7–12.

Akbar M, Aldinger G, Krahmer K, et al. Custom stems for femoral deformity in patients less than 40 years of age: 70 hips followed for an average of 14 years. Acta Orthop 2009;80:420–425.

Aldinger G, De Pellegrin M, Kusswetter W. The personalized hip prosthesis. Ital J Orthop Traumatol 1988;14:429–433.

Boudrieau RJ. Miniplate reconstruction of severely comminuted maxillary fractures in two dogs. Vet Surg 2004;33:154–163.

Crosse KR, Worth AJ. Computer-assisted surgical correction of an antebrachial deformity in a dog. Vet Comp Orthop Traumatol 2010;23:354–361.

Drygas KA, Taylor R, Sidebotham CG, et al. Transcutaneous tibial implants: A surgical procedure for restoring ambulation after amputation of the distal aspect of the tibia in a dog. Vet Surg 2008;37:322–327.

Egloff DV, Varadi G, Narakas A, et al. Silastic implants of the scaphoid and lunate. A long-term clinical study with a mean follow-up of 13 years. J Hand Surg Br 1993;18:687–692.

Eufinger H, Wehmoller M. Individual prefabricated titanium implants in reconstructive craniofacial surgery: Clinical and technical aspects of the first 22 cases. Plast Reconstr Surg 1998;102:300–308.

Fitzpatrick N, Smith TJ, Pendegrass CJ, et al. Intraosseous transcutaneous amputation prosthesis (ITAP) for limb salvage in 4 dogs. Vet Surg 2011;40:909–925.

Groth MJ, Bhatnagar A, Clearihue WJ, et al. Long-term efficacy of biomodeled polymethyl methacrylate implants for orbitofacial defects. Arch Facial Plast Surg 2006;8:381–389.

Guillou RP, Frank JD, Sinnott MT, et al. *In vitro* mechanical evaluation of medial plating for pantarsal arthrodesis in dogs. Am J Vet Res 2008;69:1406–1412.

Guillou RP, Demianiuk RM, Sinnott MT, et al. *In vitro* mechanical evaluation of a limited contact dynamic compression plate and hybrid carpal arthrodesis plate for canine pancarpal arthrodesis. Vet Comp Orthop Traumatol 2011;25:408–417.

Harrysson OLA, Cansizoglu O, Marcellin-Little DJ, et al. Direct metal fabrication of titanium implants with tailored materials and mechanical properties using electron beam melting technology. Mater Sci Eng C 2008;28:366–373.

Haslauer CM, Springer JC, Harrysson OLA, et al. *In vitro* biocompatibility of titanium alloy discs made using direct metal fabrication. Med Eng Phys 2010;32: 645–652.

Kiatisevi P, Witoonchart K, Pattarabanjird N, et al. Palliative limb salvage using a retrograde nail-cement composite after intercalary resection of a distal femoral osteosarcoma: A case report. J Orthop Surg (Hong Kong) 2009;17:383–387.

Klika AK, Murray TG, Darwiche H, et al. Options for acetabular fixation surfaces. J Long Term Eff Med Implants 2007;17:187–192.

Kumar AR, Bradley JP, Harshbarger R, et al. Warfare-related craniectomy defect reconstruction: Early success using custom alloplast implants. Plast Reconstr Surg 2011;127:1279–1287.

Kusumoto N, Sohmura T, Yamada S, et al. Application of virtual reality force feedback haptic device for oral implant surgery. Clin Oral Implants Res 2006;17:708–713.

Langenbach A, Marcellin-Little DJ. Management of concurrent patellar luxation and cranial cruciate ligament rupture using modified tibial plateau levelling. J Small Anim Pract 2010;51:97–103.

Levine B. A new era in porous metals: Applications in orthopaedics. Adv Engin Biomat 2008;10:788–792.

Liptak JM, Pluhar GE, Dernell WS, et al. Limb-sparing surgery in a dog with osteosarcoma of the proximal femur. Vet Surg 2005;34:71–77.

Liska WD, Marcellin-Little DJ, Eskelinen EV, et al. Custom total knee replacement in a dog with femoral condylar bone loss. Vet Surg 2007;36:293–301.

Lundberg M, Hagberg K, Bullington J. My prosthesis as a part of me: A qualitative analysis of living with an osseointegrated prosthetic limb. Prosthet Orthot Int 2011;35:207–214.

MacDonald TL, Schiller TD. Limb-sparing surgery using tantalum metal endoprosthesis in a dog with osteosarcoma of the distal radius. Can Vet J 2010;51: 497–500.

Marcellin-Little DJ, Harrysson OLA, Cansizoglu O. In vitro evaluation of a custom cutting jig and custom plate for canine tibial plateau leveling. Am J Vet Res 2008;69:961–966.

Marcellin-Little DJ, Cansizoglu O, Harrysson OLA, et al. In vitro evaluation of a low-modulus mesh canine prosthetic hip stem. Am J Vet Res 2010a;71: 1089–1095.

Marcellin-Little DJ, Sutherland BJ, Harrysson OLA, et al. In vitro evaluation of free-form biodegradable bone plates for fixation of distal femoral physeal fractures in dogs. Am J Vet Res 2010b;71:1508–1515.

McKee WM, May C, Macias C, et al. Pantarsal arthrodesis with a customised medial or lateral bone plate in 13 dogs. Vet Rec 2004;154:165–170.

Mulier JC, Mulier M, Brady LP, et al. A new system to produce intraoperatively custom femoral prosthesis from measurements taken during the surgical procedure. Clin Orthop Relat Res 1989;249:97–112.

Oka K, Moritomo H, Goto A, et al. Corrective osteotomy for malunited intra-articular fracture of the distal radius using a custom-made surgical guide based on three-dimensional computer simulation: Case report. J Hand Surg Am 2008;33:835–840.

Osagie L, Figgie M, Bostrom M. Custom total hip arthroplasty in skeletal dysplasia. Int Orthop 2012;36:527–531.

Raaijmaakers M, Gelaude F, De Smedt K, et al. A custom-made guide-wire positioning device for hip surface replacement arthroplasty: Description and first results. BMC Musculoskelet Disord 2010;11:161.

Robertson DD, Walker PS, Granholm JW, et al. Design of custom hip stem prostheses using three-dimensional CT modeling. J Comput Assist Tomogr 1987;11: 804–809.

Robinson RP, Clark JE. Uncemented press-fit total hip arthroplasty using the Identifit custom-molding technique. A prospective minimum 2-year follow-up study. J Arthroplasty 1996;11:247–254.

Scholz M, Wehmoller M, Lehmbrock J, et al. Reconstruction of the temporal contour for traumatic tissue loss using a CAD/CAM-prefabricated titanium implant-case report. J Craniomaxillofac Surg 2007;35: 388–392.

Singare S, Yaxiong L, Dichen L, et al. Fabrication of customised maxillo-facial prosthesis using computer-aided design and rapid prototyping techniques. Rapid Prototyping J 2006;12:206–213.

Sotereanos N, Sewecke J, Raukar GJ, et al. Revision total hip arthroplasty with a custom cementless stem with distal cross-locking screws. Early results in femora with large proximal segmental deficiencies. J Bone Joint Surg Am 2006;88:1079–1084.

Sporer SM, Della Valle C. Porous metal augments: Big hopes for big holes. Orthopedics 2010;33:651.

Sullivan J, Uden M, Robinson KP, et al. Rehabilitation of the trans-femoral amputee with an osseointegrated prosthesis: The United Kingdom experience. Prosthet Orthot Int 2003;27:114–120.

Swanson AB, de Groot Swanson G, et al. Carpal bone titanium implant arthroplasty. 10 years' experience. Clin Orthop Relat Res 1997;342:46–58.

Tadros M, Costantino PD. Advances in cranioplasty: A simplified algorithm to guide cranial reconstruction of acquired defects. Facial Plast Surg 2008;24: 135–145.

Vinnars B, Adamsson L, Af Ekenstam F, et al. Patient-rating of long term results of silicone implant arthroplasty of the scaphoid. Scand J Plast Reconstr Surg Hand Surg 2002;36:39–45.

Walker PS, Nunamaker D, Huiskes R, et al. A new approach to the fixation of a metacarpophalangeal joint prosthesis. Eng Med 1983;12:135–140.

Wirtz DC, Schiffers N, Pandorf T, et al. Critical evaluation of known bone material properties to realize anisotropic FE-simulation of the proximal femur. J Biomech 2000;33:1325–1330.

Wohlers T. *Additive Manufacturing and 3D Printing State of the Industry, Annual Worldwide Progress Report*. Fort Collins, CO: Wohlers Associates, 2011.

Yocham GD, Sanderson C, Rounds P, et al. Central tarsal implant in a racing greyhound. J Am Vet Med Assoc 1988;193:840–842.

Zardiackas LD, Parsell DE, Dillon LD, et al. Structure, metallurgy, and mechanical properties of a porous tantalum foam. J Biomed Mater Res 2001;58:180–187.

Index

Note: Page numbers in **bold** refer to tables; those in *italics* refer to figures.

Advances in Small Animal Total Joint Replacement, First Edition. Edited by Jeffrey N. Peck and Denis J. Marcellin-Little.
© 2013 John Wiley & Sons, Inc. Published 2013 by John Wiley & Sons, Inc.